Emergency Care of Children and Young People

Dedication

This book is dedicated to our children, Izzy Wood, and Will and Henry Porter, all of whom have recently used children's emergency services!

Emergency Care of Children and Young People

EDITED BY

Karen Cleaver & Janet Webb
School of Health and Social Care
The University of Greenwich
London
UK

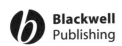
Blackwell
Publishing

Blackwell Publishing editorial offices:
Blackwell Publishing Ltd, 9600 Garsington Road, Oxford OX4 2DQ, UK
 Tel: +44 (0)1865 776868
Blackwell Publishing Inc., 350 Main Street, Malden, MA 02148-5020, USA
 Tel: +1 781 388 8250
Blackwell Publishing Asia Pty Ltd, 550 Swanston Street, Carlton, Victoria 3053, Australia
 Tel: +61 (0)3 8359 1011

First published 2007 by Blackwell Publishing Ltd

ISBN: 978-1-4051-0110-3

Library of Congress Cataloging-in-Publication Data
Emergency care of children and young people / edited by Karen Cleaver & Janet Webb.
     p. ; cm.
  Includes bibliographical references and index.
  ISBN: 978-1-4051-0110-3 (pbk. : alk. paper)
  1. Pediatric emergency services—Great Britain. 2. Hospitals—Emergency services—Great Britain. 3. Pediatric nursing—Great Britain. I. Cleaver, Karen. II. Webb, Janet, 1961–
  [DNLM: 1. Emergencies—nursing—Great Britain. 2. Adolescent—Great Britain. 3. Child—Great Britain. 4. Emergency Service, Hospital—Great Britain. WY 154 E5206 2007]
  RJ370.E418 2007
  618.92'0025—dc22

                                                        2006100270

A catalogue record for this title is available from the British Library

Set in 9.5/12pt Palatino
by Graphicraft Limited, Hong Kong
Printed and bound in Singapore
by Fabulous Printers Pte Ltd

The publisher's policy is to use permanent paper from mills that operate a sustainable forestry policy, and which has been manufactured from pulp processed using acid-free and elementary chlorine-free practices. Furthermore, the publisher ensures that the text paper and cover board used have met acceptable environmental accreditation standards.

For further information on Blackwell Publishing, visit our website:
www.blackwellnursing.com

Contents

Contributors

Louise Bunn Nurse Practitioner, Minor Injuries Unit, Plymouth

Karen Chandler Senior Lecturer in Children's Nursing, Department of Family Care & Mental Health, University of Greenwich

Karen Cleaver Head of Department, Family Care & Mental Health, University of Greenwich

Priscilla Dike Senior Lecturer in Midwifery, Department of Family Care & Mental Health, University of Greenwich

Rebecca Hoskins Nurse Consultant, Bristol Royal Infirmary, and Senior Lecturer in Emergency Care, University of West of England

Janet Kelsey Senior Lecturer in Children's Nursing, Faculty of Health and Social Work, University of Plymouth

Gill McEwing Senior Lecturer in Children's Nursing, Faculty of Health and Social Work, University of Plymouth

Dr Olive McKeown Senior Lecturer in Mental Health, Department of Family Care & Mental Health, University of Greenwich

Ann Rich Senior Lecturer in Children's Nursing, Department of Family Care & Mental Health, University of Greenwich

Camille Roddam Community Children's Nurse/Specialist Nurse in Diabetes, Queen Elizabeth NHS Trust, Woolwich

Pat Rose Senior Lecturer in Practice Learning, School of Health and Social Care, University of Chester

Jean Shepherd Senior Lecturer in Children's Nursing, Department of Family Care & Mental Health, University of Greenwich

Lesley Wayne Nurse Practitioner, Minor Injuries Unit, Plymouth

Janet Webb Principal Lecturer/Professional Lead, Child Health & Welfare, Department of Family Care & Mental Health, University of Greenwich

Preface

The editors of this book have experience of paediatric emergency care spanning more than two decades. During this time, a number of changes to the provision of paediatric emergency services have occurred, and having evolved from being a 'Cinderella service' it is now a recognised speciality. For both of us, our decision to work in this setting stemmed from our experiences as general nurses working in accident and emergency departments. Like many nurses working in this setting, we enjoyed the unpredictability and diversity of the workload. The variety and diversity meant that as nurses working with children, our workload day to day could involve the assessment and treatment of minor injuries, care of the critically ill child who is medically unwell and caring for the child who had sustained serious and life-threatening injuries following major trauma. There were also the numerous attendances for minor ailments, acute illnesses (not life threatening) and the need to be ever vigilant to the possibility of child abuse and or neglect, whatever the reason for attendance.

As nurses working in this field, we have long been aware of how difficult it can be to locate information and, more latterly, evidence specific to the care of children in this setting. It therefore became our 'mission' to compile a book which would provide an informative and evidence-based review of the basis and fundamental principles of the emergency care of children and young people.

Against this background, Chapter 1 briefly sets the scene by providing an overview of the context of children's emergency services and considers childhood and family life in the UK, and how this may influence decisions about access to health care, specifically emergency services. Chapter 2 considers some of the general principles of assessing and managing the care of children in the accident and emergency setting, and in recognition that practitioners also need to work within an ethical and legal framework, Chapter 3 follows on with an overview of the ethical and legal issues that have implications for assessment, interventions and outcomes for children in the emergency care setting. The chapter considers the relevant legislative frameworks, namely The Children Act 1989, The Human Rights Act 1998 and the Children Act 2004.

All practitioners working within the emergency care setting not only have a responsibility and duty to ensure quality and safety of care but also have a responsibility to work together with other agencies to help safeguard children from harm. Indeed, the welfare of children is paramount, as enshrined within both the 1989 and 2004 Children Acts. With this in mind, issues around the safeguarding of children are discussed in Chapter 4, which is concerned with child protection and the roles and responsibilities of the emergency care practitioner, the starting point being that child protection is everyone's responsibility. Hospital emergency departments are often the first place where injured children come into contact with the health services. It is important that those children who are vulnerable, victims of, or at risk of, abuse or neglect do not pass through these departments unrecognised. The recognition of a vulnerable child, a child in need and a child in need of protection from harm depends greatly on the skills of the practitioner in this setting. Thus, child protection concerns and recognition of abuse and neglect are discussed within the context of current policies, guidelines and legislation. Potential child protection issues are also highlighted in subsequent chapters in relation to assessment particularly of a child presenting with an injury.

In recognition of the particular needs of young people, Chapter 5 has been devoted to examining some of the challenges faced by this population group, and the consequences for the provision of accident and emergency care to them. There is a perception that adolescence is a healthy stage in our life-cycle; however, the onset of puberty and other associated changes, both physically and emotionally, mean that this age group are still vulnerable, but in a different way from infants and young children. Their propensity for experimentation means they remain vulnerable to (serious) accidental injury, but also to the use of drugs and alcohol. Both these substances in turn can increase risk taking behaviour, and also make young people less inhibited, often resulting in sexual intercourse, and thus the associated concerns arising from this in terms of unwanted pregnancies and sexually transmitted infections. However, the biggest health challenge facing young people is mental health, with the prevalence of self-harm amongst this age group increasing. These factors are discussed and the needs of young people fully considered in this chapter.

Minor injuries account for a significant proportion of children attending emergency departments and minor injury units (MIUs). More significant injuries and conditions need to be excluded and the appropriate management and subsequent outcomes are dependent on an accurate assessment. The assessment needs to take account of the child's age and stage of development as well as the injury itself, as these have implications for the treatment and management of the injury and therefore subsequent outcome of the child's visit and overall experience. Thus, Chapter 6 is concerned with the assessment, intervention and outcome of children attending with a minor injury. A differentiation between a minor injury and a more serious injury is given and the evidence base for care and treatment of minor injuries is provided. Chapter 7 provides an overview of factors to consider when assessing and managing children's pain.

It is worth noting here that children are more susceptible to injury as they are naturally inquisitive and learn by exploring (Child Accident Prevention Trust, 2004), with 275 children aged under 15 dying as a result of injury and poisoning in the UK in 2004, with over 2 million children taken to hospital following an accident (Child Accident Prevention Trust, 2006). Furthermore, trauma is the leading cause of death and disability over 1 year of age (European Resuscitation Council & Resuscitation Council UK, 2004). It is therefore imperative that A & E practitioners are able to recognise the deteriorating child in order to intervene at an early stage. Chapter 8 considers the key considerations in recognising the seriously ill child whose condition is deteriorating, requiring rapid intervention. The ABC approach is used as a framework for the assessment and management of the seriously ill child whether the physiological deterioration is the result of major trauma from injury or an acute medical condition with or without an underlying chronic condition.

A recommendation of the National Service Framework (DoH, 2004) is that professionals should be appropriately trained, with knowledge and competence to provide care to the acutely seriously ill child. Chapter 9 is thus concerned with the resuscitation of a child who has sustained a cardiopulmonary arrest and the skills required of the emergency care practitioner. It discusses the sequences for both basic and advanced paediatric life support based on the Resuscitation Council UK (2006) guidelines. Consideration in relation to the care of the parents and family is also addressed.

The book then moves on to consider commonly encountered paediatric problems. Chapter 10 examines the needs of children who attend with respiratory illness/disease, which accounts for a significant number of attendances to the emergency department. The prevalence of respiratory illness in children is partly due to anatomical and physiological factors, as well as infants' and young children's vulnerability to infection due to reduced immunity. Children who present with respiratory distress may have one of a number of underlying problems ranging from infection to asthma, to substance misuse involving inhalation of 'class A drugs' or other harmful substances. These diverse causes of respiratory illness are considered and methods of treatment outlined, having reviewed the anatomical and physiological differences in the infant's and young child's respiratory tract.

Fever phobia is a reported phenomenon and reflects the anxieties that both parents and health care professionals have in relation to this symptom. This therefore often results in aggressive treatment of fever. However, such anxieties arise from people's concerns that convulsion may result from an untreated fever, or the fever may be indicative of meningitis. The emergency management of meningitis can influence the outcome in terms of both survival, and subsequent quality of life. Factors to consider when assessing a child's temperature and managing their fever are therefore reviewed and an overview of the emergency management of meningitis is provided in Chapter 11.

Children and young people with sickle cell disease (SCD) face many challenges, particularly when a crisis occurs. These are extremely painful and may also be life threatening if splenic sequestration has occurred. Although many paediatric units usually make provision for families whose children have SCD to access the in-patient services directly, a proportion of children and young people are seen in the emergency department, some of whom may have a less than positive experience due to prejudices and racial stereotyping. The experiences of one mother, whose son received good care and who is highly satisfied with the services provided, recounts from her perspective what it is like to have a child who suffers from SCD, and the value that she has placed on having access to prompt emergency services. These are discussed in Chapter 12.

The number of children being diagnosed with Type 1 diabetes is increasing and age at diagnosis is also younger than before. Initial diagnosis often occurs in the A & E department following a referral from primary care. A referral may have been made as either the diagnosis is suspected, or where symptoms are not necessarily suggestive but on further investigation following arrival in the emergency department are found to be caused by Type 1 diabetes. Chapter 13 focuses on two case studies that illustrate such presentations, which follow on from a brief overview of the physiological basis of Type 1 diabetes.

The book aims to provide a contemporary basis for the emergency care of children for a range of practitioners working in this setting, and in so doing draws on a range of evidence to provide what we hope is an informative basis for care. It is, however, not intended to be a definitive base for practice. Whilst it addresses the main principles of care and addresses assessment, intervention and management of care of common presentations in the emergency setting, it should be used in conjunction with other sources of evidence such as national and local policies and protocols.

Since starting out on this book so much has changed, and will continue to change. We hope, however, that readers of this book will 'dip in' and use this as a resource for informing their practice. All our colleagues who have contributed to the book have undertaken extensive reviews of the literature, and each chapter has an extensive reference list, drawing on a wide range of research and other evidence from a range of disciplines.

A note about terminology: the book addresses the needs of children and young people within the emergency care setting. Where the term child is used this applies to all ages from 0 to 18 years. The term emergency department is used throughout, but it is recognised that emergency care is delivered in a number of alternative settings, in particular minor injury units, walk-in centres and nurse-led clinics; where the term emergency care is used, this equally applies to other settings.

Throughout the text, 'Department of Health' has been abbreviated to DoH. We are aware that the accepted abbreviation is now DH.

Karen Cleaver
Janet Webb

References

Child Accident Prevention Trust (2004) *Children and Accidents*. Fact-sheet. www.capt.org.uk/faq. Last accessed 16/02/2006.

Child Accident Prevention Trust (2006) *Child Accident Facts*. Fact-sheet. www.capt.org.uk/faq. Last accessed 16/02/2006.

Department of Health (2004) *National Service Framework for Children, Young People and Maternity Services*. DoH, London.

European Resuscitation Council and Resuscitation Council UK (2004) *European Life Support Course: Provider Manual for Use in the UK*. RC UK, London.

Resuscitation Council UK (2006) *Resuscitation Guidelines 2005*. RC UK, London.

Acknowledgements

We wish to acknowledge the infinite help and patience of Steve and Colin and all our family and friends – too many to mention – notably those who looked after our children while we reviewed and prepared this manuscript. Many thanks! We would also like to thank all the contributing authors for their hard work and commitment.

Table of Cases

Table of Statutes

Chapter 1 Setting the Scene: The Context of Emergency Care for Children and Young People

Karen Cleaver and Janet Webb

Children and family life in the UK

The numbers of children in the UK are declining as a proportion of the population, currently accounting for around 20% of the UK's population (Office for National Statistics (ONS) 2005a) with 14.8 million children under the age of 20 years recorded in the 2001 census (ONS 2004). The majority of children (88%) live in England and Wales, although proportionally Northern Ireland and the major conurbations in Scotland, England and Wales are where most of the UK's children live (ONS 2004). Boys outnumber girls as live births and continue to outnumber females until aged 45 years where this trend then reverses (Platt 1998). The multi-cultural nature of UK society is reflected amongst our children; young people from minority ethnic backgrounds account for 10% of children under the age of 20, of which young people from India and Pakistan account for the highest numbers of ethnic minority children, with black African children being the group where the largest increases in the population have been noted at census (ONS 2004).

Social change during the 20th century has led to a number of variations in the family life of children and young people in the UK. For example the mean age of motherhood has risen during the latter part of the 20th century. More children were born to older mothers at the end of the 1990s than at the beginning, with evidence that qualified women are more likely to delay childbearing, have fewer children and return to full-time employment than unskilled women (Dex & Joshi 1999). Paradoxically, though, the UK has one of the highest rates of teenage pregnancy in the European Union, with the adverse affects on both the mother and child well

documented (Social Exclusion Unit 1999). One result of this paradox is the increasing reliance on the provision of day care for children, and increasing registration of 3–4-year-olds at pre-schools.

Social change has also affected family composition. Changes in attitudes as well as legislation around divorce have meant that we have seen a dramatic rise in the divorce rate in the UK. Although this has stabilised over the past decade, more than one in four children will experience parental divorce by the age of 16 (Rodgers & Pryor 1998). This has coincided with an increase in the number of lone parent families; it is estimated that 2.7 million children (20%) are living within lone parent families (Haskey 1998). Both these factors have led to changes in family structures, with 'couple families' most likely to be found amongst Indian-headed households (92%), followed by Pakistani/Bangladeshi families (85%) and white families (79%). It is acknowledged that lone motherhood is more prevalent amongst black families, representing just under half of black-headed households (ONS 2004).

Children's health and well-being

In the 2001 census 99% of children rated their health 'good' (90%) or 'fairly good' (9%), and overall childhood remains a healthy period of our lives. The ONS (2004) provides information on aspects of children's health, revealing that (perhaps contrary to expectations) improvements are evident. For example asthma, eczema and hay fever are amongst the commonest 'chronic' diseases of childhood, but rates would seem to be decreasing, particularly for asthma where there has been a steady decline during the 1990s. Childhood cancer rates remain the same, accounting for only 0.5% of all cancers, although deaths from cancer in childhood are high at around 20%. One area where concerns remain is around mental health, with 1 in 10 children reported as having a mental health problem (ONS 2005b). It is of note that incidence is highest amongst children from lone parent families and in families where neither parent is working. Mental health problems (with the exception of autism) are also associated with low educational achievement in both the child and parent. This pattern in respect of socio-economic circumstances and mental health, is also reflected in other aspects of child health; the links between deprivation, poverty, social exclusion and health are well documented; in children this is particularly evident when looking at data relating to accidents and accidental deaths (Platt 1998). There are also concerns around childhood obesity that have been widely reported, as well as the declining uptake of the MMR vaccination.

An increasingly mobile global population has resulted in an increase in the numbers of children whose families are refugees or seeking asylum. These families have particular health needs, and many have experienced traumatic episodes in their lives as a result of war/conflict and its consequences, including persecution, torture, sexual and economic exploitation and absolute poverty. Concerns also remain around child protection and child protection practices. Despite numerous public inquiries into high profile cases of child abuse and neglect, questions remain about the effectiveness of inter-agency working in the safeguarding of children and the protection of children at risk, comprehensively illustrated by the Laming Report (Laming 2003) and the Bichard Inquiry Report (Bichard 2004).

Legislative and policy context

The arrival of the 21st century has coincided with significant reforms in relation to children's services in their wider sense, with the publication of *Every Child Matters* (DfES 2004), *The National Service Framework for Children, Young People and Maternity Services* (NSF) (DoH 2004a), and the Children Act 2004 (Parliament 2004). All share the same fundamental principles which were origin-

ally enshrined within the underlying philosophy of the Children Act 1989 (Parliament 1989), namely that the welfare of children is paramount. These recent reviews of policy and legislation have largely been driven by recent public inquiries, established in the wake of significant concerns relating to the extent to which children and young people are safeguarded and their interests protected, for example into the death of Victoria Climbié (Laming 2003), and the deaths of children undergoing corrective heart surgery at Bristol Royal Infirmary (Kennedy 2001).

Drawing as it does on previous and current recommendations around good practice, the NSF will shape the future ten years of the provision of children's health services. The main aim and focus of this NSF is to bring about a cultural change (Hainsworth 2004), with services being designed and delivered around children, their families and their needs rather than around the needs of the organisations or professionals (Smith 2004), reflecting the stated principles of the NHS Plan (DoH 2000). Standard 7 addresses hospital services and makes a number of recommendations for practice that equally apply to emergency departments as they do to in-patient children's wards.

The Laming Inquiry (2003) into the death of Victoria Climbié, and the recommendations arising from this, have influenced key aspects of the NSF, particularly around safeguarding children. This is further underpinned by the Children Act 2004 in which there is a refusal to separate child protection from wider policies to improve children's lives. It emphasises universal services as a prerequisite for more targeted interventions. It has many positive elements such as the introduction of the five outcomes required for children's positive development; the emphasis on early intervention; a determination to support parents and carers; and an acknowledgement of both the need for 'workforce reform' as well as the current contribution of child care professionals (DoH 2004a).

Emergency services for children

While the specific needs of children attending for emergency care are now more widely recognised, this has not always been the case. During the 1980s a survey by the British Paediatric Association (1985) identified a number of short-comings in the provision of paediatric accident and emergency services. This included lack of dedicated/separate paediatric areas, lack of specialist facilities such as toys and play areas and lack of paediatric trained staff – both doctors and nurses. During the early 1990s debates emerged about the appropriateness of staffing accident and emergency departments with children's trained nurses (Davis 1991; Webb & Cleaver 1991). However by the end of the 1990s increases in the numbers of appropriately trained staff were evident (Audit Commission 2001), with the Healthcare Commission (2005:6) finding that in the average department, 6% of nurses are children's trained, although recruitment of nurses to this speciality remains a challenge (Elston & Thornes 2002; Salter & Maconochie 2004).

While other enhancements have also been noted (Healthcare Commission 2005), a review by an intercollegiate working party in 1999 made 32 recommendations for the future provision of accident and emergency services for children (Royal College of Paediatrics and Child Health 1999) which were to be implemented by 2004. On reviewing progress, Salter and Maconochie (2004) note that children's emergency services are now largely located on the same site as in-patient services, but a quarter of departments seeing more than 18 000 children annually did not have separate triage facilities. They concluded that overall there is considerable room for improvement, and that a number of the initial recommendations were yet to be achieved. Concerns are also evident in relation to assessment and management of paediatric pain, the quality of information and communication and, in particular, the requirements for adolescents still need to be fully ascertained and addressed (Healthcare Commission 2005; Salter and Stallard 2004).

The provision of emergency services has been subject to scrutiny and review following the publication of the NHS Plan (DoH 2000) reinforced by the publication *Reforming Emergency Care* (DoH 2001) and the imposition of the target for 4-hour waiting times. Recent reports,

while acknowledging that there are areas for improvement remaining, have hailed these reforms a success (DoH 2004b; Healthcare Commission 2005). The need to ensure that all patients attending hospital based emergency services are seen, treated and discharged within four hours means that for many practitioners working in these areas, a key element of their role is ensuring the 'through flow' of patients (Byrne & Heyman 1997). Mobilising patients through the department efficiently requires practitioners to undertake an initial assessment, and involves a form of triage. Generally this is undertaken by nurses, with national triage scales increasingly being implemented, including the use of the 'Manchester Triage System' – for a useful review of nurse triage see Woolwich (2000).

Access to hospital based care for children and young people usually follows self-referral to emergency departments, minor injury units or NHS Direct (the latter referring children on for emergency hospital based care). Only a minority of consultations in primary care lead to hospital referral (ONS 2004). This is a key factor for families who are geographically or socially isolated, and for those recently arrived in the UK, who can gain access to healthcare 'round the clock'. Prior to the introduction of the NHS the purpose of a 'casualty' department had been to provide medical care for those who were unable to afford a general practitioner (Sanders 2000). Thus it was anticipated that with the introduction of the NHS providing free, universal access to health care for all, patients would seek consultations initially from their GPs. Evidently, though, this has not been the case, with ever increasing numbers of patients, reflected in both adult and paediatric attendances. Children now account for between one third and one quarter of all attendances, the ONS (2004) reporting that 3.5 million children attend emergency departments annually.

This reported figure suggests an increase in attendances, and is borne out in some research studies. For example, a study by Boyle *et al.* (2000) found clear evidence that the numbers of children attending as a proportion of the local childhood population had increased, while the proportion of children admitted had declined from 56% to 32%. Reasons for this decline in the number of admissions as a proportion of attendance are not given, but it is possible that improved ambulatory care and community children's nursing services mean that there is enhanced support for children and families at home. As might be expected there is evidence that children living in areas where social deprivation is high are more likely to make use of hospital based emergency services (Beattie *et al.* 2001). However, there is evidence that children and young people from minority ethnic groups, while able to access primary care, receive less secondary care (Saxena *et al.* 2002).

Recent research which has examined trends in paediatric attendances for emergency care reveal that the majority of children attend following trauma, with just over a quarter attending with 'medical' problems (Armon *et al.* 2001; Hendry *et al.* 2005), with 79% of all attendees in Hendry *et al.*'s (2005) study being triage category 4. It is evident from the literature that a number of patients who attend hospital based emergency services do so with minor injuries and illnesses that could be managed in primary care settings. This has over the years led to debates around what constitutes an appropriate attendance. Murphy (1998a) provides a review of the literature on inappropriate attendance and identifies the huge discrepancy in determining the proportions of visits that are justified, these ranging from 6–80%. There is no agreed definition as to what constitutes an inappropriate attendance, but themes in the literature have been identified. These include non-accidents and non-emergencies, patients with pre-existing symptoms (having lasted more than 24 hours), and conditions that could be adequately managed by a GP, the latter also expressed as not requiring hospital care. Lack of knowledge on behalf of the patients as to the services provided by GPs is also seen as a contributory factor (Murphy 1998a; Sanders 2000). All of the studies reviewed by these authors related to the attendance of adults, primarily because there is limited research which has examined inappropriate attendance in children (Prince & Worth 1992). This could be because

children are perceived differently from adults, with medical personnel reluctant to categorise children as 'trivia', even when they attend with complaints that would normally be categorised as such (Dingwall & Murray 1983). One small-scale study which has examined inappropriate attendance of children identified that one third of children's attendance at one accident and emergency department was considered to be inappropriate (Prince & Worth 1992). The highest proportion of inappropriate attendance was related to the age of the child (higher amongst younger children); social class and geographical location to the hospital were also contributory factors, but there was no correlation with availability of the family's GP.

Studies that have explored parental decision making in relation to their unwell child have found that parents use their own system of triage to determine the appropriate service for their children. A number of factors influence this decision making – namely perceived expertise of the centre, access and parental expectations (Cooper *et al.* 2003; Woolfenden *et al.* 2000). However there can be considerable differences between a patient's (lay) perspective of what constitutes an emergency and those of health care professionals (MacFaul *et al.* 1998; Murphy 1998a). In their study, which examined 887 admissions over a three-week period, MacFaul *et al.* (1998) found that 99% of parents were of the opinion that admission was needed; this corresponded with 71% of admissions judged as necessary by consultant paediatricians, while GPs viewed 88% of the admissions to be necessary. Convulsions and recall of past illnesses were associated with a high need for admission score on the part of parents. Comments from the completed questionnaires also revealed how parents found admission to be beneficial in putting their minds at rest, enabling them to feel more confident at continuing with the care of their unwell child at home soon after admission.

Increasingly though, it is recognised that reasons for inappropriate attendance are complex, and as Byrne *et al.* (2003) found, frequent attendees are a psychosocially vulnerable group, reporting poorer mental health, and low levels of social support. In recognition of these complex issues, we would concur with writers (Byrne *et al.* 2003; Hendry *et al.* 2005; Murphy 1998b; Sanders 2000; Steel 1995; Walsh 1995) who have argued that the label inappropriate belongs to the service rather than the patient. Indeed a number of studies have identified that there is an association with deprivation scores and children's attendances at emergency departments (see for example Hendry *et al.* 2005).

In response, hospital based emergency departments are providing primary care, employing GPs and nurse practitioners, as both have been found to be effective at identifying those who could be managed by primary care practitioners at triage (Dale *et al.* 1995a) and reducing rates of investigation, prescription and referral (Dale *et al.* 1995b). As a consequence there has been an increase in the number of emergency departments providing designated primary care services, with an associated increase in the numbers of nurse practitioners, although variations are evident in terms of the scope of services they offer, with wide interpretations and understandings of the role (Dolan *et al.* 1997).

Although Dale *et al.*'s studies included children, the extent to which children are currently managed by GPs and nurse practitioners located in emergency departments is unclear, with some evidence that, within hospital based services, children's nurses working in the emergency department were (reluctantly) perceived by colleagues as the 'experts' in relation to children (Cleaver 2003), although Jones's (1996) study suggests that there is some benefit where children's nurses have developed this role. Key to the development of expertise within the context of paediatric emergency care and development of the role of nurse practitioners is multidisciplinary education (Cleaver 2003; Crouch 2000), which it is hoped this book will contribute towards.

References

Armon, K., Stephenson, T., Gabriel, V., MacFaul, R., Ecleston, P., Werneke, U. & Smith, S. (2001) Determining the common medical presenting problems to an accident and emergency department. *Archives of Disease in Childhood*, **84**, 390–392.

Audit Commission (2001) *Acute Hospital Portfolio. Review of National Findings: Accident and Emergency.* Audit Commission, London.

Beattie, T.F., Gorman, D.R. & Walker, J.J. (2001) The association between deprivation levels, attendance rate and triage category of children attending a children's accident and emergency department. *Emergency Medical Journal*, **18**(2), 110–111.

Bichard, M. (2004) *The Bichard Inquiry. An Independent Inquiry Arising from the Soham Murders Chaired by Sir Michael Bichard.* The Stationery Office, London.

British Paediatric Association (1985) *Children's attendances at A & E departments: Report by the Joint Committee of the British Paediatric Association and the British Association of Paediatric Surgeons.* BPA, London.

Boyle, R., Smith, C. & McIntyre, J. (2000) The changing utilisation of a children's emergency department. *Ambulatory Child Health*, **6**, 39–43.

Byrne, G. & Heyman, R. (1997) Understanding nurses' communication with patients in accident and emergency departments using a symbolic interactionist perspective. *Journal of Advanced Nursing*, **26**, 93–100.

Byrne, M., Murphy, A.W., Plunkett, P., McGee, H.H., Murray, A. & Bury, G. (2003) Frequent attenders to an emergency department: A study of primary health care use, medical profile, and psychosocial characteristics. *Annals of Emergency Medicine*, **41**, 309–318.

Cleaver, K. (2003) Developing expertise – the contribution of paediatric accident and emergency nurses to the care of children, and the implications for their continuing professional development. *Accident & Emergency Nursing*, **11**, 96–102.

Cooper, C., Simpson, J.M. & Hanson, R. (2003) The district hospital emergency department: Why do parents present? *Emergency Medicine*, **15**, 68–76.

Crouch, R. (2000) Primary Care: The A & E dimension. In: *Accident & Emergency. Theory into Practice.* B. Dolan & L. Holt (eds). Bailliere Tindall, London.

Dale, J., Green, J., Reid, F., Glucksman, E. & Higgs, R. (1995a) Primary care in the accident and emergency department: I. Prospective identification of patients. *British Medical Journal*, **311**, 423–426.

Dale, J., Green, J., Reid, F., Glucksman, E. & Higgs, R. (1995b) Primary care in the accident and emergency department: II. Comparison of general practitioners and hospital doctors. *British Medical Journal*, **311**, 427–430.

Davis, R. (1991) Letters. *Nursing Times*, **24**, 2.

Department for Education and Skills (2003) *Every Child Matters.* The Stationery Office, London (available at: http://www.dfes.gov.uk/everychildmatters).

Department of Health (2000) *The NHS Plan: A plan for investment; A plan for reform.* The Stationery Office, London.

Department of Health (2001) *Reforming Emergency Services.* The Stationery Office, London.

Department of Health (2004a) *The National Service Framework for Children, Young People and Maternity Services.* DoH. London (on line at www.publications.doh.gov.uk/nsf/children).

Department of Health (2004b) *Transforming Emergency Care in England.* The Stationery Office, London.

Dex, S. & Joshi, H. (1999) Careers and motherhood: Policies for compatibility. *Cambridge Journal of Economics,* **23,** 641–659.

Dingwall, R. & Murray, T. (1983) Categorisation in A & E departments: 'Good' patients, 'bad' patients and children. *Sociology of Health & Illness,* **5,** 127–148.

Dolan, B., Dale, J. & Morley, V. (1997) Nurse practitioners: the role in A & E and primary care. *Nursing Standard,* **11**(17), 33–38.

Elston, S. & Thornes, R. (2002) *Children's Nursing Workforce July 2002. A report to the Royal College of Nursing and the Royal College of Paediatrics and Child Health.* RCN/RCPCH, London.

Hainsworth, T. (2004) The NSF for children, young people and maternity services. *Nursing Times,* **10**(40), 28–30.

Haskey, J. (1998) One-parent families and their dependent children in Great Britain. In: *Private Lives & Public Responses,* R. Ford & J. Millar (eds). Policy Studies Institute, London.

Healthcare Commission (2005) *Acute Hospital Portfolio Review. Accident & Emergency.* Commission for Healthcare Audit and Inspection, London.

Hendry, S., Beattie, T.F. & Heaney, D. (2005) Minor illness and injury; factors influencing attendance at a paediatric accident and emergency department. *Archives of Disease in Childhood,* **90,** 629–633.

Jones, S. (1996) An action research investigation into the feasibility of experienced registered sick children's nurses (RSCN's) becoming children's emergency nurse practitioners (ENP's). *Journal of Clinical Nursing,* **5**(1), 13–21.

Kennedy, I. (2001) *Learning from Bristol: the report of the public inquiry into children's heart surgery at the Bristol Royal Infirmary 1984–1995.* The Bristol Royal Infirmary Inquiry, London.

Lord Laming (2003) *The Victoria Climbié Inquiry. Report of an Inquiry by Lord Laming.* The Stationery Office, London.

MacFaul, R., Stewart, M., Werneke, U., Taylor-Meek, J., Smith, H.E. & Smith, I.J. (1998) Parental and professional perception of need for emergency admission to hospital: prospective questionnaire based study. *Archives of Disease in Childhood,* **79,** 213–218.

Murphy, A. (1998a) 'Inappropriate' attenders at accident and emergency departments I: definition, incidence and reasons for attendance. *Family Practice,* **15,** 23–32.

Murphy, A. (1998b) 'Inappropriate' attenders at accident and emergency departments II: health service responses. *Family Practice,* **15,** 33–37.

Office for National Statistics (2004) *The Health of Children and Young People.* ONS, London.

Office for National Statistics (2005a) *Population Trends.* Winter 2005 No 122. ONS, London.

Office for National Statistics (2005b) *Survey of the Mental Health of Children and Young People.* ONS, London.

Platt, M.J. (1998) Child Health Statistics Review. *Archives of Disease in Childhood,* **79,** 523–527.

Prince, M. & Worth, C. (1992) A study of 'inappropriate' attendances to a paediatric accident and emergency department. *Journal of Public Health,* **14,** 177–182.

Rodgers, B. & Pryor, J. (1998) *Divorce and Separation: The outcomes for children.* Joseph Rowntree Foundation, York.

Royal College of Paediatrics and Child Health (1999) *Accident and emergency services for children: a report of a multidisciplinary working party.* RCPCH, London.

Salter, E. & Stallard, P. (2004) Young people's experience of emergency medical services as road traffic accident victims: a pilot qualitative study. *Journal of Child Health Care,* **8**(4), 301–311.

Salter, R. & Maconochie, I.K. (2004) Implementation of recommendations for the care of children in UK emergency departments: national postal questionnaire survey. *BMJ,* doi:10.1136/bmj.38313.580324.F7 (published 3 December 2004).

Sanders, J. (2000) A review of health professionals' attitudes and patients' perceptions on inappropriate accident and emergency attendances. The implications for current minor injury service provision in England and Wales. *Journal of Advanced Nursing,* **31,** 1097–1105.

Saxena, S., Eliahoo, J. & Majeed, A. (2002) Socioeconomic status and ethnic group differences in self reported health status and use of health services by children and young people in England: cross sectional study. *British Medical Journal,* **325**(7363), 520.

Smith, F. (2004) The NSF for Children, Young People and Maternity Services: an overview. *Paediatric Nursing,* **16**(8), 30–32.

Social Exclusion Unit (1999) *Teenage Pregnancy.* HMSO, London.

Steel, J. (1995) Inappropriate – the patient or the service? *Accident & Emergency Nursing*, **3**, 146–149.

Walsh, M. (1995) The health belief model and the use of accident and emergency services by the general public. *Journal of Advanced Nursing*, **22**, 694–699.

Webb, J. & Cleaver, K. (1991) The child in casualty. *Nursing Times*, **87**, 26–31.

Woolfenden, S., Ritchie, J., Hanson, R. & Nossar, V. (2000) Parental use of a paediatric emergency department as an ambulatory care service. *Australian, New Zealand Public Health*, **24**, 204–206.

Woolwich, C. (2000) Nurse Triage. In: B. Dolan & L. Holt (eds) *Accident & Emergency. Theory into Practice.* Bailliere Tindall, London.

Chapter 2 **Principles of Emergency Care for Children and Young People**

Lesley Wayne, Louise Bunn and Janet Webb

Introduction

This chapter outlines the approaches that may be used in the assessment and care management of children within the accident and emergency setting. It is firstly important to understand that the child's perception of their presenting problem or injury (and sometimes their family's perception) may differ greatly from that of practitioners. This may be illustrated by the child who complains of pain or injury from a relatively insignificant event; or one who frequently attends with parents requesting a 'check over' with every minor scrape or bump. The important issue is never to be complacent about a child's attendance until a full assessment of the presenting problem and their unarticulated needs has been undertaken. The reason for the attendance and the strange environment of the emergency department can cause the child anxiety and distress. Therefore, more time is needed in comforting and reassuring children than may be necessary with adults. Time and effort invested in securing and maintaining the trust and confidence of a child will facilitate a smoother, less traumatic progress through treatment and care. It is therefore important that nurses caring for children possess a range of skills in order to manage the child's care within this setting (RCN 1998).

With this in mind, this chapter will firstly outline the general principles of assessing children with emphasis on the need to make a brief assessment of the child's cognitive and physical development, whilst also considering the child's and family's levels of anxiety and their coping mechanisms. Pointers to communicating with children and their families and managing situations through the use of play and distraction are given. As in any setting, documentation of initial and ongoing assessment along with documentation of subsequent interventions and outcomes is vital. However, as well as gaining information directly related to the presenting injury/illness the visit to the department provides opportunity for the practitioners to assess other issues which may have implications for the child's welfare and safety. Documentation is therefore discussed with an example of an assessment format which lends itself to this context.

The principles of assessing children

Assessment of the severity of the child's presenting illness/injury and the need for treatment is vital. This, however, needs to be done simultaneously with an assessment of the child's developmental age and cognitive skills. The practitioner's skill in assessing these and achieving a good relationship with the child and their family are essential to information gathering. It should be remembered that the emergency department may be the child's first experience of a hospital environment (RCN 1998). Furthermore, children can react in many ways to an unplanned hospital visit (Morcombe 2001). Whilst some children are only mildly apprehensive of this encounter, for others the visit might be a desperately unhappy, frightening experience whatever the reason for their attendance. This may present a picture of a screaming, uncooperative child or a quiet, withdrawn and unhappy one (Dolan 1997; Lanning 1985). Additionally, children of different ages have different verbal and cognitive abilities, thus the assessment must also take into account behaviours that indicate upset or anxiety; the strategies used to elicit children's descriptions of these concepts vary with the child's age. Differences in physiological responses and parental/family responses based on the age of the child presenting must not be overlooked during the assessment. Indeed, emergency care practitioners are in a position to reduce adverse psychological effects that may be experienced as a result of the attendance. Failure to treat a child sensitively, according to their age and stage of development, may result in long-lasting psychological effects (Morcombe 2001).

Establishing a good rapport

Numerous reports and policy documents have, since the Platt Report (Ministry of Health 1959), stressed the need for specialist paediatric staff trained in assessing and implementing care appropriate to the developmental stage of the child. More recently this is reflected in the *National Service Framework for Children, Young People and Maternity Services* (DoH 2004). Furthermore, the assessment itself and the subsequent treatment and care of the child are dependent on both the child and his parents/carers having a trusting relationship with all the staff of the department. The basis for establishing a good rapport and forming that trusting relationship is communication.

The use of the following techniques might be considered too time-consuming to be of benefit. They may be considered inappropriate for use in a busy emergency department. However, we would like to stress this is not our experience. Investment in time here is well spent and will be advantageous initially and in the future, assisting the practitioner in establishing a good rapport with the child and family.

1   Assess the child's initial reaction to you and the environment. Children's knowledge and understanding is based not only on their age, social background and culture but also on life experiences. This can be very limited when a child first attends an emergency department, or very vivid if a previous traumatic visit has occurred (RCN 1998).
2   Be especially aware of the child's, and your own, body language. Communication with children should be age related and relies upon a careful choice of words and often a good deal of action. Children tend to use non-verbal communication, both in the way that they express themselves and in the way in which they interpret information from others. Awareness of eye contact, facial expression, gesture, body posture and movement are essential to achieving a high level of communication. Children are imaginative and respond well to play so the practitioner can enhance understanding through demonstrations. Fear too can be dissipated through play (Burr 2005; DoH 2004; Hart & Bossert 1994; Smith 1995).
3   Use a gentle approach, a soft tone of voice, and also engage the parent in conversation. It usually helps to talk to the parent/carer first and then involve the child. It may sometimes be necessary to appear to ignore the child in order to observe their behaviour.
4   Get down to the child's level as towering above them will often frighten them.
5   Address the child by his usual name. It sometimes helps to discuss something personal to the child such as a toy.
6   When dealing with the child who is reluctant to interact with you, place a physical barrier between yourself and the child; engaging in play activities by yourself or with the assistance of the parent or a colleague will enable you to distance yourself. These actions will usually appeal to the inquisitive nature of the child who will be unable to resist the 'invitation' to play.

Having established a relationship you are subsequently able to proceed with your assessment or examination of the injury itself using the following strategies:

*   A description of the proposed assessment and treatment is essential. Explanation and/or demonstration of the intended assessment and treatment procedures should be appropriate to the child's level of understanding. Cognitive ability will vary with each child but remember children may regress in stressful situations.
*   Use cartoons, pictures and photographs, dolls or soft toys to support verbal explanations. The child's and parent's level of understanding can be checked by requesting them to feedback the information.

- Use age-appropriate language (Dolan 1997). Assess the child's cognitive developmental stage and beware of ambiguity, e.g. 'that's a bad cut', might be interpreted by the child as meaning that he/she is a 'bad' person and is to blame for their injury (remember, pain is often perceived as a punishment by children).
- Where appropriate elicit the child's help in all activities.
- Continue to involve the parents in conversation.
- Take your time and wait for replies.
- Never force an issue.
- Be thoughtful and honest.

Assessment, triage and documentation

It is recognised that history-taking and assessment are usually carried out simultaneously and include obtaining and documenting information about:

- The social context of the child, name of the person accompanying the child, who has parental responsibility including details of whether they are present or need to be contacted/aware that the child is attending the department
- The presenting problem and history of injury
- Assessment of the child's pain using an appropriate pain assessment tool (Moor 2001; RCN 1998)
- Details of any medication, including analgesia, already administered by parents/carers
- Known allergies.

As well as gaining information directly related to the injury, the assessment and triage process enables the opportunity to check on immunisations, developmental progress and the feeding and sleeping patterns of the child. Whilst this may not be directly related to the reason for attendance itself, this assessment may have implications for the overall welfare of the child. Additionally the assessment and ordered documentation of an injury will assist the practitioner/triage nurse in recognising injuries that are not consistent with the presenting history and may alert child protection concerns. Any child protection concerns should be discussed, docu-

mented and advice sought in accordance with local protocols and national policy for safeguarding children (Chapter 4 has further information).

Documentation

We cannot emphasise enough the importance of clear, factual, accurate and contemporaneous note-taking whatever the outcome of the initial triage assessment. Indeed, in all aspects of emergency care, documentation is as vital as the treatment given; it is the basis for communication, continuity and quality care (Dent 2005). It is essential (and a requirement under professional codes of conduct) that records can be understood and used by the many different professionals who might be involved in treating the child (Rodden & Bell 2002; Dent 2005). Records are also subject to professional and legal obligations and reference to your notes may be required in the future, even several years hence. Sadly, involvement in litigation is a possibility and if this occurs you will be thankful that you have an accurate, documented history of events. Moreover, the approach to record-keeping that Courts of Law adopt is that 'if it is not recorded it has not been done' (NMC 2005). Records should follow a logical and methodological sequence which in this context includes initial assessment and triage findings, relevant clinical findings, outcomes and decisions made, information given to the child and family and any drugs or other treatment prescribed and given. Numerous factors which contribute to effective record-keeping and formats may vary; our format based on Guly (1996) (see Table 2.1) meets contemporary professional requirements, is logical and also lends itself to the context of emergency departments and the assessment of children (GMC 1995; NMC 2005).

Play: a therapeutic tool

Play is 'an expression of the child's understanding of his/her world and represents their attempts to master the environment' (Le Vieux-Anglin & Sawyer 1993). Thus play is vital and its importance should not be dismissed. During play the child takes command which positively reinforces their sense of self-control. It is, though, often neglected by health care professionals

Table 2.1 Suggested format for documentation

1	Presenting complaint	The child's reason for attendance
2	History of presenting complaint	How, when and where the injury occurred/when the illness started, any treatment given, the administration of first aid, wound care and analgesia.
3	Past medical history	Underlying medical conditions, previous injuries, e.g. fractures, involvement of other health or social care professionals.
4	Current medication	Prescribed and self-administered.
5	Known allergies	
6	Tetanus and immunisation status	
7	Dominant hand	Recorded for all limb injuries.
8	Social history and context	Who the child is accompanied by, who has parental responsibility and do they need to be contacted, which pre-school/nursery/school they attend, name of health visitor/school nurse, general practitioner, social worker support, siblings, any sporting activities etc.
9	Assessment of the presenting condition or injury and clinical examination findings	This should follow an accepted logical progression. If it is an injury we find it appropriate to use the medical model of look, feel, move (Guly 1996). It is, however, recognised that the accident and emergency practitioner needs to focus on the child as an individual not just the injury that they present with, thus the medical model is used in this context. **Assessment of level of pain** – document here and on a pain assessment tool. **Remember** that in order to deliver the care that is appropriate for the child and their family (and exclude the possibility of neglect or abuse) it is necessary at this point to assess the child's cognitive and physical abilities and decide whether these are conversant with their expected developmental stage. Be aware that children are likely to regress in a strange environment and under stressful circumstances. The expert on the child is their parent, so consult them, listen and document the parent's assessment of, or concerns about, the presenting problem. *Aides-mémoire* on child development are useful to have available, e.g. the book *Accidents and Child Development* (Child Accident Prevention Trust 2000).
10	Provisional diagnosis	
11	Plan	Decisions made and outcome i.e. further investigations, such as x ray or proposed treatment including the involvement of the child and family. Initiating the prescription and administration of pain relief according to local policies. The reduction of the child's anxieties through the use of play. The provision of information related to triage, the process of care delivery and any potential delay in treatment. The provision of information related to the prevention of accidents or first aid treatment. Contacting the child's next of kin or other relatives. **Remember** that throughout the assessment and treatment period the presence of a parent will reassure an anxious child and provide the practitioner with the opportunity to clarify details, obtain an in-depth history and give advice to the parent. Separation will only increase anxiety and cooperation might be lost.
12	Confirmed diagnosis	
13	Treatment	Actions actually performed, e.g. cleansing, exploration and closure of wound and dressing applied.
14	Outcome of treatment and care	Referrals and discharge, record of the advice given. Any re-education of parents/families and information of other health care facilities available.

Remember! Confidentiality must be maintained according to local and national policies. Where there is an issue of child protection, you must act at all times in accordance with local and national policies (NMC 2005).

(Webster 2000), especially in the emergency care setting. However, the provision of play facilities is extremely important, as play is the means by which a child learns and is able to express his fears and come to terms with what is happening, and, helpfully, can help to fill the waiting time more constructively. It is often suggested that limited environmental space (such as that of an emergency department) and possible restrictive movement of the child restricts play. However, play should be inventive using imagination. It should suit the needs of the child and take account of their surroundings.

Bolig (1990) suggested seven criteria necessary for normal play in that play must be:

- Voluntary
- Internally motivated
- Pleasurable and relaxed
- Active with motion and cognition
- Organism rather than object-dominated
- Unique and unpredictable
- Have an element of pretence.

Garvey (1977) described different types of play:

- Play with motion and interaction – active experiences that also provide sensory stimulation
- Play with objects – use of objects to explore and manipulate the environment
- Play with language – use of word games to enhance language development
- Play with social materials – use of pretending and make-believe to explore relationships between objects, actions and people
- Play with rules – setting limits or constraints of play to formalise it or to provide an object to play against
- Ritualised play – controlled, generally rhythmic repetition.

A working knowledge of growth and development is fundamental in order for the professional to instigate meaningful play therapy (Taylor *et al.* 1999). Strategies chosen will not only be closely linked with the individual's development but will also consider the application of treatment. Remember too that children have vivid imaginations and can fantasise about hospitals and what happens in them, particularly if this is their first visit. One of their main fears is of the unknown, and it is therefore important that the child is prepared for the experience (McClowry & McLeod 1990). Strategies which can be used in the emergency department include:

- Dolls, soft toys etc. are ideal for the explanation and demonstration of treatments and procedures.
- The child can be encouraged to imagine and rehearse the forthcoming situation.
- Adolescents may be helped by the use of puzzles, diagrams and drawings.

Using play in this way not only helps the child's understanding, but has the added advantage of acting as a relaxation tool and distraction technique. It also helps to allay the parents' fears and anxieties, enabling them to assist the child, and ultimately you. We would emphasise that time spent initially will reap reward; the child, through gaining control, will be more cooperative, reducing the stress for all involved.

Play as distraction

Distraction techniques allow children to use their imagination and in doing so draw their focus away from the injury, especially when associated with pain (McCaffery & Beebe 1989). Cooperation can be gained by the use of specific distraction techniques. Among our favourites are:

- Bubbles, glitter sticks, music/story tapes, puzzles, storybooks and water play
- The use of fantasy e.g. imagery is also a useful technique but can be difficult to employ in an emergency situation.

Box 2.1   Scenario utilising therapeutic play and distraction to aid communication and compliance

Jason is a four-year-old boy whose mother is extremely anxious and protective of her child. She tells you that he will scream, resist examination and treatment: 'On visits to the GP they wrap him up and get on with it, because he doesn't understand'.

Box 2.1 (Continued)

Presenting complaint

A facial wound to his left cheek sustained when walking into a door handle 30 minutes ago. There was no loss of consciousness, no vomiting, no drowsiness, no apparent headache, no visual disturbance or abnormal gait to indicate dizziness.

Past medical history

His mother tells you that he has learning disabilities and attends the local child development centre. She advises you that he has a developmental delay regarding his speech.

- Medication – none
- Allergies – none known
- Tetanus status – up to date.

On examination

Jason is uncooperative; it is therefore necessary for the nurse practitioner to build a rapport with him and gain his trust.

The following was found to work: An explanation was given to his mother informing her how we were going to gain Jason's trust and confidence through play. He remained at a distance from the nursing staff, constantly running around. He was observed to lack concentration for any significant time. Parallel play was commenced involving the nurse practitioner (NP) and a colleague. This gradually gained his attention. Jason subsequently became intrigued and involved in the play as he gained trust in the staff. As this trust increased, staff were free to progress to therapeutic play, incorporating the intended examination and procedure (Collier & MacKinley 1993; Le Vieux-Anglin & Sawyer 1993; Somerville 2001; Visintainer & Wolfer 1975).

Greater cooperation is gained by encouraging the child to participate in the examination and therapeutic procedures, e.g. 'Pooh Bear' (a great favourite of ours) may be incorporated into the play scenario. The intended procedure is then rehearsed using 'Pooh' as the patient. 'Conversations' between 'Pooh' and the practitioner can be used to reinforce the information being given and build a rapport with the child. The child is encouraged to carry out the intended procedure, e.g. washing and closure of wounds. All these pointers allow you to give the child a degree of control and autonomy, enabling them to be involved in any choices to be made regarding their treatment (DoH 1998; Somerville 2001).

Jason became involved in washing 'Pooh's wound' spontaneously and progressed to cleaning his own wound with the assistance of the NP. He subsequently complied with assessment and treatment while sitting on his mother's knee and being distracted by his mother blowing bubbles.

Treatment and discharge

Jason's wound was closed using tissue adhesive; he did not cry. He was discharged with his mother who was given routine wound care advice. Jason was rewarded for his good behaviour with a colouring book, sticker and bravery certificate.

Alert: Assessing injuries in children can be challenging. There are many possible reasons why children may not cooperate with a physical examination/assessment as an adult would:

- Pain
- Fear
- Shyness
- Lack of understanding due to age of development.

Thorough assessment and adequate pain relief facilitates management of minor childhood injuries (Young *et al.* 2005).

Conclusion

Clearly assessing children and young people in the emergency department can be challenging, thus practitioners require different skills than those used when assessing adults. As Young *et al.* (2005) note, children may not cooperate during an initial assessment or physical examination as an adult would. Reasons include pain, fear, shyness or a lack of understanding of what the practitioner is requesting. An understanding of the child's developmental age is therefore important in assessing their needs and the assessment should focus on wider issues related to the child's welfare as well as the presenting illness/injury. Communication strategies should be used according to the child's age and stage of development and establishing a good rapport helps to make an accurate assessment of the child's presenting illness or injury. A logical format for documentation is required which lends itself to a more holistic assessment of the child and family, of which an example has been given within this chapter. The use of play is as important in the accident and emergency setting as anywhere else where children are cared for and is invaluable as a therapeutic tool and distraction technique. Practitioners have a responsibility to develop specialist skills to enable them to assess and manage pain effectively according to national policy and local protocols thereby improving the outcomes for the child and delivering care as advocated in the NSF (DoH 2004).

References

Bolig, R. (1990) Play in health care settings: a challenge for the 1990's. *Children's Health Care*, **19**(4), 229–233.

Burr, S. (2005) Volunteering serious fun. *Paediatric Nursing*, **17**(3), 30–32.

Child Accident Prevention Trust (CAPT) (2000) *Accidents and Child Development, Guidelines for Practitioners*. CAPT, London.

Collier, J. & MacKinley, D. (1993) Play preparation guidelines for the multidisciplinary team. *Child Health*, October, 123–125.

Dent, K. (2005) Record Keeping – just for the fun of it? *Paediatric Nursing*, **17**(1), 18–20.

Department of Health (1998) *Seeking consent: working with children*. DoH, London.

Department of Health (2004) *National Service Framework for Children, Young People and Maternity Services*. The Stationery Office, London.

Dolan, K. (1997) Children in accident and emergency. *Accident Emergency Nursing*, **5**(2), 88–91.

Garvey, C. (1977) *Play*. Harvard University Press, Cambridge, Massachusetts.

General Medical Council (1995) *Duties of a Doctor*. GMC, London.

Guly, H.R. (1996) *History Taking, Examination and Record Keeping in Emergency Medicine*. Oxford University Press, Oxford.

Hart, D. & Bossert, E. (1994) Self-reported fears of hospitalized school-age children. *Journal of Pediatric Nursing*, **9**(2), 83–90.

Lanning, J. (1985) Paediatric trauma, emotional aspects. *AORN Journal*, **42**(3), 345–351.

Le Vieux-Anglin, L. & Sawyer, E.H. (1993) Incorporating Play Interventions into Nursing Care. *Pediatric Nursing*, 19(5), 459–463.

McCaffery, M. & Beebe, A. (1989) *Pain: Clinical Manual for Nursing Practice*. Mosby, London.

McClowry, S.G. & McLeod, S.M. (1990) The psychological responses of school-age children to hospitalisation. *Children's Health Care*, **19**(3), 155–161.

Ministry of Health (1959) Ministry of Health and Central Service Council. *The welfare of children in hospital. Report of the Committee* (Chairman Sir H. Platt). HMSO, London.

Moor, R. (2001) Pain assessment in A & E: a critical analysis. *Paediatric Nursing*, **13**(2), 20–24.

Morcombe, J. (2001) Reducing Child Anxiety in the A & E Department. *Understanding Mental Health*. http://www.defeatdepression.org/pdf/aandedept.pdf (accessed August 2005).

Nursing and Midwifery Council (2005) *The NMC code of conduct: standards for conduct performance and ethics*. NMC, London.

Rodden, C. & Bell, M. (2002) Record keeping: developing good practice. *Nursing Standard*, **17**(1), 40–42.

Royal College of Nursing (RCN) (1998) *Nursing Children in the Accident and Emergency Department*, 2nd edn. RCN, London.

Smith, F. *et al.* (1995) *Children's Nursing in Practice: The Nottingham Model*. Blackwell Science, Oxford.

Somerville, L. (2001) Children Love Surprises . . . but (Conference Report, presented at NSW OTA Annual Conference, April 2001) *ACORN*, Winter, 34–36.

Taylor, J., Muller, D., Whattley, L. & Harris, P. (1999) *Nursing Children. Psychology, Research and Practice*, 3rd edn. Stanley Thornes, Cheltenham.

Visintainer, M.A. & Wolfer, J.A. (1975) Psychological preparation for surgical pediatric patients: The effect on children's and parents' stress responses and adjustment. *Pediatrics*, **56**(2), 187–201.

Webster, A. (2000) The facilitating role of the play specialist. *Paediatric Nursing*, **12**(7), 24–27.

Young, S.J., Barnett, P.L. & Oakley, E.A. (2005) Bruising, abrasions and lacerations: minor injuries in children 1. *MJA Practice Essential Paediatrics*, **182**(11), 588–592.

Chapter 3 Legal and Ethical Emergency Care of Children

Pat Rose

Introduction

In this chapter, we will be exploring the range of laws, codes and recommendations that inform children's emergency care. This will be done through examining key Articles of the Human Rights Act 1998 (henceforth referred to as this/ the Act). This Act underpins all UK law related to the functioning of public authorities such as the NHS, and was designed to protect individuals from the power of the State (Plant 2000). The European Convention on Human Rights and Fundamental Freedoms (henceforth to be referred to as 'the Convention'), was adopted by the Council of Europe in 1950. It was drafted by a senior civil servant in the UK, and the UK was the first State to ratify it. This means that prior to the passing of the UK Human Rights Act 1998, all new UK law took into account the Convention Articles, and in establishing case law, UK judges made decisions in line with the Convention. For many years, it was felt that a UK Act was therefore unnecessary. The problem, however, was that if someone felt their rights had been breached, they had to take the case to the European Court of Human Rights. Now that the UK has its own Act, cases can be heard in the UK.

Some laws relating to health care differ between Scotland, England, Wales and Northern Ireland. However, the requirement to abide by the Convention was included as part of the devolution of power legislation (Horton 2000); therefore the issues discussed in this chapter apply equally to all the UK countries. Some of the 18 Articles within the Act apply directly to health care provision, and some, though not directly applicable, raise issues for health care professionals.

Before discussing the relevant Articles and the issues they raise, it is important to differentiate between law, codes and recommendations as each arises from a different source, and carries different implications. The place of ethics in informing decision making also needs to be considered.

Law is defined as 'a rule enacted or customary in a community and recognised as enjoining or prohibiting certain actions and enforced by the imposition of penalties' (*Concise Oxford Dictionary*). Enacted rules are the Acts of Parliament, such as the Children Act 1989, 2004, the Access to Medical Records Act 1990, the Misuse of Drugs Act 1971, and of course the Human Rights Act 1998. Customary law, also known as case law, is a ruling made by a judge where an Act is open to interpretation. Examples of case law relevant to health care provision, which will be discussed within this chapter, include *Donoghue* v. *Stevenson* [1932] AC 562, which ruled on duty of care, and *Gillick* v. *West Norfolk and Wisbech AHA and the DHSS* [1985] 3 All ER 402, which ruled on consent to medical treatment by a minor. Enjoining law is that which carries a penalty if the action is not carried out, for example seat belts must be worn in a car. Prohibitive law is that which carries a penalty if the action is carried out, for example if a driver exceeds the speed limit. The law that informs health care practice is a mixture of enjoining and prohibitive law as will become evident as the chapter progresses.

Codes are the sets of rules governing behaviour in specific contexts. For nurses the Nursing and Midwifery Council (NMC) *Code of Professional Conduct: Standards for Conduct, Performance and Ethics* (NMC 2004) is the primary statement of professional behaviour. For doctors it is the 'Duties of a Doctor' contained within *Good Medical Practice* (General Medical Council (GMC) 2001), and other professions have their codes. Whilst these codes are not law, they are usually required by law. For example, the NMC is required by the Nursing and Midwifery Order 2001 (Article 3(2)) to establish standards of conduct for nurses. Any breach of a professional code carries a penalty imposed by the professional body as opposed to the Courts.

Recommendations arise from many sources and their influence is often linked to their source. For example, government bodies such as the Department of Health make recommendations based on the findings of standing committees, commissioned research and interpretation of government policy. The Audit Commission makes recommendations based on its findings. Recommendations may be national, such as those of the National Institute for Health and Clinical Excellence (NICE) that arise from research evidence, or local, such as those of the Healthcare Commission (CHI) that arise from 'inspection' of individual NHS trusts. Of particular significance however are the standards for hospital services for children (Department of Health (DoH) 2003) contained in the *National Service Framework for Children, Young People and Maternity Services* (DoH 2004). This document applies to all areas where children are cared for in hospital and makes frequent specific mention of accident and emergency departments. All these recommendations carry weight and are expected to be implemented. Failure to implement them, by an individual employee, may constitute a breach of contract, and result in disciplinary action, and, for an organisation, may result in a penalty such as loss of income, or loss of managerial autonomy.

Some recommendations arise from charities and pressure groups and whilst they carry less weight in terms of risk of penalty if not acted on, they often have the weight of public opinion behind them. A prime example of this is the way in which the recommendations of Action for Sick Children (formerly the National Association for the Welfare of Children in Hospital) revolutionised care of children in hospital because of pressure from parents, for example resident parents, separate accident and emergency facilities

for children, and care for children by suitably qualified staff.

It is sometimes difficult to differentiate between law, codes and recommendations as the imperative to abide by each, and the penalties for failure to do so, may seem equally stringent. Indeed, there is often no practical difference between the three. Nevertheless, within all legislation, codes of practice and recommendations, the overriding concern is for the welfare of the child, and health care professionals must act in the best interests of the child. However, one problem for health care professionals is that there is such a plethora of law, codes and recommendations, often contradictory, that it is difficult to find a way through the jungle and make the right decision. And, of course, the imperative to make the right decision is not primarily in order to avoid penalty, but first and foremost, in order to provide the best possible care for children and their families. Ethics, or the study of right and wrong behaviour, is often used to justify difficult decisions. By applying ethical principles – such as the best interests of the child; the promotion of personal autonomy; the greatest good and least harm to the greatest number – staff can account for decisions made in the face of unclear or contradictory law, codes and recommendations.

This chapter provides a review of key legislation, and other codes and recommendations, explores their relationships, explains how they have been interpreted, and highlights the decisions staff may be called upon to make when caring for a child in an emergency department. This will be done by examining in detail seven of the Articles of the Act. The Articles omitted relate to issues that are not usually encountered by health care professionals such as slavery, fair trial and freedom of assembly.

Each section begins with a list of the ethical and legal issues discussed within it. The Article is then quoted, and where indicated by '. . .' the Article continues, usually to give exceptions to the right concerned. Where this occurs, the relevant content is summarised in the first paragraph of the discussion. Some themes, such as consent, confidentiality and duty of care, become threads running through more than one section. It is particularly in the case of these threads that contradictions may arise, which lend themselves to the application of ethical principles.

Article 2: the right to life

Related ethical and legal issues:

- Duty of care
- Withdrawing and withholding treatment.

> Everyone's right to life shall be protected by law. No one shall be deprived of his life intentionally . . .

The right to life is a fundamental principle of British society. The only lawful exceptions to this are: where people have been convicted of a capital crime (not applicable anywhere in the UK since 1999); self-defence; the lawful arrest or prevention of escape of a person lawfully detained; and the quelling of riot or insurrection.

The right to life is of course based on the assumption that the value of life overrides all other considerations. Indeed, in the language of religion, the sanctity of life is a universal human principle and it is this principle that underpins the duty of care incumbent on all health care professionals.

In making decisions regarding the giving or withholding of life sustaining treatment, the Royal College of Paediatrics and Child Health (RCPCH 2004) discuss the issue of duty of care. They suggest that the duty of care has two elements. First, the professional duty to sustain life and to restore patients to health, to which they add that even if a child cannot be restored to health, there is 'an absolute duty to comfort and to cherish the child and to prevent pain and suffering' (Para 2.3.1.1). Second, the legal duty, in which any treatment or care given with the primary intention of causing death is unlawful. The dilemma arises however when withholding or withdrawing treatment will result in the death of the child even though that was not the primary intention. In emergency care, because the past health status of the patient is often initially unknown, and because the prognosis

may initially be unpredictable, all patients are actively treated in respect of their presenting symptoms. It is often much later in the course of their treatment, generally after they have left the department, that the efficacy of further treatment comes into question. Nevertheless, there are occasions when the decision must be made, for example when a child arrives in cardiac and/or respiratory arrest. Full resuscitation is commenced, but when it becomes clear that the child is not responding, the decision is taken to withdraw this intervention and death ensues. The commoner causes of this type of catastrophic collapse include sudden infant death, drowning, smoke inhalation, severe dehydration and overwhelming infection.

In health care there have been cases presented to the Courts where withdrawal of medical treatment has been permitted and has led to the natural death of the person concerned. The case from which this precedent arose was that of Tony Bland, a young man who was severely crushed in the Hillsborough football disaster where too many fans poured into the back of a fenced stand and those at the front could not escape the crush. Tony Bland was left in a persistent vegetative state, his cardiovascular system was functioning but he had no detectable voluntary neurological function and could not take nutrition orally. It was deemed that artificial feeding was a medical intervention that was futile in terms of improving his condition and could therefore be terminated (*Airedale NHS Trust* v. *Bland* [1993] 1 All ER 821). The precedent set was that if intervention does not help a patient, and indeed may be burdensome to the patient, it may be withdrawn even if that results in the patient's death. This precedent applies both to children and adults.

The decision to withhold or withdraw intervention is particularly difficult in the case of babies and children in an emergency department, partly because they are at the beginning of their life, partly because of the overwhelming devastation the loss of a child causes to a family, and to society as a whole. The precedent described above is difficult to apply in this setting as it seems very early in the course of the child's care to be making such a profound decision. Thus, in acute situations the RCPCH (2004) recommends that it is always necessary to give life-sustaining treatment first and to review this when enough information and/or a more experienced opinion are available.

Those caring for children in an emergency department need to understand the ethical principles relating to the withholding or withdrawing of life sustaining treatment in children. In discussing the decision making process, the RCPCH (2004) provides a guide to the five circumstances where withholding or withdrawing treatment might be considered. Those relevant to the emergency care of children are:

- **The no hope / no chance situation.** A child brought to an emergency department may have suffered such extensive trauma or overwhelming infection that despite all medical intervention, life cannot be sustained. In these circumstances treatment is simply delaying death. The RCPCH suggest that to persist with futile treatment may be deemed an assault as it does not serve the best interests of the child. This is supported by case law, for example the case of a 16-month-old child with muscular atrophy, who was on a ventilator (Re C, a minor [1997] 40 BMLR). In this case the doctors wanted to try the child off the ventilator, and if she could not manage, then not put her on again. They argued that if she could not breathe unaided she would never be able to do so. The parents, orthodox Jews, wanted their daughter's life preserved at all costs. The Court however ruled that doctors could not be compelled to give useless treatments, and agreed that in this case ventilation would not help the child regain the ability to breathe (McHale *et al.* 2001).
- **The no purpose situation.** Treatment may be withheld or withdrawn if it is deemed likely that the child will be left so profoundly impaired that it would not be reasonable to expect her or him to bear it. For example, an infant may be brought to an emergency department having suffered an apparent sudden infant death. It may be evident from the

history and condition of the infant that whilst full resuscitation may establish some degree of cardio-respiratory function, the infant would inevitably be left with such profound cerebral palsy that life would be unbearable. In this case treatment should not be commenced. Other circumstances where this decision may need to be made in an emergency department include drowning, severe and extensive burns, and severe head injury.

There are cases where the decision whether to treat a child or not is exceptionally difficult to make. Woods (2001) describes these cases as having certain features in common:

- Very difficult decisions are to be made about treatment versus non-treatment.
- There is a high degree of ethical uncertainty and unease.
- Disagreement between health care professionals and parents are based on medical need versus parental beliefs and values.
- Legal means are used to reach a conclusion.
- The case receives media attention.
- There is a degree of public sympathy for the parents.

She goes on to discuss the two opposing viewpoints inherent in these cases. First, there is the 'rights of parents' viewpoint. This position assumes that parents know what is best for their child and will choose the best. The opponents of this view suggest that parents do not always know what is best for their child, particularly when they may not understand an illness, or what medicine has to offer in the way of help. They also suggest that not all parents always have their child's best interests at heart, and cite cases of child neglect and other abuse at the hands of parents to support this view. Thus, they argue that the child has the right to the best that medicine can offer, regardless of the parents' views.

The second viewpoint is described by Woods (2001) as the 'responsibilities and duties of doctors' viewpoint. The underlying assumption here is that, on the basis of their knowledge and experience, doctors know best and the public trust them to recommend the right course of treatment.

Opponents of this view argue that the public are becoming increasingly knowledgeable about health and treatment choices, the use of alternative therapies is increasing, and that quality of life is gaining precedence over sanctity of life.

In cases of conflict between parents and health care professionals, if time allows the Court becomes the arbiter. The decision usually supports the medical view, whether it be to give or to withhold or withdraw treatment. In the emergency department, where immediate decisions have to be made, it becomes paramount that the multidisciplinary team and the parents can come to agreement about the best course of treatment and care for the child. Woods (2001) suggests that it may fall to the nurse to put the views of parents to doctors, and vice versa. Whether this is the case or not, it is important that the guidelines for decision making (as described above) are strictly adhered to, and the reasons for the ultimate decision are clearly documented.

Article 3: the right to humane treatment

Related ethical and legal issues:

- Holding still, restraining and containing
- Treatment as a deterrent.

> No one shall be subjected to torture or to inhuman or degrading treatment or punishment.

Strictly speaking, this Article applies to the prohibition of torture. There are no exceptions to this, and rightly so. It is almost impossible to imagine torture, or degrading or inhuman treatment happening to children in an emergency department, but issues for health care professionals are raised by this Article. Consider the following scenario:

Box 3.1

Tracey is 12 years old. She has been rushed to the accident and emergency department after taking a deliberate overdose of paracetamol, which she of course does not realise the full danger of. As part of her treatment Tracey is required to drink the charcoal. She refuses and fights vigorously

when it is held to her lips. Finally, with the help of her father and two male nurses, she is held down, her nose held and the charcoal poured into her. She spits it out, and eventually the nurses give up. Next, Tracey is subjected to venepuncture to establish the baseline paracetamol level in her blood. This is done without the use of anaesthetic cream, as a matter of policy, as it is felt to be a deterrent to the child repeating the overdose.

Leaving aside the issue of consent for the time being, this scenario warrants analysis in the light of Article 3 of the Act. Clearly, Tracey is not being tortured, although she may perceive her treatment in this way. However, one has to question whether the way in which the administration of charcoal was carried out is degrading and inhuman treatment. Inhuman is defined as: 'brutal; unfeeling; barbarous' (*Concise Oxford Dictionary*) whilst degrading has been defined in law as 'that which arouses in the victim a feeling of fear, humiliation, anguish and inferiority capable of humiliating and debasing the victim' (*Ireland* v. *UK* [1978] 2 EHRR 25). It seems clear, using these definitions, that Tracey could experience fear, humiliation and anguish though the treatment could only be classed as inhuman if it were carried out in a brutal and unfeeling way. Barbarism is associated with lack of civilisation, a charge that could not easily be brought against emergency care staff. Thus, whilst probably not inhuman, the question remains as to whether the treatment was degrading to the point that her right under this Article was violated.

In defence of their actions, the nursing staff would probably refer to their code of ethics (NMC 2004) that places on them a duty of care. In addition, the staff may refer to the professional guidelines on the restraint of children. Literature is available regarding the safe handling of children (Collins 1999; Robinson and Collier 1997), and the Royal College of Nursing (RCN 1999) provides guidance on restraining, holding still and containing children, which the DoH (2003: 3.23) states should be adhered to. Four general principles in good decision making are recommended:

- An ethos of caring and respect for the child's rights where restraint, holding or containing without the child's consent, are a last resort and not a first line of intervention
- Openness about who decides what is in the child's best interest in relation to restraint, holding and containing, and clear mechanisms for staff to be heard if they disagree with the decision
- A policy relevant to the client group and setting which sets out when holding, restraint or containing may be necessary and how it may be done
- Sufficient numbers of staff who are trained and confident in safe and appropriate techniques and alternatives to restraint, holding and containing.

This guidance suggests that all emergency departments that care for children need to implement a policy on restraint, holding and containment, and ensure staff are appropriately trained, perhaps within the annual programme of moving and handling training. In relation to our scenario, if these were not in place, this might strengthen Tracey's case that this right was violated.

This scenario illustrates the way in which one law, the right not to be treated in a degrading way, may appear to contradict other law and ethical principles, namely duty of care and the best interests of the child. This also illustrates why professional guidelines are so important to professional practice.

The possibility of the treatment being inhuman or degrading is not the only issue this scenario raises. The other issue is that of inhuman or degrading punishment. Punishment has two functions, one of reparation and one of deterrent. It is the deterrent aspect of punishment that is of concern here. Tracey is subjected to venepuncture without anaesthetic cream as a deterrent to her taking another overdose. Clearly it is not the venepuncture itself that is the punishment, but the lack of anaesthetic cream. Punishment is a process of inflicting a penalty for an offence. By taking an overdose, Tracey has offended against a society that values life. Thus, it could be argued that she needs to be punished in order to deter

her from such behaviour in the future, in much the same way as any parent punishes the offences of children in order to socialise them. Parents, and those who care for children, are permitted to punish children in order to impose discipline. However, there are two questions which must be asked in the case of Tracey's punishment. First, the appropriateness of the punishment, and secondly the right of health care professionals to administer it. It is a longstanding principle of children's health care that children should not be threatened with medical treatment as a punishment. Indeed, unless the reason for Tracey's overdose is resolved, she may repeat the behaviour, but hide the fact for fear of punishment, thus putting her at greater risk. In considering the right of the staff to administer this punishment, those charged with the care of children are not allowed to engage in physical punishment. Venepuncture without anaesthetic cream in this circumstance is clearly a physical punishment and therefore not permitted.

It is the intention behind the choice not to use anaesthetic cream in this case that is the problem. There are legitimate reasons to carry out venepuncture without anaesthetic in children in the emergency department. These include:

- Urgent venepuncture where it would be dangerous to wait for anaesthetic cream to take effect, e.g. in giving fluids to a dehydrated child, or antibiotics to a child suspected of having meningococcal infection
- Use of an un-anaesthetised site when venepuncture of anaesthetised sites fails and venepuncture has become urgent
- Confirmation from a competent child that they will cooperate without anaesthetic
- Advice from a parent that waiting for anaesthetic cream to take effect will cause the child more distress than immediate venepuncture without anaesthetic.

In the context of this Article of the Act, this scenario demonstrates that it may be legitimate to carry out degrading procedures where there is no alternative and in order to save life or reduce suffering. However, regardless of whether it is inhuman and degrading or not, it is not legitimate for staff to use any health care intervention as a form of punishment.

Article 5: the right to freedom

Related ethical and legal issues:

- Mental health care
- Notification of infectious diseases
- Competence to practise
- Negligence
- Children as subjects of research.

> Everyone has the right to liberty and security of person. No one shall be deprived of his liberty save in the following cases . . .

Most of the exceptions to this right apply to people being deprived of their liberty because they have committed a crime. One exception relates to detention of a minor by lawful order for educational purposes, i.e. compulsory attendance at school, and there are two other exceptions, that may have relevance for the staff in children's emergency care, which will be discussed here.

Liberty is a relatively easy concept to understand. It means freedom from captivity. There are two circumstances relevant to emergency care where children may be lawfully deprived of their liberty. First, under the Mental Health Act 1983, detention is permitted if a mental disorder warrants hospital treatment and the person concerned is a danger to her/himself and/or society. This applies to both children and adults, though in the case of a child, detention should be a last resort. Secondly, certain infectious diseases must be notified to the local Public Health Department and, in exceptional circumstances, people suffering from a highly infectious disease, such as cholera, may be lawfully detained to prevent spread to others if they refuse to be treated in isolation voluntarily.

Security of the person is a little more complex than the concept of liberty. A dictionary definition of 'secure' is 'untroubled by danger or fear; safe against attack', and security is defined as 'a secure condition or feeling' (*Concise Oxford Dictionary*). Thus, security of the person could be

defined as: being, and feeling, safe from danger or attack. Not only must the parents and children be safe, they must also feel safe if their security is to be ensured whilst they are in the accident and emergency department. To ensure this the staff must be above reproach and demonstrate competence in their practice.

The NMC (2004) requires that a nurse must maintain professional knowledge and competence and other professions have similar requirements (GMC 2001). In the care of children in an emergency setting it is difficult to establish what level of knowledge, skill and competence is expected of the staff. The Government have set out recommendations for the basic level of skills and knowledge for all those whose work brings them into contact with children and young people (HM Government 2005); however each profession will have its own expected levels for the competent practice of that profession.

Competence is closely associated with the concept of negligence. When a person suffers harm because of incompetent care the person providing the care would be classed as negligent. In addressing the issue of negligence and the definition of competence, the case of *Bolem* v. *Frien Barnet HMC* [1957] 2 All ER 118, established that 'when you get a situation that involves the use of some special skill or competence . . . the standard of the ordinary skilled man exercising and professing to have that special skill' would be the level expected. The difficulty for staff in accident and emergency is that different departments within the hospital have different views as to who would be the ordinary skilled professional exercising and professing to have the special skills required. Using nursing as an example, the recommendation is that there should always be a children's nurse on duty in areas where children are cared for (DoH 1991). This implies that the children's nurse has the special skills required to nurse children. This is reinforced by the NMC (2005) who state that by virtue of the common foundation programme nurses will have knowledge and skills transferable to a range of care situations and that outside their branch specialism they may 'act as a care giver, under the supervision of a suitably qualified nurse'.

However, not all emergency departments abide by this recommendation. In a study of all the accident and emergency and minor injuries departments in one UK region it was found that only 18% confirmed that a children's nurse was on duty all the time (Playfor 2000). Furthermore, in a study of the beliefs and ideas held about children by accident and emergency nurses in one department, one of the themes emerging from interview data was the belief that children's nurses had no role in an accident and emergency department as the general staff were experienced with children (Partridge 2001). This suggests that, in this department at least, the ordinary skilled professional would be the general or adult nurse in the department. Rather worryingly, however, in the same study another theme to emerge was that the staff felt fearful of caring for children generally, seriously ill children, resuscitation situations and in cases of rapid deterioration. If a nurse is afraid of caring for children, this may suggest a lack of competence, thus putting children at risk of danger, rather than ensuring their security.

Thus, whilst recommendations, and perhaps common sense, might suggest that nurses competent to care for children in the emergency department would have the skills of a qualified children's nurse, this is neither the practice, nor the belief of many nurses within this field. The legal view has yet to be tested as no case of negligence against an NHS trust has been brought in this context. Nevertheless, as nurses have a responsibility to ensure their own competence, those working in an emergency department without a children's nursing qualification need to consider how they would justify that they are competent should the need arise. The situation differs little in relation to doctors. The Department of Health (1991) recommends that there should always be medical staff trained and experienced in caring for children present in an emergency department, yet Playfor (2000) found this to be the case in 47% of the departments she studied. The RCPCH (1999) recommends that there should always be a doctor trained in advanced paediatric life support, and nurses trained in paediatric basic life support.

Playfor (2000) found that in 14% of departments there was no regular paediatric resuscitation training. Again, this could lead parents to fear for the security of their children in the emergency department.

A different aspect of safety and security of children in emergency care relates to their participation in research. More and more students, from all professional disciplines, are studying at higher levels and undertaking placements where they may wish to conduct research studies. Added to that, the drive towards evidence based practice means that more qualified health care professionals are seeking to undertake research. Thus, patients in every setting may be invited to participate in research studies, and this includes children in emergency departments.

It is a recognised standard of ethical practice that informed consent is obtained from participants in research studies. However, it is one thing to ask children to agree to an intervention that may help them get better, but quite another to ask them to agree to an invasion of their person, or privacy, that may lead to improved care for future children. The RCPCH Ethics Advisory Committee (2000) has provided comprehensive guidelines for the ethical conduct of research involving children. One of the most important aspects is that the potential benefit must be weighed against the potential risk. They classify risk as:

Minimal, causing no physical pain, e.g.

- Questioning, observing or measuring children, in a sensitive way and with consent
- Collecting urine
- Using blood collected as part of treatment.

Low, causing brief physical pain, tenderness, and bruising, e.g.

- Venepuncture
- Injections
- Mucous membrane scrapings.

High, e.g.

- Biopsy of internal organs
- Arterial puncture
- Cardiac catheterisation.

The RCPCH Ethics Advisory Committee (2000) argue that it is only ethical to use children as participants in research if the risk is minimal, or if the child concerned is likely to benefit directly from the research. Higher risk research is therefore only permitted when the child is suffering from a very serious condition. In all research involving children, the consent of parents must be obtained and if the child can understand what is proposed then their consent or agreement must also be obtained (DoH 2001a,b). When a child is brought to an emergency department in a serious condition, the time needed to assess the risk and benefit of potentially risky research, and discuss this fully with the parents, will be superseded by the need to treat the child. Therefore, it could be argued that this is not a suitable environment to conduct anything other than minimal risk research involving children if the safety and security of the children is to be ensured. However, the RCPCH Ethics Advisory Committee (2000) argue that if emergency care to children is to be improved then research is necessary. However they acknowledge that to obtain consent in an emergency situation may be impractical and put the well-being of the child in jeopardy. They go on to state that provided 'the specific approval of a research ethics committee has been obtained for the project overall, it would be ethical to carry out research on children on such occasions of extreme urgency without obtaining consent. It is possible, however, that it would still be unlawful if the research were not expected to benefit the child in question'. Thus they suggest that research on children in need of emergency care can be carried out if it is therapeutic to the child.

Article 8: the right to privacy

Related ethical and legal issues:

- Confidentiality
- Consent.

> Everyone has the right to respect for his private and family life, his home and his correspondence . . .

This is the Article that enshrines in law the right to confidentiality. This right applies equally to adults and children of all ages. Indeed it was this principle that Tony Blair, as the UK Prime Minister, used in refusing to say whether his one-year-old child, Leo, had received the then controversial mumps, measles, rubella (MMR) vaccine. Blair argued that giving this information was a breach of Leo's right to have his medical records remain confidential. Department of Health (2001b) guidance states, 'if children refuse to share information with parents, health care professionals must normally respect their wishes'. There are, however, exceptions to the right to privacy, which the staff must be aware of. Consider the following scenario:

Box 3.2

Mary is 12 years old. She is brought to the emergency department by her mother with a history of dizziness, vomiting and disorientation, having just returned home from a gym party. Mary's mother is very upset and extremely worried. She wonders if Mary has food poisoning. Mary is very agitated and on examination, the staff begin to suspect that she may be suffering from drug abuse. In respect for Mary's privacy, they invite Mary's mother to go to the visitors' room for a cup of tea, saying that she will be more help to Mary when she is calmer. Once she has gone, the nurse asks Mary if she has taken drugs. Although she initially protests her innocence, Mary eventually admits that someone gave her a tablet. She begs the staff not to tell her mother, and promises that she has learnt her lesson and will never do it again.

The question now is whether Mary has a right to privacy in relation to this incident, and if not, who needs to be told. Within the Act there are four exceptions to the right to privacy that should be considered here:

- Public safety
- Prevention of disorder or crime
- Protection of health or morals
- Protection of the rights and freedoms of others.

These exceptions are echoed by the NMC (2002:5.3), which confirms that disclosures of confidential information may be made in the public interest, or if required by law or a court order.

Clearly, if someone is giving or selling drugs to a 12-year-old girl, a crime has been committed, and there is a risk to public safety and to the rights and freedoms of others, as other children may be at risk. Thus, the police need to know about this incident. Once the police are involved, Mary's parents would inevitably know, as the police cannot interview Mary without a parent present. Thus, whilst in this case it would be the police informing the parents, this would occur as a direct result of the staff informing the police. Clearly, Mary would feel the staff had breached her trust in this circumstance.

In taking drugs, Mary is putting her health at risk, and by breaking the law, is at risk morally too. She has however promised that she has learned her lesson, and will never do this again. It is the detailed knowledge of child development that will help the nurse decide whether Mary's health and morals will be at risk if her parents are not told. Issues such as peer pressure and pushing of boundaries are features of adolescence that Mary is only just confronting. In addition, at the age of 12 she is only just at the stage of moral development where right and wrong are considered in the light of social norms as opposed to self-interest (Kohlberg 1984). Thus, despite Mary's protests, it may be deemed imperative to tell her parents in order to protect her health, morals and development.

Substance abuse is of course very serious. It may be however, that a child reveals that he or she has been involved in an illegal or dangerous activity that could be perceived as somewhat less serious. Perhaps a child reveals that he has stolen a packet of sweets from a shop, or one sweet from a school friend. Maybe a child reveals that he or she has sustained an injury by playing in an unsuitable area, a building site for example. In any scenario where a child reveals something, and asks that it be kept from parents, the health care staff must decide, based on the provisions of the Act, whether it would be legal and/or ethical to breach that confidence, and if so, who needs to know. They must then be able to justify the decision should they be called to do so. Clearly an understanding of the cognitive development of children would be necessary in justifying any decision to breach the confidentiality of a child.

The issue of privacy is also linked to the concept of consent. As a general rule, it is the responsibility of parents, or those who have parental responsibility, to consent to the treatment of children under the age of 16 years, thus it is self-evident that they must be given information about their child's condition. The Family Law Reform Act 1969 assumes minors of 16 and 17 years are as competent as adults to give consent, and therefore must equally be given information. There are reasons why someone of 16 years or over may not be able to consent to treatment. They include:

- Learning disability
- Physical disability that prevents communication of a decision to consent or not consent
- Mental illness
- Reduced consciousness.

In the case of young people of 16 or 17 years, in these circumstances, the parents may consent, whereas for those of 18 years and over, no one can consent on their behalf and the health care professionals must base their decisions on the patient's best interests. Children and young people are advised by the Department of Health (2001a) to find out the following information from health care professionals:

- Why they think the treatment will be good for you
- What sort of things it will involve
- What benefits they hope will result
- How good the chances are of you getting such benefits
- Whether there are any alternatives
- Whether there are any risks
- Whether the risks are large or small
- What may happen if you don't have the treatment.

The Department of Health (2001b) acknowledge that in an emergency there may not be time to give a child all the information they may need; however, the guidance makes it clear that time must be spent giving children information if their life is not at risk.

Although 16 years is the age at which young people can consent to medical treatment without question, there are circumstances when the competence of a child under 16 years may need to be considered. Consider the following scenario:

Box 3.3

John is 15 years old. He is brought to the emergency department by a teacher because he has fallen during an adventure outing with the school. He has a severe graze to his leg. The graze needs be cleaned up and a dressing applied but no sutures are necessary. In addition, because there is considerable debris in the wound, and John has not yet had a booster, the senior house officer has prescribed a tetanus toxoid injection. John's parents cannot be contacted. His mother is spending the day shopping, and his father is at work on a building site. Neither has their mobile phone switched on.

In this scenario, the health care professionals must decide whether any treatment has to be given straight away, or whether it can wait until the parents can be contacted to consent. If the decision is that treatment must be given they must then assess whether John is competent to consent, or whether they must make decisions that are in his best interests. In deciding whether treatment must be given immediately the health care professionals must ask whether delay may endanger life, or cause further suffering. In this case, whilst the situation is not immediately life threatening, there is a risk of further suffering in the form of infection, including tetanus, if the wound is not cleaned up and dressed. Indeed, delay would make the cleaning process more difficult and cause more pain or discomfort.

As it is the role of nursing staff to clean and dress or close simple wounds, it is the nursing staff who must gain consent. Usually, oral consent

is satisfactory where a general anaesthetic is not involved, because the patient can withdraw their consent at any time if they decide they do not want an aspect of the treatment.

The guidelines for assessing the competence of a minor to consent to treatment are known as the Fraser Guidelines, and arose from the *Gillick* v. *West Norfolk and Wisbech AHA and the DHSS* [1985] 3 All ER 402 (HL). Mrs Victoria Gillick, a Roman Catholic with five daughters, became concerned because, in the drive to reduce teenage pregnancies, the Department of Health and Social Security issued guidance stating that in some circumstances it would be lawful for GPs and family planning clinics to give contraceptive advice to sexually active young people under the age of 16, and in some cases prescribe the contraceptive pill, without the knowledge or consent of the parents (Dimond 2005). Mrs Gillick decided to challenge this guidance although none of her daughters was seeking such advice at the time. Mrs Gillick wrote to the health authority asking for an assurance that, if any of her daughters did go to a doctor for contraceptive advice or the pill, she would be informed and no such advice or treatment would be given without her consent. The health authority declined to give that assurance and Mrs Gillick challenged that decision through the Courts. Appeal and counter appeal resulted in the case coming before the highest Court in the country, the House of Lords. Here the Lords ruled that in certain circumstances a young person under 16 years could be given contraceptive advice and treatment. At the House of Lords hearing, Lord Fraser gave guidelines that have been applied successfully to other circumstances in which children under 16 years may give consent to treatment. These guidelines have become known as the Fraser Guidelines and are as follows:

- The young person will understand the professional's advice.
- The young person cannot be persuaded to inform their parents.
- The young person is likely to begin, or to continue having, sexual intercourse with or without contraceptive treatment.

- Unless the young person receives contraceptive treatment, their physical or mental health, or both, are likely to suffer.
- The young person's best interests require them to receive contraceptive advice or treatment with or without parental consent.

A young person who is deemed competent under the Fraser Guidelines is sometimes known as 'Gillick competent' although this phrase is losing favour as it is felt by some that Mrs Gillick's name should not be connected to a concept that is the very opposite of what she was trying to achieve.

Returning to the scenario, at the age of 15, John is likely to have had many wounds that would have needed cleaning and dressing. Whilst this may be a more severe wound, John is likely to be able to understand what cleaning and dressing it would entail. He is also likely to understand that infection may result if the wound is not cleaned. Thus, it could be argued that he is competent under the Fraser Guidelines. In addition, if the process became too uncomfortable, he would be able to ask that it be stopped. John's oral consent would therefore be likely to be acceptable (DoH 2001a), but it should be witnessed by two members of staff, and the factors leading to the decision that he is competent documented. This is in case anything untoward happens and the treatment of a minor without parental consent is questioned.

If John had been 5 years old, rather than 15, the situation might have been different. It is very unlikely that a 5-year-old can ever be deemed competent to consent to treatment. In these circumstances, staff must act without consent to achieve the best interests of the child. In this case, that would probably mean cleaning and dressing the wound without consent, or with the consent of the teacher if authorised to give it. Parents are often asked to sign a form authorising teachers, or other carers, to take medical decisions, and they may do so if they wish (DoH 2001b). In this case the person authorised by the parents should be given sufficient information to make the decision about the particular need the child has, but not be given information that is unrelated to it.

Assuming John's wound has been successfully cleaned and dressed, the next part of his treatment is the tetanus injection. The situation is a little different here. In cleaning a wound, the process is non-invasive and foreign bodies are removed; however, giving the vaccine is an invasive procedure in which a toxoid is introduced. Nurses may be a little more dubious about doing this without parental consent. In assessing John's competence to consent, the nurse would have to be sure that John understood the nature of the disease against which the vaccine provides protection, the way in which the vaccine works, and the way in which it is administered. He would also have to assure staff that he knew his history in terms of protection against tetanus. He would have to be able to say whether he had received the childhood course of immunisations, and whether he had suffered any adverse effects. Tetanus is a rare condition and it is highly unlikely that any of the nurses, let alone John, would have encountered it. He is also unlikely to have studied human biology to the degree that he could understand how a toxoid vaccine works. However, the requirement is not that he understands pathology and immunology, merely that he understands in the same way that a person over 16 years would understand. This is where knowledge of child development will assist the nurse. The nurse must decide if John has achieved adult cognitive development, or whether he is an immature 15-year-old. In terms of his own history, the teacher may have confirmation that he has had childhood immunisations but this is not usually a condition of children being able to attend school trips. The teacher may also have been given information about John's medical history, such as allergies and adverse reactions to drugs.

John may be quite happy to submit to the injection, and he and his teacher may be able to confirm his past immunisation record, but it is not imperative that the vaccination is carried out immediately. Thus the safest course of action if he refuses it, or there is any doubt about his competence to consent, is for the teacher to be given a letter to John's parents, explaining the circumstances, and asking that he be brought back to the department that evening for the injection. In the case of a non-competent child, this should always be done. The school nurse, or health visitor in the case of pre-school children, also needs to be aware that the vaccine was not administered in case the parents fail to bring the child back and follow-up in the community is needed.

Article 9: the right to freedom of thought

Related ethical and legal issues:

- Refusal of treatment
- Spiritual care.

> Everyone has the right to freedom of thought, conscience and religion; this right includes freedom to change his religion or belief, and freedom, either alone or in community with others and in public or in private, to manifest his religion or belief, in worship, teaching, practice and observance.

The limitations to this right are similar to those of Article 8, i.e.

- Public safety
- Protection of health or morals
- Protection of the rights and freedoms of others.

In an emergency setting, there are two possible circumstances in which the health care professional may need to consider this right.

First, where the parents say that it is against their religion for a child to have the recommended treatment or care. Giving a blood transfusion to a practising Jehovah's Witness is a common example. When this circumstance arises the best interests of the child is the prime consideration. If the treatment is essential, and urgent, it must be given without parental consent. If however, there is time to seek legal advice prior to giving the treatment, this should be done. The Courts will invariably rule in favour of treatment, unless they receive expert advice that there is another equally effective alternative that is acceptable to the parents. In the case of Jehovah's Witnesses, and the rule about blood transfusions,

the current situation is that whilst believers are no longer excommunicated from the faith if they have a blood transfusion, they are expected to acknowledge that they have done wrong and seek forgiveness, or they will be deemed to have left the faith of their own volition (Jehovah's Witnesses 2000). Thus, whilst members of this faith might protest that they do not want their child to have a transfusion, they usually accept that they will be overruled if necessary. Similar circumstances to this may arise in respect of other treatments, and other religions. It is also important to remember that a person does not have to give a reason for withholding consent to treatment. They can merely say 'it is against my beliefs'. The right to hold personal beliefs is protected in the same way as religious beliefs by this Article.

Consider the following scenario:

> **Box 3.4**
>
> Peter is 15 years old. For the past two years he and a group of his friends have been vegetarian and believe in using alternative therapies. Peter attends the emergency department with a serious fractured femur that needs manipulation under anaesthetic. Peter has refused analgesia, and when his parents sign the consent form, he protests. He says that it is against his beliefs to have an anaesthetic because it will introduce poison to his body.

In deciding whether Peter can be treated without consent, the first decision is whether he is Fraser competent. This would mean ascertaining whether he really understands the implications of leaving a fractured femur untreated, in the same way that a person over 16 years would understand. Assuming he is competent, the next consideration is whether the limitations to the right to practise his beliefs apply. Clearly there is no risk to public safety if Peter is not treated. There is a risk to Peter's health, but as a competent person, he understands this and accepts the risk. The next question is whether he would be harmed morally if the fracture was left untreated. It would be difficult to argue that he would. Finally, the rights and freedoms of others must be considered and once again, it would be difficult to argue that they would be infringed. Thus, it seems that Peter must be left untreated.

However, there are other actions the staff may take to try to secure legal consent. It may be that Peter does not fully understand the relationship between traditional and alternative therapies, or the real risks of analgesia and anaesthetic. If these were fully explained he might consent. If this is not successful, the case could be referred to the Court who may rule that Peter does not have the right to refuse treatment despite being Fraser competent. The precedent for this ruling was set in the Court of Appeal who ruled in the case of a 16-year-old girl who was refusing treatment. The Court said that whilst the Family Law Reform Act 1969 gave the girl the right to consent, it did not give her the right to refuse treatment (re W (a minor) (medical treatment) [1992] All ER 627). Of course, these possible courses of action may take too long. If a child such as Peter needs immediate treatment to save his life, or prevent serious or long-term suffering, the treatment could be given without the child's consent and the case referred to above could be used in defence should the child wish to take action in the future.

There are two possible twists to this type of scenario. First, Peter's parents may hold the same beliefs as Peter and refuse consent. In this case, the above actions could be taken in the same way. Secondly, the parents may hold these beliefs and refuse consent but Peter may not share his parents' beliefs and may consent himself. In this case, his consent would be valid.

The second circumstance where the nurse may need to respect the rights enshrined in this Article of the Act is when a child and family may need to practise a ritual of their belief system as part of the process of caring for the sick child. For example, they may wish to pray with or around the child, have the child anointed or blessed in some way by a minister of religion, or carry out a ritual healing of some type. In these circumstances, unless there is a risk to the health of the child, or to public order, the child and family must be facilitated to practise their beliefs, in private, or in public as appropriate.

Article 10: the right to freedom of expression

Related ethical and legal issues:

- Racism, sexism and the abuse of staff
- Professional judgement
- Whistleblowing.

> Everyone has the right to freedom of expression. This right shall include the freedom to hold opinions and to receive and impart information and ideas without interference by public authority . . .

The limitations to this right are similar to those of Articles 8 and 9, i.e.

- Public safety
- Protection of health or morals
- Protection of the rights and freedoms of others.

In this Article, these limitations are described as duties and responsibilities that arise out of the exercise of freedom of expression, and reference is also made to the importance of the protection of the reputation of others and disclosure of information received in confidence.

Freedom of expression is closely linked to freedom of thought, but it goes one step further in that thoughts, in the form of beliefs and values, can be kept private to the person holding them; freedom of expression is about making thoughts public. Whilst there is no restriction on what any UK citizen may believe, there are some restrictions on the expression of those beliefs, for example, a person may hold negative beliefs about people from certain cultural, racial or socio-economic groups, and may say so, but may not incite others to espouse to those beliefs. In the emergency care setting, it is unlikely that members of the public would engage in such activity. The more likely scenario is that a young person or parent may give expression to their beliefs by refusing to receive care from staff in the groups they hold negative views about, for example, refusing to be cared for by a male nurse, or a black nurse.

In the case of a competent adult, this situation is relatively easy to deal with. Care is offered, but the patient does not have a choice about who delivers the care. Refusal to receive care from a particular health care professional is a refusal to receive the care offered and the department does not have to offer alternative care. However in the case of a girl not wanting to receive intimate care from a male member of staff, an alternative is often arranged (RCN 1993).

In the case of parents or children refusing care from a particular health care professional on the grounds of their colour or race, for example, a judgement would need to be made as to the urgency of the case. It may be possible to refer the child to out-patients, or the GP, to give necessary care. However, if the care is urgent the staff must consider whether to acquiesce to the demand for a different member of staff, however distasteful that may be, in order to give the child, who may not even understand what is going on, the care needed. If this is deemed inappropriate, either on principle, or because the only person with the necessary expertise is the person being refused, then this must be regarded as refusal to consent to treatment and the staff would have to follow the processes discussed earlier and either act without consent, or secure consent through the legal system. It is important in making this type of decision to remember that the member of staff whom the family do not want caring for them has a right not to be discriminated against under Article 14 of the Act, and every department needs a robust policy for protecting staff from discrimination.

The right to freedom of expression does not apply only to children and their parents. It also applies to the staff. When working in a professional capacity, the staff sometimes have to make judgements that balance their own views with the policies of their employers. Professional people are entitled to use their professional judgement and make decisions that are not in keeping with the employer's policies, guidelines and recommendations; however, should harm come to a patient in these circumstances, the employer would not necessarily accept vicarious liability and the member of staff would have to rely on their own professional insurance for any ensuing legal fees or compensation claims. The increasing emphasis on evidence-based practice, and the availability of information to the public through the internet, makes it increasingly difficult for health care professionals to rely solely on clinical judgement in making decisions about treatment and care.

The issue of whistle blowing is closely linked to freedom of expression. If a member of staff suspects malpractice on the part of a colleague there is a duty to make that known in order to protect the public (GMC 2001; NMC 2004). Despite this, staff are still reluctant to make their concerns known. For example, in respect of an incident occurring in 1994, the nurses reporting to the Shipman Inquiry in 2001 gave the reasons for failing to make their concerns known in respect of one patient as:

- The NHS culture at the time dictated that doctors should not be challenged.
- The overdose of morphine was a terrible mistake rather than deliberate.
- It was the place of someone else to prompt an investigation.
- It was not their place to raise suspicions (Harrison 2003).

One of the difficulties in making the decision whether to express concerns is that there is equally a duty not to express views that might damage the reputation of anyone who is not guilty of malpractice. Elaine Chase gives a vivid account of the devastating effect on her life and career when her name was falsely linked with the deaths of 18 children (Parish 2002). Thus, health care professionals and their managers need to make careful and informed judgements, ideally supported by verifiable evidence.

It is not only cases of suspected malpractice that must be reported. Nurses, for example, are required to make known any concerns about the environment for care (NMC 2004). This raises the issue of how far nurses can condone facilities that are not in keeping with recommendations, for example in terms of separate waiting, play and treatment areas for children, and availability of appropriately qualified staff (DoH 2003).

Article 14: the right not to be discriminated against

Related ethical and legal issues:

- Discrimination
- Gagging clauses.

The enjoyment of the rights and freedoms set forth in this Convention shall be secured without discrimination on any ground such as sex, race, colour, language, religion, political or other opinion, national or social origin, association with a national minority, property, birth or other status.

Discrimination means treating a person less favourably than another in a similar situation. This Article of the Act prohibits discrimination in the fulfilment of the freedoms set out in the Act. Thus, we have already established that under Article 5 of the Act, the right to security may include being treated and cared for by appropriately qualified and competent staff. Whilst it is probably safe to say that there is a nurse and doctor qualified in the care of adults on duty at all times, the evidence from one health region suggests that this may be the case for children in only 18% of departments (Playfor 2000). Furthermore, this evidence suggests that 24% of departments may not have regular paediatric resuscitation training, and 53% may not always have a doctor with paediatric experience on duty. It could therefore be argued that in emergency departments where adults have appropriately qualified staff always available, and children do not, the children are being discriminated against on the grounds of age (which under the Act could be defined as an 'other status') in terms of their right to security (see Article 5).

In circumstances where staff have any concerns about practice or care provision, this must be disclosed. However, one of the key issues identified as making staff reluctant to come forward is the fear of discrimination. Harrison (2003) describes a number of cases where this has occurred, and it is one of the reasons why the Public Interest Disclosure Act 1998 was passed.

This Act explicitly outlaws discrimination and victimisation of whistleblowers, and the imposition of gagging clauses by employers. The Department of Health (NHS Executive 1999) has made recommendations regarding the policies and procedures that need to be in place to comply with the provisions of the Act. In the emergency department, as in any practice setting, staff need to be aware of these policies.

Conclusion

This chapter has provided an examination of ethical and legal issues facing health care professionals caring for children in emergency departments. It is important to remember that law is dynamic and each time a judge makes a decision regarding controversial legal issues, the law may change. Likewise, new law may be enacted by parliament. In response to changes in law, the Department of Health, regulatory bodies and professional organisations may issue new guidelines for practice. Whilst this chapter was accurate at the time of writing, the reader is reminded to keep up-to-date with changes in law, recommendations and professional guidelines that may impact on legal and ethical emergency care for children.

References

Collins, P. (1999) Restraining children for painful procedures. *Paediatric Nursing*, **11**(3), 14–16.

Department of Health (1991) *Welfare of Children and Young People in Hospital*. HMSO, London.

Department of Health (2001a) *Consent. What you have a right to expect. A guide for children and young people*. DoH, London.

Department of Health (2001b) *Consent. What you have a right to expect. A guide for parents*. DoH, London.

Department of Health (2003) *Getting the Right Start: National Service Framework for Children. Standard for Hospital Services*. DoH, London.

Department of Health (2004) *National Service Framework for Children, Young People and Maternity Services*. DoH, London.

Dimond, B. (2005) *Legal Aspects of Nursing*, 5th edn. Longman, London.

General Medical Council (2001) *Good Medical Practice*, 3rd edn. GMC, London.

Harrison, S. (2003) Speak up . . . if you dare. *Nursing Standard*, **17**(18), 12–13.

HM Government (2005) *Common Core of Skills and Knowledge for the Children's Workforce*. DfES, London.

Horton, R. (2000) Health and the UK Human Rights Act 1998. *Lancet*, **356**(9236), 1186–1188.

Jehovah's Witnesses (2000) *Statement to the media*. Public Affairs Office. www.ajwrb.org/basics/jwpressrelease6-14-00.jpg.

Kohlberg, L. (1984) *The Psychology of Moral Development*. Harper and Row, New York.

McHale, J., Gallagher, A. & Mason, I. (2001) The UK Human Rights Act 1998: implications for nurses. *Nursing Ethics*, **8**(3), 223–233.

NHS Executive (1999) *The Public Interest Disclosure Act 1998: Whistleblowing in the NHS*. Health Service Circular HSC 1999/198.

Nursing and Midwifery Council (2004) *The NMC code of professional conduct: standards for conduct, performance and ethics*. NMC, London.

Nursing and Midwifery Council (2005) *Providing nursing care for patients outside branch specialism*. http://www.nmc-uk.org/nmc/main/advice/providingCareForPatientsOutsideBranchSpecialism.html.

Parish, C. (2002) Coming to terms. *Nursing Standard*, **17**(14–15), 12–13.

Partridge, T. (2001) Children in accident and emergency: seen but not heard? *Journal of Child Health Care*, **5**(2), 49–53.

Plant, N. (2000) Up in the air. *Nursing Times*, **96**(37), 32–33.

Playfor, S. (2000) Accident and emergency services for children within the Trent region. *Emergency Medicine Journal*, **128**(3), 164–168.

Robinson, S. & Collier, J. (1997) Holding children still for procedures. *Paediatric Nursing*, **9**(4), 12–14.

Royal College of Nursing (1993) When can nurses refuse to care? *Nursing Standard*, **7**(41), 32–33.

Royal College of Nursing (2003) *Restraining, Holding Still and Containing Children and Young People: Guidance for Good Practice*. RCN, London.

Royal College of Paediatrics and Child Health (1999) *Accident and Emergency Services for Children*. RCPCH, London.

Royal College of Paediatrics and Child Health Ethics Advisory Committee (2000) Guidelines for the ethical conduct of medical research involving children. *Archives of Disease in Childhood*, **82**, 177–182.

Royal College of Paediatrics and Child Health (2004) *Withholding and Withdrawing Life Sustaining Treatment in Children: A Framework for Practice*, 2nd edn. RCPCH, London.

Woods, M. (2001) Balancing rights and duties in 'life and death' decision making involving children: a role for nurses? *Nursing Ethics*, **8**(5), 397–408.

Useful websites

British Medical Association – the professional organisation for UK doctors, www.bma.org.uk

Charity Choice – an online directory of UK charities listing over 850 charities in the category of 'children and youth', www.charitychoice.co.uk

Department of Health – of the UK Government, www.dh.gov.uk

General Medical Council – the regulatory body for UK medicine, www.gmc-uk.org

Healthcare Commission – the UK body responsible for audit and inspection of health care providers, www.healthcarecommission.org.uk

Health Professions Council – the regulatory body of professions allied to medicine, www.hpc-uk.org

National Institute for Health and Clinical Excellence – the agency responsible for making 'best practice' recommendations, www.nice.org.uk

Nursing and Midwifery Council – the regulatory body for UK nursing, www.nmc-uk.org

Royal College of Nursing – the professional organisation for UK nurses, www.rcn.org.uk

Royal College of Paediatrics and Child Health – the body responsibly for postgraduate education, continuing education and setting standards of paediatric and child health medical practice, www.rcpch.ac.uk

Chapter 4 Safeguarding and Protecting Children: The Roles and Responsibilities of the Emergency Care Practitioner

Janet Webb

Introduction – child protection work – prevention and early intervention

Over the last 30 years in the United Kingdom the issue of child abuse and what to do about it has been the subject of considerable political and media interest (Corby 2006; Parton 2004). Most accounts of the background to child protection work begin with Henry Kempe and his 'discovery' of the child battering syndrome in the early 1960s, as if the problem did not exist before this or had somehow lain dormant. Similarly, sexual abuse is often described as having been discovered in Britain at the beginning of the 1980s. However, child abuse is not a new phenomenon, nor is public or state concern about it (Corby 2006; Howarth 2001; Reder & Duncan 2004).

Recently the roles of professionals involved in safeguarding children, and the priorities and focus of child protection policy and practice have shifted in important ways, with the publication of a series of Department of Health (DoH) research projects (DoH 1995a) providing the starting point for a re-evaluation of approaches to child protection work (Corby 2006). Additionally, the activities of social workers, health care workers, and other professionals involved in the field have been the focus of political and media interest following the Laming Inquiry into the death of Victoria Climbié, which raised fresh concerns about child protection policy and practice (Laming 2003), leading to a further review of policies and practices.

The Laming Inquiry into the death of Victoria Climbié revealed poor practice within and between social services, the police and the health sector. Indeed, Lord Laming's (2003) report provided 108 recommendations for tightening up the child protection system; 22 of the recommendations related to the acute sector, with accident and emergency services being one of the many areas criticised by Lord Laming. It is evident from this report and a number of others preceding this, that professionals cannot carry out child protection responsibilities in isolation from everyone else because, if they do, a child in danger is more at risk of slipping through the net (Wright 2002).

There is a body of evidence which indicates that unless there is confirmation of abuse and neglect, families experiencing problems may not always receive the services their children would benefit from (Cleaver et al. 1999; DoH 1995a; Laming 2003; Powell 2003; Scottish Executive 2002). Yet it is recognised that preventative work is important with early intervention to improve outcomes (DoH 2004; Dubowitz 1989; Ennals 2003; Powell 2003; Thyen et al. 1995). Preventative activity in child protection work encompasses primary prevention (policies and activities that repress the development of risk factors for child abuse), secondary (early idenification of risk factors associated with abuse and neglect or early intervention) and tertiary (therapy, rehabilitation and intergenerational work) (Powell 2003). Staff in the emergency department setting are more likely to be involved at primary and secondary levels. It is therefore important that practitioners are able to recognise and respond to early indicators of a vulnerable child, child abuse and neglect, whilst recognising that risk factors are contributing rather than determining factors (Belsky 1993; Browne & Stevenson 1988; Powell 2003).

Regrettably, though it may never be possible to fully prevent and eradicate child abuse, better knowledge and more informed multi-agency and interprofessional working practices will help in its reduction (Howard 2004). In this context this chapter will consider the roles and responsibilities of practitioners working within emergency departments in relation to safeguarding children and child protection work, and what practitioners should do within the context of current debates, policy and legislation.

Understanding the terms – defining child abuse, safeguarding children and child protection

Child protection is the decisive action taken to protect children and young people from harm (DoH 1991) and it is part of safeguarding and promoting welfare (HMG 2006). Safeguarding and promoting the welfare of children are the contemporary terms used to describe 'the process of protecting children from abuse and neglect, preventing the impairment of their health and development, and ensuring they are growing up in circumstances consistent with the provision of safe and effective care which is undertaken so as to enable children to have optimum life chances and enter adulthood successfully' (HMG 2006). Section 10 of the Children Act 2004 refers to ensuring the well-being of children and this 'requires local authorities and other agencies to cooperate with a view to improving the well-being of children in relation to the 5 outcomes first set out in *Every Child Matters*' (HMG 2006). It is argued that 'all children deserve the opportunity to achieve their full potential' as 'set out in five outcomes that are key to children and young people's well-being':

- Stay safe
- Be healthy
- Enjoy and achieve
- Make a positive contribution
- Achieve economic well-being (DfES 2003; HM Government 2006).

However, whilst practitioners need to be aware of these outcomes, within the context of the emergency department their focus is on the safety and health of children.

Child abuse itself is difficult and complex to define; it could for example be argued that the abuse of children is a misuse of power and trust by adults. It could also be described as being about what is acceptable in a given culture in a given time; thus an ever changing socially constructed phenomenon. Furthermore, myths and stereotypes exist about children, child abuse and the perpetrators of abuse, influencing personal values and beliefs, which in turn if not acknowledged can determine how a child is assessed and the effectiveness, or not, of subsequent interventions. It is therefore worth considering one's own values and beliefs about abuse and remembering that the perpetrators of abuse have often experienced adverse situations in childhood themselves, with the long-term effects of abuse having untoward ramifications, which can last all their lives. There are approximately 12 million children in England and Wales, with 50 to 100 children dying each year as a result of the consequences of abuse or neglect. Most abuse occurs within the family and by somebody known to the child. Notably, however, of the total child population 3 to 4 million children are considered to be 'vulnerable' (DoH 2003).

A note on terminology: the legal definition of a child is anyone up to the age of 18 as identified in the Children Act 1989 and the Children (Scotland) Act 1995. Therefore, in this context and in relation to safeguarding children the term child/children is used to cover babies, children and young people in this age range.

It is also worth noting that the *National Service Framework for Children, Young People and Maternity Services* (NSF) (DoH 2004) covers all babies, children and young people, and child/children is frequently used as a shorthand to cover all under 19s. The delivery of the NSF is interwoven with *Every Child Matters: Change for Children* which is a new approach to the well-being of children and young people from birth to age 19 (DoH 2003). However, agencies have different statutory responsibilities for children and young people of different age ranges, and services are commissioned accordingly. The NSF aims to improve the age-appropriateness of services and base this around the needs of the individual young person and their family, including, in particular, planning appropriately for transition to adulthood. This may mean that some children receive services from children's service providers for a longer period than others. Thus, the practitioner should take this into account when making referrals to other agencies and professionals.

Box 4.1   Vulnerability – what constitutes a vulnerable child?

George lives in poverty. He has poor attachment experiences, long-standing established behavioural problems, is falling behind at school and about to be excluded. He has many unresolved separations and poor social skills. He lives with a single parent and has a younger sibling who has a disability.

George is disadvantaged because he has a number of stressors (Daniel *et al.* 1999). Not only is he vulnerable because of poor attachment experiences, but he has also experienced a number of unresolved separations. He is falling behind at school and about to be excluded, thus he is already at risk of suffering from developmental delay or interruption. He has experienced many negative life events, which are also likely to increase his vulnerability. There is a powerful interaction between vulnerability and adversity as it may be that the more vulnerable the child, the more they are affected by adverse experiences. Equally the greater the persistent adversities the more likely they are to render a child vulnerable (Daniel *et al.* 1999).

Thus vulnerability can be defined as those innate characteristics of the child, or those imposed by their family circle and wider community which might threaten or challenge healthy development (Daniel *et al.* 1999). Within the context of safeguarding children and thus child protection it could be argued that there is a continuum of vulnerability. All children are vulnerable to some extent as the younger they are the more depend-

ent they are on adults to ensure their safety. However, factors that might render a child vulnerable to abuse and neglect and/or to not weathering ordinary adversities and veering off a healthy developmental path can be separated into:

- Some intrinsic characteristics in the child which might render them more vulnerable
- Those vulnerabilities imposed by parents' views or expectations of the child.

Alongside these general factors, the particular age of the child and developmental stage may render the child particularly vulnerable.

Research informs us about the combinations of stresses which are likely to render a particular child more vulnerable. If those children who are particularly vulnerable are identified early, it is likely that subsequent interventions can be focused more precisely, so as to harness any potential for resilience within the child and within his or her close environment (Daniel *et al.* 1999). This has implications for staff in emergency departments to pick up on cues which indicate vulnerability in a child and ensure they make referrals to the appropriate agencies.

In work with children, the term 'vulnerable' has been used to describe:

- Characteristics of groups of children who may be more at risk from a range of social and health problems than others
- Individuals for whom a number of factors have combined to place them at risk, this includes children and young people with a disability who are particularly vulnerable to abuse/neglect (Watson 1989)
- Children who have suffered or who are considered likely to suffer abuse from their carers in the future.

It should not be assumed that children who are socially 'vulnerable' to life risks have also been abused or are the most at risk of child abuse. However, there are some children who appear to be particularly vulnerable to different types of risk and more vulnerable to abuse. Thus the practitioner should be able to recognise and develop the skills to recognise children who are most vulnerable. There are different types of vulnerabilities that children face, thus it is important to identify whether children are at risk of abuse or at risk more generally. In this context it is helpful to use the terms from the Children Act 1989 and *Working Together* (HM Government 2006) which are 'children in need' and 'children in need of protection' or children whose needs require 'safeguarding' from harm. Children defined as being 'in need' under section 17 of the Children Act 1989, are 'those whose vulnerability is such that they are unlikely to reach or maintain a satisfactory level of health or development, or their health and development will be significantly impaired, without the provision of services, plus those who are disabled' (HM Government 2006).

Some children are in need because they are suffering or are likely to suffer significant harm and are therefore in need of protection from abuse and or neglect and may require more urgent intervention. HM Government (2006) states that

> *'abuse and neglect are forms of maltreatment of a child. Somebody may abuse or neglect a child by inflicting harm, or failing to act to prevent harm. Children may be abused in a family or in an institutional or community setting; by those known to them, or more rarely by a stranger. They may be abused by an adult or adults or another child or children'.*

Harm is defined as 'ill treatment (including sexual and non-sexual abuse), impairment of health (physical and mental) or impairment of development' (Children Act 1989 S.32(2)). It is these definitions that apply to professional practice in relation to recognising concerns and protecting children, and as is evident from the definitions, children may be abused or neglected by inflicting harm or by knowingly not preventing harm. It is also important to recognise that children may be abused in a family or in an institutional or community setting, usually by those known to them, and only occasionally by a stranger. The need for early recognition of a child at risk of harm or significant harm is therefore absolutely essential, with emergency practitioners potentially at the front line in such a key area of work.

Constituents of abuse

Browne (2002) notes that in the 1980s three forms of child maltreatment were identified: physical, sexual and psychological or emotional abuse. Each type of maltreatment is characterised into 'active' or 'passive' forms of abuse.

Active abuse involves violent acts that represent the exercise of physical force, causing injury or forcibly interfering with personal freedom. Passive abuse refers to neglect, which can only be considered violent in the metaphorical sense, as it does not involve physical force. Nevertheless, it can cause both physical and emotional injury including non-organic failure to thrive in young children (Browne 2002).

'Child abuse and neglect' are today generic terms encompassing all ill treatment of children including serious physical and sexual assaults as well as cases where the standard of care does not adequately support the child's health or development. HM Government (2006) sets out definitions and examples of the four broad categories of abuse, which are used for the purpose of registration on the child protection register. These are:

- Physical abuse
- Emotional abuse
- Sexual abuse
- Neglect.

Physical abuse

Physical abuse may involve hitting, shaking, throwing, poisoning, burning or scalding, drowning, suffocating, or otherwise causing physical harm to a child. Physical harm may also be caused when a parent or carer feigns the symptoms of, or deliberately induces, illness in a child whom they are looking after. This unusual and potentially dangerous form of abuse is now described as fabricated or induced illness in a child.

Physical injury as a result of abuse is the actual or likely injury to a child, or failure to prevent physical injury (or suffering) to a child, including deliberate poisoning, suffocation and injury.

Physical abuse can lead directly to neurological damage, physical injuries and disability, or at the extreme – death. Harm may be caused to children both by the abuse itself and by the abuse taking place in a wider family or institutional context of conflict and aggression. Physical abuse has been linked to aggressive behaviour in children, emotional and behavioural problems and educational difficulties.

Emotional abuse

Emotional abuse is the persistent emotional maltreatment of a child such as to cause severe and persistent adverse effects on the child's emotional development. It may:

- Convey to children that they are worthless or unloved, inadequate, or valued only insofar as they meet the needs of another person
- Feature age or developmentally inappropriate expectations being imposed on children
- Involve causing children frequently to feel frightened or in danger, e.g. witnessing domestic violence
- Involve serious bullying causing children frequently to feel frightened or in danger
- Involve the exploitation or corruption of children.

Some level of emotional abuse is involved in all types of ill treatment of a child, though emotional abuse may occur alone.

There is increasing evidence of the adverse long-term consequences for children's development where they have been subject to sustained emotional abuse. Emotional abuse has an important impact on developing a child's mental health, behaviour and self-esteem. It can be especially damaging in infancy. Underlying emotional abuse may be as important, if not more so, than other forms of abuse in terms of its impact on the child. Domestic violence, mental health problems and parental substance misuse may be features in families where children are exposed to such abuse.

Sexual abuse

Sexual abuse involves forcing or enticing a child or young person to take part in sexual activities, whether or not the child is aware of what is happening. The activities may involve physical contact, including penetrative (e.g. rape or buggery) or non-penetrative acts. They may include non-contact activities, such as involving children in looking at, or in the production of, pornographic material or watching sexual activities, or encouraging children to behave in sexually inappropriate ways. It is the actual or likely exploitation of a child or adolescent in sexual activities they do not truly comprehend or to which they are unable to give informed consent or that violates social taboos of family roles.

Disturbed behaviour including self-harm, inappropriate sexualised behaviour, sadness, depression and loss of self-esteem have all been linked to sexual abuse. Its adverse effects may endure into adulthood. The severity of impact on a child is believed to increase the longer the abuse continues, the more extensive the abuse and the older the child. A number of features of sexual abuse have also been linked with severity of impact, including the extent of premeditation, the degree of threat and coercion, sadism and bizarre or unusual elements. A child's ability to cope with the experience of sexual abuse, once recognised or disclosed, is strengthened by the support of a non-abusive adult carer who believes the child, helps the child understand the abuse and is able to offer help and protection.

Neglect

Neglect involves the persistent failure to meet a child's basic physical and/or psychological needs, likely to result in the serious impairment of the child's health or development. It may involve a parent or carer failing to provide adequate food, shelter and clothing, failing to protect a child from physical harm or danger, or the failure to ensure access to appropriate medical care or treatment. It may also include neglect of, or unresponsiveness to, a child's basic emotional needs.

Severe neglect of young children is associated with major impairment of growth and intellectual development. Persistent neglect can lead to serious impairment of health and development and ensuing long-term difficulties with social functioning, relationships and educational progress. Neglect can, in extreme cases, also result in death.

All of the above categories are used for both intrafamilial and extrafamilial abuse and neglect, perpetrated by someone inside or outside the child's home. Mixed categories are also recorded, registering more than one type of abuse and or neglect occurring to a child.

It is important to note that victims of child maltreatment are unlikely to be subjected to only one type of abuse (Browne 2002), for example both physical and sexual abuse are always accompanied by emotional abuse, which include verbal assault, threats of sexual or physical abuse, close confinement, for example locking a child in a room, withholding food and other aversive treatment (Browne & Herbert 1997). Furthermore, within each type of abuse there is a continuum of severity ranging from mild to life threatening.

As an emergency care practitioner it is important to have an awareness that there are many causal factors involved in child abuse and neglect. Poverty, social isolation, family breakdown and poor parent–child relationships are associated with all forms of child abuse and neglect and have been cited as risk factors for child sexual abuse. Additionally Finkelhor and Baron (1986) suggest that a third of sexually abused children have previously been physically abused, indicating that a number of common factors are involved (Bergner *et al.* 1994; Browne 2002). It is, however, important to state that it is **not** the practitioner's role to diagnose child abuse, but it is imperative that you are:

- Alert to the possibility of abuse and neglect
- Able to recognise, and know how to act upon, indicators that a child's welfare or safety may be at risk
- Familiar with these and any additional local procedures
- Able to access immediately contact details of the named or designated professionals from whom advice can be sought (HM Government 2006; London Child Protection Committee 2003).

Dimond (2002) notes that providing a diagnosis of child abuse is a weighty matter, the ramifications of which can be enormous. The DoH (1999) also states that the difficulties of assessing the risk of harm should not be underestimated. It is imperative that everyone who deals with allegations and suspicions of abuse maintains an open and inquiring mind. Suspected concerns should be referred on for appropriate management and the assessment made and any interventions documented. Opportunities for interventions in some cases may be sparse and when concerns are detected it is essential that steps are taken. This could be a vital part of the jigsaw in providing evidence or just recognising a vulnerable child at risk of abuse. It is also important to remember that abuse can happen in all strata of society; practitioners must remain objective and non-prejudiced, setting aside social and societal stereotypes.

Recognition and response

The starting point would be that in the course of an interaction with a child and/or family you suspect that a child is suffering from or likely to suffer from significant harm. Practitioners are responsible for acting if they have reason for concern, or reason to suspect that a child is at risk of harm, or in need of protection. Staff should alert appropriate personnel and refer to the local child protection procedures for local guidance in how to proceed.

In relation to recognising and responding to concerns it might be useful to undertake the following activity:

- Identify which of the following scenarios might be suspected as abuse or neglect and those which would not give cause for concern
- Decide the risk level for each scenario
- Decide whether you think the threshold for 'significant harm' has been reached.

Recognition, risk indicators and intervention

With the above scenarios in mind it is worth considering the factors that are frequently found in cases of child abuse or neglect. However, it must also be remembered that their presence is not proof that abuse has occurred but:

	Scenario	Abuse or neglect	Risk level	Significant harm?
1.	Lewis aged 19 months has a laceration on his scalp sustained when his older brother threw a toy. He also has bruising to both shins and knees and over his left temple.	Yes/No	High Moderate or Low	Yes/No
2.	Jessica aged 21 months has a history of a painful left arm, no history of trauma. She also has bruising on her buttocks and the back of her legs.	Yes/No	High Moderate or Low	Yes/No
3.	Amy aged 3 months has a history of not moving her left arm. On examination her arm is swollen and tender above the elbow. A fracture of her left humerus is diagnosed.	Yes/No	High Moderate or Low	Yes/No
4.	An adult patient informs you that her 8-year-old boy has been left alone at home.	Yes/No	High Moderate or Low	Yes/No
5.	You receive a telephone call from a member of the public who informs you that when he got home from work he found his partner agitated and confused. She told him their 2-month-old baby had an evil spirit inside him, which she has to remove. The baby is asleep.	Yes/No	High Moderate or Low	Yes/No

- Must be regarded as indicators of the possibility of significant harm
- Justifies the need for careful assessment and discussion with designated/named/lead person, manager or in the absence of the above an experienced colleague
- May require consultation with and/or referral to the social service department.

The absence of such indicators does not mean that abuse or neglect has not occurred.

Children of concern or risk indicators

In an abusive relationship the child may

- Appear frightened of the parents
- Act in a way that is inappropriate to her/his age and development (though full account needs to be taken of different patterns of development and different ethnic groups)
- Have significant health concerns e.g. chronic illness, disability and mental health
- Have poor attachment/bonding with parents
- Sustain injuries that do not compare with the story given.

The parent or carer may

- Persistently avoid the child health services and treatment of the child's episodic illnesses or
- Frequently visit emergency departments
- Have unrealistic expectations of the child
- Frequently complain about/to the child and may fail to provide attention or praise (high criticism/low warmth environment)
- Be absent
- Be misusing substances
- Persistently refuse to allow access on home visits
- Be involved in domestic violence
- Have physical ill health
- Suffer mental ill health
- Not meet the child's physical, social, health or developmental needs
- Be immature/young parents

- Evidence family dysfunction
- Raise concerns about their social situation/environment.

There is also a potential risk to children when individuals, previously known or suspected to have abused children, move into the household.

However, it must be noted that the above is for guidance only and not meant to be exhaustive or definitive. Not all parents experiencing adversity abuse or neglect their children. The specific signs that are potentially concerning are listed below. However, with regard to the above scenarios they should all be considered a cause for concern until further questions are asked and answered and if concerns still remain then these should be acted on. For example, in scenario 1 the injuries to 19-month-old Lewis are compatible with a toddler of that age in terms of bruising to his legs. It is important to find out the age of the brother; if he is 3 then the fact that he threw a toy when his mother was out of the room because Lewis was being 'annoying' would be plausible. If the brother was 16 then this would generate different concerns. The issue is whether or not the story is plausible but might require child development advice or advice about accident prevention or whether the story is raising further concerns. Scenario 2 should raise concerns, as children of this age do not normally bruise themselves in this area.

Recognising physical abuse

The following are often regarded as indicators of concern:

- An explanation which is inconsistent with an injury. In scenario 3, it is unlikely that a 3-month-old, who will not be very mobile, can injure themselves in the upper arm. One must question how the injury occurred.
- Several different explanations provided for an injury.
- Unexplained delay in seeking treatment.
- The parents or carers are uninterested or undisturbed by an accident or injury.
- Parents are absent without good reason when their child is presented for treatment.

- Repeated presentation of minor injuries or illnesses (which may represent a 'cry for help' and if ignored could have a more serious outcome or lead to a more serious injury).
- Family use of different doctors and accident and emergency departments.
- Reluctance to give information or mention previous injuries.

Bruising

Children can and do have accidental bruising, but the following must be considered as concerning unless there is evidence or an adequate explanation provided:

- Any bruising to a pre-crawling or pre-walking baby with no adequate explanation.
- Bruising in or around the mouth, particularly in small babies which may indicate force feeding – notably a torn frenulum without adequate explanation and a delay in seeking treatment. In accidental circumstances the parents are likely to seek immediate medical care.
- Two simultaneous bruised eyes, without bruising to the forehead. This is rarely accidental although a single bruised eye can be accidental or abusive.
- Repeated or multiple bruising on the head or on sites unlikely to be injured accidentally in this way. These sites include upper arms, thighs, buttocks.
- Variation in colour possibly indicating injuries caused at different times.
- The outline of an object, e.g. a key, belt marks, hand-prints, hair brush.
- Bruising or tears around or behind the earlobe(s) indicating injury by pulling or twisting.
- Bruising around the face.
- Grasp marks on small children or fingertip bruising.
- Unexplained bruising on the arms, buttocks or thighs may be an indicator of sexual abuse.

Bite marks – either human or animal

Bite marks can leave clear impressions of the teeth. Human bite marks are oval or crescent shaped. Those over 3 cm in diameter are more likely to have been caused by an older child or adult. A medical assessment or opinion should be sought where there is any doubt over the origin of the bite.

Burns and scalds

It can be difficult to distinguish between accidental and non-accidental burns and scalds and this will always require experienced medical assessment/opinion. However, any burn with a clear outline may be suspicious. These include:

- Circular burns from cigarettes (but may be friction burns if along the bony protuberance of the spine).
- Linear burns from hot metal rods or electrical fire elements.
- Burns of uniform depth over a large area.
- Scalds that have a line indicating immersion or poured liquid. For example a child getting into hot water of its own accord will struggle to get out and cause splash marks and children pouring a hot liquid over themselves will move out of the way. There will be splash marks; and bilateral scalds of the same size are suspicious.
- Old scars indicating previous burns/scalds which did not have appropriate treatment or adequate explanation.
- Scalds to the buttocks of a small child, particularly in the absence of burns to the feet are indicative of dipping into a hot liquid or bath.

Fractures

Non-mobile children rarely sustain fractures and there are grounds for concern if:

- The history provided is vague, non-existent or inconsistent with the fracture type
- There are associated old fractures
- Medical attention is sought after a period of delay when the fracture has caused symptoms such as swelling, pain or loss of movement
- There is an unexplained fracture in the first year of life.

Scars

A large number of scars or scars of different sizes or ages, or on different parts of the body may be concerning and indicative of abuse.

See Table 4.1 which compares accidental with non-accidental injury.

Recognising emotional abuse

It is argued that emotional abuse may be difficult to recognise especially in the emergency department. It is not as clear-cut as the signs of physical abuse. Additionally the signs are usually behavioural (thus difficult to determine over a short period of time such as a visit to an emergency department). The manifestations of emotional abuse might also indicate the presence of other kinds of abuse. The following should however be concerning:

- Unrealistic expectations of the baby or child
- Blaming a baby or young child for apparent untoward behaviour, for example claiming that a baby has soiled its nappy on purpose in order to irritate its parents
- Making undermining comments to a baby even though the baby cannot verbally understand, such as suggesting that the baby is ugly or has a bad temper. Such comments will invariably continue as the baby grows older.

The following may also be indicators of abuse:

- Developmental delay
- Abnormal attachment between a child and parent/carer e.g. an anxious attachment, indiscriminate or no attachment
- Aggressive behaviour towards others
- Scapegoated within the family
- Frozen watchfulness, particularly in preschool children – unnatural stillness in a child and anxious preoccupation with an adult's (parent's) movement may be found alongside reluctance to play and lack of spontaneity and exploration
- Low self-esteem and lack of confidence
- Difficulty in relating to others – often seen as a loner or appearing withdrawn
- Failure to thrive – loss of weight, slowness in reaching the development milestones, lethargy, tiredness, withdrawal or very aggressive tendencies may all point to a history of ill treatment

Table 4.1 Signs and symptoms of child abuse

Characteristics of accidental injuries	Characteristics of non-accidental injuries
Bruises are likely to be: • few and scattered • no pattern • frequent • same colour and age Burns and scalds are likely to be: • treated • easily explained Injuries are likely to be: • minor and superficial • quickly treated • easily explained Fractures are likely to be: • arms and legs • seldom to the ribs except for road traffic accidents (rare in very young children) • rarely due to brittle bone syndrome	Bruises are likely to be: • frequent • patterned, e.g. finger and thumb marks • old and new in same place (note colour) • in unusual positions Burns and scalds are likely to have: • a clear outline • splash marks around burn • unusual position, e.g. back of hand • indicative shapes, e.g. cigarette burns, bar of electric fire Suspicious injuries are likely to be: • bite marks • finger nail marks • large and deep scratches • incisions, e.g. from razor blades Fractures are likely to be: • numerous and healed at different times • always suspicious in babies under 2 years of age Sexual abuse may result in: • unexplained soreness • bleeding or injury to genital or anal areas • sexually transmitted diseases Physical abuse (non-accidental injury) entails soft tissue injury to the skin, eyes, ears and internal organs, as well as to ligaments and bones. Burns and scalds are included. Most of this abuse is short term and violent, though it may be repetitive.

• Excessive crying – may provoke parental abuse
• Attitude of the parents is important – they may handle the child in an unfeeling or mechanical way, or cause unnecessary delay in seeking medical advice. On the other hand the mother may express undue anxiety.

Recognising sexual abuse

This is unlikely to be diagnosed within the context of an emergency department although there are some physical and behavioural signs that should raise concern within the context of assessment of the child's overall welfare and safety. It is important to understand that boys and girls of all ages may be sexually abused but are often afraid of saying anything due to both guilt and fear. Thus recognition can be difficult unless the child discloses and is believed.

Some physical indicators associated with this form of abuse include:

• Pain or itching of the genital area
• Blood on underclothes
• Pregnancy in a younger girl where the identity of the father is not disclosed
• Physical symptoms such as injuries to the genital or anal area, bruising to the buttocks, abdomen and thighs, sexually transmitted disease, presence of semen on vagina, anus, external genitalia or clothing.

Some behavioural indicators associated with this form of abuse include:

- Inappropriate sexualised conduct
- Sexually explicit behaviour, play or conversation, inappropriate to the child's age and stage of development
- Continual and inappropriate or excessive masturbation
- Self-harm – eating disorder, self-mutilation and suicide attempts
- Involvement in prostitution or indiscriminate choice of sexual partners
- An anxious unwillingness to remove clothes, e.g. sports events or medical examination although this may also be related to cultural norms or physical difficulties.

Recognising neglect

Evidence of neglect is built up over a period of time and can cover different aspects of parenting. However, part of the jigsaw may be recognised in an emergency setting and interventions instigated as a result.

Indicators and concerns include:

- Failure of the parents to meet the basic essential needs e.g. hygiene, feeding, clothes, warmth or medical care
- A child who is listless, apathetic and unresponsive with no apparent medical cause
- Failure to grow and develop within normal expected pattern possibly with accompanying weight loss
- The child thrives away from the home environment (difficult to assess in an emergency department environment)
- Child frequently absent from school
- Child left with adults who are intoxicated or violent
- Child abandoned or left alone for excessive periods.

The unborn child

In some circumstances professionals within the different agencies are able to anticipate the likelihood of significant harm with regard to an expected baby. Accident and emergency staff should be alert to such issues, for example domestic violence is known to have occurred or the prospective parent discloses, or it is known, that they are misusing substances in a way that is likely to significantly impact on the baby's safety or development. Concerns should be addressed as early as possible in order to provide sufficient time for full assessment and support to help enable the prospective parents to provide safe care or plan to ensure the safety of the baby following birth.

The legislative framework

The legislative framework for protecting children in England and Wales is embodied in the Children Act 1989 and the Children Act 2004 (Parliament 1989, 2004). The significant statute for Scotland is the Children (Scotland) Act 1995 (Parliament 1995). The guiding principles for both these Acts are the same, notably they make children's welfare a priority and this is the paramount consideration. To this end it is considered that wherever possible the best place for children to be brought up and cared for is within their own family.

The two Sections of the Act that emergency care practitioners need to be aware of pertain to Sections 17 and 47. The former requires local authorities to provide services for children and families in need. A child is considered to be in need if:

- He is unlikely to achieve or maintain, or to have the opportunity of achieving or maintaining, reasonable standard of health or development without the provision for him of services by a local authority
- His health or development is likely to be significantly impaired, or further impaired, without the provision for him of such services
- He is disabled (a child is disabled if he is blind, deaf or dumb or suffers from mental disorder of any kind or is substantially and permanently handicapped by illness, injury or congenital deformity or other such disability as may be prescribed).

Section 47 of the Children Act 1989 (Parliament 1989) concerns the duty of local authorities to assess and investigate situations where there are suspicions that a child has suffered significant harm (or could in the future) from lack of care or a deliberate act by her/his carers. If the child is considered to be at risk of significant harm, section 47 of the Act provides a number of options, as follows.

An **Emergency Protection Order** enables the applicant (usually social services) to remove a child to a safe environment or to prevent the removal of a child from a safe environment. The order lasts for 8 days but can be challenged after 74 hours by parents/carers.

However, the Court will need to be satisfied that:

- There is reasonable cause to believe that the child is likely to suffer significant harm
- Access to the child is being frustrated when the applicant has reasonable cause to believe that access is required as a matter of urgency.

The key feature is the need to balance the protection requirements of the child and the legitimate interests and responsibilities of the parents/carers.

A **Child Assessment Order** is a time limited order enabling social services to undertake or arrange for an assessment of a child to be undertaken without the consent of the parent or care giver. This assessment considers the child's physical, emotional and psychological well-being.

However, the Court needs to be satisfied that the applicant has reasonable cause to suspect the child is suffering or likely to suffer significant harm but is not at immediate risk. It is unlikely that such an assessment can be made in the absence of such an order due to lack of cooperation, and the Court will not grant a Child Assessment Order if there are grounds for an Emergency Protection Order. It must be noted though that a Child Assessment Order does not permit the assessment of a mature child if he/she refuses to consent to such a medical or psychiatric examination/assessment.

Contemporary policy and legislation

The Laming Inquiry into the death of Victoria Climbié was one of a number of drivers that set the stage for the national framework for change and the implementation of the *National Service Framework for Children, Young People and Maternity Services* (NSF) (DoH 2004). This is underpinned by the Children Act 2004 in which there is a refusal to separate child protection from wider policies to improve children's lives (DfES 2003).

The NSF appears to be building on the underlying philosophy of the Children Act 1989 (Parliament 1989) in that the children's welfare is paramount as well as building on the recommendations from both the Kennedy and Laming inquiries. It is a ten-year strategy that recognises that change will not happen overnight. It sets standards for the first time for children's health and social care. In this context it is Standard 5 which has particular relevance as this is concerned with safeguarding and promoting the welfare of children and requires that: 'All agencies work together to prevent children suffering harm and to promote their welfare, provide them with services they require to address their identified needs and safeguard children who are being or who are likely to be harmed'.

The Children Act 2004

The Children Act 2004 (Parliament 2004) secured Royal Assent on 15 November 2004. The Act is the legislative spine on which it is intended to build the reforms of children's services, and has established:

- A Children's Commissioner to champion the views and interests of children and young people
- A duty on Local Authorities to make arrangements to promote cooperation between agencies and other appropriate bodies (such as voluntary and community organisations) in order to improve children's well-being (where well-being is defined by reference to the five outcomes), and a duty on key partners to take part in the cooperation arrangements
- A duty on key agencies to safeguard and promote the welfare of children
- A duty on local authorities to set up Local Safeguarding Children Boards and on key partners to take part (these replace Area/Local Child Protection Committees or ACPC/ LCPCs)
- The provision for indexes or databases containing basic information about children and young people to enable better sharing of information

- A requirement for a single Children and Young People's Plan to be drawn up by each local authority
- A requirement on local authorities to appoint a Director of Children's Services and designate a Lead Member
- The creation of an integrated inspection framework and the conduct of Joint Area Reviews to assess local areas' progress in improving outcomes
- Provisions relating to foster care, private fostering and the education of children in care.

The Children Act 2004 (Parliament 2004) gives a focus and status to children's services, strengthening but not replacing existing legislation.

Working Together

Working Together (DoH 1999; HM Government 2006) is the concept advocated for child protection work as it cuts across the normal boundaries of single discipline working (Pearce 2003). The above legislation is framed within this concept thereby providing emergency care practitioners with a commonly recognised and adopted framework to work within; it is a key reference point and the most recent policy document should be available within the emergency setting.

Assessment issues in child protection and implications for emergency care practitioners

It is an accepted principle that good assessment is the foundation of sound child protection work and planning. The research over the last ten years suggests, however, that it is questionable whether agreement exists as to what constitutes good assessment at various stages in the child protection process, whether it actually happens in practice and whether assessment is subsequently linked with effective intervention. There is also evidence that in the absence of clear guidelines subjective evaluations of levels of risk emerge (Giller *et al.* 1992). Without a framework for assessment decisions are more likely to be

guided by value judgements rather than by policy documentation or research findings. Giller *et al.* (1992) also found that the registration of a child on the child protection register itself did not guarantee thorough assessment and planning. Indeed, practitioners should be aware that the registration of a child on the child protection register does not guarantee protection. If they have a concern they should act on it whether the child is on the child protection register or not. Experience has identified that it is possible to be lulled into a false sense of security assuming that somebody else will do something without a referral about the existing concern being made; the implications of this for practice include the following:

- Misleading assumptions about other colleagues' meanings and activities can lead to confusion, antagonism and lack of cooperation. As a result, children and families may not receive the protection and help they need.
- Health care professionals need to understand each other's roles and functions and what their particular assessment could contribute to safeguarding and promoting children through the new assessment framework.
- All those involved in the assessment of children and families are involved in the promotion of the welfare of children and their protection from significant harm.
- There needs to be a common understanding in each case and at each stage of the work of how children and families will be involved in child protection processes and what information should be shared with them.
- Attention should be paid to what children say, how they look and how they behave.
- Attention is sometimes focused on the most visible or pressing problems and other warning signs are not appreciated.
- There should be a presumption of openness.

Assessment and the Common Assessment Framework

In safeguarding and promoting the welfare of children in need (or in need of protecting) it is important to ascertain with the family whether a child is in need and how that child and family might best be helped. The effectiveness with which a child's needs are assessed will be key to the effectiveness of subsequent actions and services and, ultimately, to the outcomes for the child. Thus practitioners need to be aware of the Common Assessment Framework which provides a common process for the early assessment to identify more accurately and speedily the additional needs of children and young people (DfES 2006; DoH 2000a).

The Common Assessment Framework aims to provide an easy-to-use assessment of the child's individual and family needs, which can be built up over time and with consent shared between practitioners. It is a framework for the ongoing assessment for all children who are vulnerable, in need and in need of protection. The framework is designed to:

- Improve the quality of referrals between agencies by making the referrals more evidence based
- Help embed a common language about the needs of children and young people
- Promote the appropriate sharing of information
- Reduce the number and duration of the different assessment processes which children and young people need to undergo (DfES 2006; DoH 2000b).

The framework is embedded within the multi-agency referral forms and should inform local child protection procedures and your own assessment. See DfES (2006) *Common Assessment Framework for Children*. Available at: http://www.everychild-matters.gov.uk/delivering services/caf/.

Professional responsibility and response – frequently asked questions

What should I do if I am concerned?
When to trigger child protection procedures?
The principles relating to all assessments and interventions should be flexible and sensitive with the welfare and safety of the child as the paramount consideration. Any concerns regarding children referred to social services should be specific in respect of any actual or potential risk. Decisions taken to implement child protection procedures may be taken on receipt of an initial referral from accident and emergency staff or at any time during the ongoing assessment of the child and family subsequent to their visit to an emergency department.

The flow chart shown outlines a suggested process to follow when child abuse is suspected for a child attending the emergency department (Figure 4.1). It is based on the Working Together Guidelines (HM Government 2006) and recommendations by Lord Laming (2003). **It is however important to stress that concerns are identified and if an assessment generates another question then it is important that the question is asked and information is gathered identifying factually what the concern is.**

The emergency care practitioner must have knowledge of the current legislation and their responsibilities therein, and as a minimum must:

- Know where the local Safeguarding Board's manual is kept
- Have a working knowledge of local policy and what it contains
- Know whether child protection policies can be accessed on the trust intranet
- Know the local policy for triggering child protection procedures
- Have information about Working Together in England and Wales or Protecting Children in Scotland, and the expectation of sharing responsibility regarding the safeguarding and protecting of children by working with other agencies
- Know who the named professionals for child protection are within the trust
- Know the designated nurse and doctor for child protection within the health authority
- Have the ability to recognise the signs and symptoms of child abuse.

In Scenario 2 above, where Jessica, aged 21 months, has a painful left arm and bruising on her

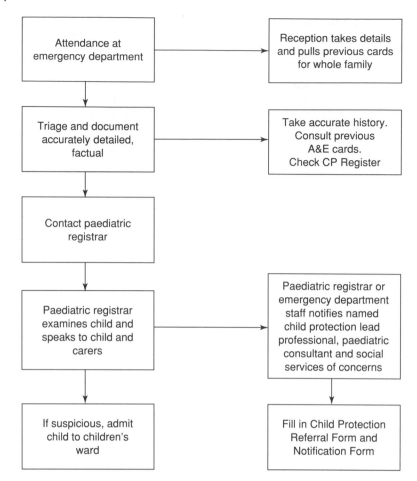

Figure 4.1 Processes to follow when there are child protection concerns for a child attending the emergency department.

buttocks and back of her legs, in all probability the practitioners are seeing a child who is the victim of a physical assault, thus it is in the child's best interests to take action and consultation with other professionals should be sought. Emergency care staff should have internal procedures which identify child protection designated/named managers or staff who are able to offer advice and decide upon the necessity for a referral to social services. Consultation may also be accomplished directly with social services; this can be without mentioning names if prior to making a formal referral.

Alert: It is important to share information with relevant individuals/professionals at all times.

How should you record your grounds for concern?

Concerns should be recorded factually in the child's notes. There should be a written record of:

- Discussions with the child
- Discussions with the parent(s)
- Discussions with managers
- Information provided to social services
- Decisions taken
- Notes/record should be clearly timed, dated and signed.

Child protection policies should follow the requirements of the Human Rights Act 1998 (Parliament 1998) and thus actions must have due regard to the individual's rights under the Act. Decisions and their reasons must be properly recorded at all stages of procedures or intervention.

With whom could or should you discuss your concern within your own agency or organisation?

Concerns should be shared with other professionals. Any communication that practitioners have with their line manager or named nurse/ lead for child protection is a legitimate interchange between professionals and such help should always be accessed. However, a formal referral or any urgent medical treatment must not be delayed by the need for consultation. Thus, if a child is suffering from a serious injury, medical attention must be provided by emergency care staff and social services and the duty consultant paediatrician must be informed. Except in cases where emergency treatment is needed, social services and the police are responsible for ensuring that any medical examinations required as part of enquiries are initiated.

An initial discussion however may take place with a colleague within the department and this initial discussion may help to make an objective assessment of:

- The needs of the child
- Whether or not the parents or carers are able to respond appropriately to the child's needs
- Whether or not the child is being adequately safeguarded from significant harm, and if the parents or carers are able to promote the child's health and development
- Whether or not action is required to safeguard and promote the child's welfare
- The reason for any referrals as either a child in need or a child in need of protection thus clarifying the source of the referral and reason
- The information that needs to be acquired – now or during a later assessment.

It will also help to:

- Explore facts and feelings
- Give meaning to the situation which distinguishes the child's and family's understanding and feelings from those of the professionals

- Reaching an understanding of what is happening, problems, strengths and difficulties, and the impact on the child (with the family wherever possible).

Should you discuss your concern with a professional from any other agency?

If it is in the child's best interest then a referral to another agency should be made. If the child is vulnerable as opposed to in 'need' (and or in 'need of protection') and would benefit from support then it would be appropriate to refer to other health professionals such as the health visitor, school nurse or general practitioner. However, if the concerns are severe enough then a referral will be made to statutory agencies, which are normally social services.

Advice may initially be sought from a colleague, line manager, designated professionals, police child protection unit, or child protection manager or advisor, about the appropriateness of a referral. If following consultation social services conclude that a referral is required, the information provided must be regarded and responded to as such. It is important that practitioners do not keep quiet about concerns, however trivial they might seem.

Should you report your concern officially? To whom?

The common route for a referral initiated by emergency department staff would be to a duty social worker employed by the local authority. The local authority provides social services and they are expected to cooperate in accordance with their policies and the legal framework and under the general guidance of the Secretary of State. Social services take a lead role in child protection work but rely on the cooperation of all other agencies involved. They have a statutory duty to coordinate and facilitate the services involved in protecting children; especially relevant to emergency department at the initial enquiry to establish whether there are genuine concerns about a child and if so they must enable appropriate meetings with other agencies within the required timeframe. They have an obligation to keep a child at home unless there is immediate danger to the child and to provide the services necessary to achieve this. Parents and others can be under the mistaken belief that social workers are about removing children from the home. This is not so, as no one has the power to remove a child from its home or parents without a court order and emergency care practitioners can help to dispel this myth.

However, referrals can also be made to the police according to the circumstances. The referral can be urgent where the child is in immediate danger, or less immediate when instant 'on the spot' decisions do not have to be made and a more thorough assessment of the situation made.

The police have immediate powers and their help may be needed in acutely dangerous situations. For example in scenario 4 there are concerns about the 8-year-old boy left alone at home or in scenario 5 where the father is concerned about his partner believing that the baby has evil spirits inside her. In these situations it would be appropriate to contact the police in order for them to visit and assess the situation in relation to the baby or child's safety. The police are involved in child protection as part of their responsibility for the prevention and investigation of crime. They have a major role in child protection procedures. They also have emergency powers not available to other agencies. They can without prior application to the court:

- Remove a child to suitable accommodation and keep them there
- Detain a child in place of protection, for example keeping a baby in hospital and not allowing the parents to remove the child
- Enter premises to search for a child in order to save life or limb.

Any child detained in police protection can be kept in a safe place within their protection for 72 hours in England and Wales and 24 hours in Scotland. This would give social services time to obtain a court order to continue the protection of the child should this be necessary. The police would inform social services as a matter of course and the child protection processes follow the same framework whichever agency is the first point of contact.

Do you have individual responsibility to make that referral?

A professional or member of the public can make a referral. Staff working in emergency departments have a responsibility to refer a child to social services when it is believed or suspected that a child under the age of 18 years or an unborn baby:

- Has suffered significant harm in that the child is experiencing or may have already experienced abuse or neglect
- Is likely to suffer significant harm in the future
- With agreement of a person with parental responsibility would be likely to benefit from family support services.

The timing of such referrals must reflect the perceived risk but should usually be within one working day of the recognition of risk. In urgent situations, out of office hours, the referral should be made to the emergency or duty social worker. At other times if the child is known to have a social worker the referral may be made directly to them. However, staff are advised to check their local child protection procedures.

In what format should you make a referral – by telephone, in writing, directly in person?

Referrals may be made by telephone or, if not immediately urgent, a written referral using an interagency referral form with a copy kept in the notes and sent to relevant professionals. All telephone referrals should be confirmed in writing within 48 hours, using the interagency referral form. Staff will need to know where these forms can be accessed and seek advice if necessary from colleagues who have specialist knowledge in child protection procedures. It can save a lot of time in the beginning if the written referral is filled in correctly at the beginning (Fraser & Nolan 2004).

The initial referral should clearly establish:

- The nature of the concern
- How and why it has arisen
- What the child's needs appear to be
- Whether the concern involves abuse or neglect and whether there is any need for any urgent action to protect the child or any other in the household.

The social worker is likely to want to discuss the assessment of the initial concern with the practitioner who has instigated the referral.

What do you think will happen when you do make a referral to another agency?

There is an expectation that any practitioner making a referral will have carefully considered the information and gathered some background information before making the referral. The immediate response to a referral from staff in the emergency department may be:

- No further action at this stage or
- Provision of services and/or
- A fuller initial assessment of needs within 7 days or sooner if the criteria for initiating S.47 enquiries are met
- A core assessment may then be completed within 35 days if indications exist that this is required
- Emergency action to protect the child
- An S.47 strategy discussion meeting where the child and or family are well known or the facts clearly indicate that an S.47 enquiry is required.

All referrals must be acknowledged within one working day and where there is to be no further action feedback should be provided to the family and referrers about the outcome of this stage of the referral. Staff are entitled to feedback as this is one way of evaluating interventions and reflecting on/developing practice.

Alert: If there is to be further assessment and/or investigation the social worker is likely to contact you again and under the Children Act 2004 (Parliament 2004) you have a duty to contribute to the ongoing assessment and provide relevant information about the child and family (HM Government 2006).

What information should you give to the parent(s)?

Except in exceptional circumstances a referral should not be made to another agency without the parents' knowledge or before they have had the opportunity to listen to and discuss the concerns. It is also advocated that it is not only the

parents who are informed but also the child. This open and honest approach is advocated as best practice and the family is more likely to cooperate with procedures, and it lessens the chance of the family becoming hostile. Practitioners often express anxieties about informing the family of referral to social services, as there is concern that actions will be seen as a betrayal of the family. However, honesty is important if child protection concerns are to be explored thoroughly, and it is important for the family to know that they can trust the professionals and that nothing is being hidden from them. If trust in the professionals is apparent then the family can be involved in any decision making and planning about the child. Furthermore, family members normally have a right to know what is being said about them and be allowed to contribute to important decisions about their lives and the lives of their children. Research has endorsed the view that honesty and openness between professionals and families develops good relationships and helps to bring about the best possible outcomes for children (DoH 1995b). Thus, the best way to approach the situation may be with another colleague and focus the interaction on the welfare of the child. The referral is about the child's best interests. Also formal referrals from named professionals cannot be treated as anonymous, so the parent will ultimately become aware of the identity of the referrer, thus support for the referrer should be part of local policy.

Caution however, should also prevail. Partnership with families does not always mean agreeing with them or accepting their version of events, as this may not be in the child's best interests. It should be remembered that not all parents have the ability to safeguard their children even with help and support. Thus whilst it is best practice to inform the parents it is not obligatory if it is felt that the child has suffered or is likely to suffer significant harm (DoH 1999, 2003; HM Government 2006), or that if you feel the child is at risk from further harm if you were to inform the parents of a referral to social services. Any written referral should make it clear whether or not the parents and/or child have been informed. If a family receives an unexpected visit from social services or another agency they are more likely to be angry and resist the support on offer. Moreover, if the social worker or other agency know that the family has not been informed, then they can manage the situation appropriately.

Thus when making referrals staff should consider the following:

- Parental consultation.
- Where practicable, concerns should be discussed with the family and agreement sought for referral to social services unless this may, either by delay or the behavioural response it prompts, place the child at risk of significant harm.
- A decision by the practitioner not to seek parental permission before making a referral to social services must be recorded and justified as to why the parents were not informed. Where a parent has agreed to a referral this must also be documented and confirmed in the referral to social services.
- If parents refuse to give permission for the referral it is advised that further advice is sought, unless this would cause undue delay. The outcome of the advice sought and discussions should be documented.

However, if having made an assessment of the situation and taken account of the parent's wishes not to refer, it is still considered that there is need for a referral then the reason for proceeding must be recorded. Social services must be told that the parent has withheld permission. However, the parent should be contacted to inform them that after considering their wish a referral has been made.

To what extent should I consider the child's wishes?

The child's view should always be considered and if the child can understand the significance and consequences of making a referral to social services they should be asked their view. The child must not be pressed for information, led, cross-examined or given false assurances of absolute confidentiality. Such actions could prejudice police investigations, especially in cases of sexual abuse. It does however remain the responsibility of the practitioner to take whatever action is required to ensure the safety of the child and any other children, whilst getting the balance between a child centred approach and ensuring safety.

Who can I share information with and what about confidentiality?

The information that you share with other agencies must be justified in the context of the child's best interests. If you can justify that at the time of your assessment there is a need to share information, then do so as long as the information you share is only relevant to the child protection issue. It is advocated that to keep children safe from harm it is essential that professionals maximise the potential to share relevant information across geographical and professional boundaries. Sharing information helps to piece the jigsaw together. The flowchart shown provides information on the processes to be followed to facilitate effective information sharing (Figure 4.2).

The main sources of relevant law with respect to information sharing and confidentiality in child protection are:

- Common law of confidence
- European Convention on Human Rights (via its introduction into English law in the Human Rights Act 1998)
- Data Protection Act 1998
- Crime and Disorder Act 1998
- Children Act 1989 (Scotland 1995)
- Children Act 2004
- The Caldicot Standards (applicable to health and social services).

Professional guidance for all health professionals is also available in *What to do if you are worried a child is being abused*. This supersedes previous guidance to doctors, nurses, midwives and health visitors (DoH 2003). The Government has also taken powers through the Children Act 2004 (Parliament 2004) to require the establishment of national standards of databases or index systems to enable practitioners to identify the child or young person (DfES 2003). Thus practitioners are expected to follow and use both local and national procedures for information sharing.

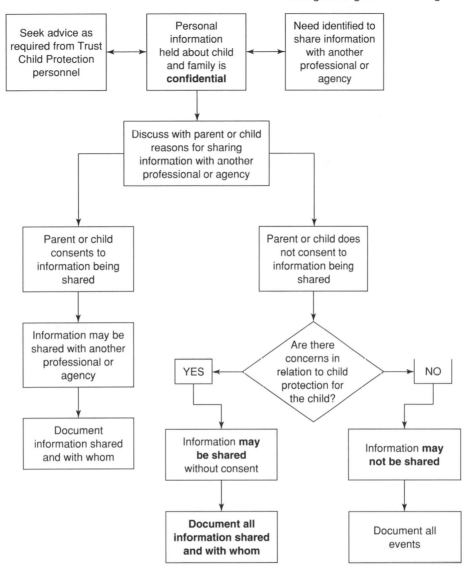

Figure 4.2   Process to follow to facilitate effective information sharing.

The overall legal position is that in general the law does not prevent individual sharing of information with other practitioners if:

- Those likely to be affected consent.
- The public interest in safeguarding the child's welfare overrides the need to keep information confidential.
- Disclosure is required under a court order or other legal obligation.

When in doubt staff are advised to consult the named professional who may in turn seek advice from the designated nurse or doctor and/or Caldicott guardian or solicitor of the Trust.

What should I document?

Document factually everything observed, said and heard in relation to the child protection concern. It is also advised that staff record the following:

- Name and date of birth of child, mother, father, partners, siblings and other significant carer
- The name and address of family if different from the child's
- Child and family's GP, health visitor, school nurse, pre-school/school, social worker
- Nature of concern e.g. injury not matching the explanation or delay in treatment; child's presentation and or carers' attitude
- Information on domestic violence, relevant mental health or learning difficulty/disability issues in the family
- Complete the multi-agency initial assessment referral form and liaison health visitor referral form
- Document all actions in the notes and keep copies of all referral forms and send copies of referral forms to relevant professionals (disclosing only child protection concerns).

Consider the following:

- What if . . . the concern was about physical abuse with evident bruising? Would there be any difference in your response?
- What if . . . it was emotional or psychological abuse? Would there be any difference in your response?
- What if . . . you thought that neglect was the issue? Would there be any difference in your response?
- What if . . . you thought that sexual abuse had occurred? Would there be any difference in your response?

There should be no difference in your actions and response whatever your concerns in relation to the child's welfare and safety.

Alert: the Child Protection Register does not protect the child. It is the actions and interventions of the professionals.

Summary of key points

- It is important to recognise and respond to concerns about a child in need.
- Do not dismiss concerns.
- Concerns must be shared with other professionals.

- A child protection advisor is available to offer guidance.
- All concerns and actions must be recorded.
- Guidance must be sought through the agency guidelines and in collaboration with other agencies.
- Refer to the *Multi-Agency Child Protection Handbook*, policy and other guidelines.
- Seek personal support.

Conclusion

The safeguarding and protection of children is the responsibility of every professional who comes into contact with children and their families. The emergency care practitioner has an important role to play in this. This chapter has covered the key issues in relation to recognising concerns, what to do and the referral process. It is vital that practitioners receive education and training about protecting children in order to keep them updated in line with national contemporary policy for practice. Furthermore it is important that they are conversant with local policy and procedures for safeguarding children. Responding to concerns and sharing information are vital to improve outcomes for children who may be at risk or are in need of protection. Indeed,

'Everybody who works with children, parents and other adults in contact with children should be able to recognise, and know how to act upon, indicators that a child's welfare or safety may be at risk. Professionals, foster carers, staff members and managers should be mindful always of the welfare and safety of children – including unborn children and older children in their work' (DoH 1999: paragraph 5.2:39).

References

Belsky, J. (1993) Etiology of Child Maltreatment: a developmental–ecological analysis. *Psychological Bulletin*, **114**, 413–434.

Bergner, R.M., Delgado, L.K. & Graybill, D. (1994) Finkelhor's risk factor checklist: a cross validation study. *Child Abuse and Neglect*, **18**(4), 331–340.

Browne, K.D. (2002) Child Abuse: defining, understanding and intervening. In: Wilson, K. & James, A. (eds) *The Child Protection Handbook*, 2nd edn. Bailliere Tindall, London.

Browne, K.D. & Herbert, M. (1997) *Preventing Family Violence*. Wiley, Chichester.

Browne, K.D. & Stevenson, J. (1988) A Checklist for completion by health visitors to identify children 'at risk' for child abuse. Report to the Surrey Area Review Committee on Child Abuse (Unpublished). In: *Early Prediction and Prevention of Child Abuse*, K. Browne, C. Davies & P. Stratton (eds). Wiley: Winchester.

Cleaver, H., Unell, I. & Aldgate, J. (1999) *Children's Needs Parenting Capacity: The Impact of Parental Illness, Problem Alcohol and Drug Use, and Domestic Violence on Children's Development*. The Stationery Office, London.

Corby, B. (2006) *Child Abuse: Towards a Knowledge Base*, 3rd edn. Open University Press, Milton Keynes.

Daniel, B., Wassell, S. & Gilligan, R. (1999) *Child Development for Child Care and Protection Workers*. Jessica Kingsley Publishers: London.

Department for Education and Skills (DfES) (2003) *Every Child Matters*. The Stationery Office, London (available online at: http://www.dfes.gov.uk/everychildmatters).

Department for Education and Skills (DfES) (2006) *Common Assessment Framework for Children*. Website: Available online at: http://www.everychildmatters.gov.uk/delivering services/caf/.

Department of Health (DoH) (1991) *The Children Act 1989 Guidance and Regulations Volume 1 Court Orders*. HMSO, London.

Department of Health (DoH) (1995a) *Child Protection – Messages from Research*. HMSO, London.

Department of Health (DoH) (1995b) *A Guide for Guardians ad Litem in Public Law Proceedings under the Children Act 198.9*. HMSO, London.

Department of Health (DoH) (1999) *Working Together to Safeguard Children: A guide to inter-agency working to safeguard and promote the welfare of children*. The Stationery Office, London.

Department of Health (DoH) (2000a) *Framework for the Assessment of Children in Need and their Families*. The Stationery Office, London.

Department of Health (DoH) (2000b) *Assessing Children in Need and their Families*. The Stationery Office, London.

Department of Health (DoH) (2003) *What to do if you are worried a child is being abused: Children's Services Guidelines*. DoI I, London.

Department of Health (DoH) (2004) *The National Service Framework for Children, Young People and Maternity Services*. DoH, London.

Dimond, B. (2002) *Legal Aspects of Midwifery*, 2nd edn. Books for Midwives Press, Oxford.

Dubowitz, H. (1989) Prevention of Child Maltreatment: What is known. *Pediatrics*, **83**, 570–577.

Ennals, P., Bernard, J., Davies, O., Bullock, R. & Tunstill, J. (2003) The will is there, but is the money? What do the proposals in the green paper on children 'Every Child Matters' mean for the professionals who will be charged with putting them into practice? Our team of experts assess the likely impact. *Communitycare.co.uk*, 14 September 2003.

Fraser, J. & Nolan, M. (2004) *Child Protection: A Guide for Midwives*. Books for Midwives Press, Oxford.

Finkelhor, D. & Baron, L. (1986) Risk factors for child sexual abuse. *Journal of Interpersonal Violence*, **1**(1), 43–71.

Giller, H. *et al.* (1992) *An Evaluation of Child Protection Procedures in four Welsh ACPC areas*. Social Information Systems.

HM Government (2006) *Working Together to Safeguard Children: A guide to interagency working to safeguard and promote the welfare of children*. The Stationery Office, London. (available online at: http://www.nelincs.gov.uk/working together).

Howard, P. (2004) Forward. In: *Child Protection: A Guide for Midwives*, J. Fraser & M. Nolan, eds. Books for Midwives Press, Oxford.

Howarth, J. (ed) (2001) *The Child's World. Assessing Children in Need*. Jessica Kingsley Publishers, London.

London Child Protection Committee (2003) *London Child Protection Procedures*. London Child Protection Committee.

Lord Laming (2003) *The Victoria Climbié Inquiry Report*. The Stationery Office, London.

Parliament (1989) *The Children Act*. HMSO.

Parliament (1995) *The Children (Scotland) Act*. HMSO.

Parliament (1998) *The Human Rights Act*. HMSO.

Parliament (2004) *The Children Act*. TSO.

Parton, N. (2004) From Maria Colwell to Victoria Climbié: Reflections on Public Inquiries into Child Abuse a Generation Apart. *Child Abuse Review*, **13**, 80–94.

Pearce, J. (2003) Training Update: Parental mental health and child protection – making the links through training. *Child Abuse Review*, **12**(2), 114–118.

Powell, C. (2003) Early Indicators of Child Abuse and Neglect: A Multi-Professional Delphi Study. *Abuse Review*, **12**, 25–40.

Reder, P. & Duncan, S. (2004) Making the Most of the Victoria Climbié Inquiry Report. *Child Abuse Review*, **13**, 95–114.

Scottish Executive (2002) *'It's everyone's job to make sure I'm alright' Report of the Child Protection Audit and Review*. Scottish Executive.

Scottish Office (1995) *Scotland's Children: A Brief Guide to the Children (Scotland) Act 1995.* The Stationery Office, Edinburgh.

Thyen, U., Thiessen, R., & Heinsohn-Krug, M. (1995) Secondary Prevention: serving families at risk. *Abuse and Neglect*, **19**, 1337–1347.

Watson, G. (1989) The abuse of disabled children and young people. In: *Child Abuse and Neglect: Facing the Challenge*, S. Rodgers, D. Heavey & E. Ashe (eds). Open University Press, Milton Keynes.

Wright, D. (2002) We Can't Do It Alone. *Community Care*, 41. www.community–care.co.uk, 25 April–1 May 2002.

Chapter 5 **Meeting the Specific Needs of Young People Attending the Emergency Department**

Jean Shepherd and Olive McKeown

Introduction

The attendance of young people or adolescents at emergency departments poses unique challenges for staff working in this setting. Although adolescence is perceived as a relatively healthy period of our lives, recent advances in medical technology mean that young people are increasingly living and surviving with life threatening or life limiting conditions. For other young people, the social pressures and changing social norms bring their own set of challenges, some of which have potential or actual detrimental effects on their health. As a consequence the use of health resources during this time of life is greater than in late childhood, particularly the use of mental health resources (MacFoul & Werneke 2001).

Increasing numbers of adolescents access accident and emergency services rather than primary health care facilities, especially for consultations around sexual health (particularly emergency contraception), mental health, self-harm and substance misuse (Hogg 1997). However, few emergency departments currently have specific provision for young people in relation to staff or facilities (RCPCH 1999). Adolescents also face an added problem where hospitals currently separate children's from adult emergency services; consequently neither service may take the lead responsibility for young people. However, the recently published National Service Framework (NSF) (DoH 2004a) has specified standards for the hospital care of children, including accident and emergency services. These standards set the framework within which acute hospital care is provided, although the lack of mandatory targets to enforce their implementation has given some cause for concern (Masterson *et al.* 2004). Against

this background, this chapter will focus on the attendance at emergency departments by adolescents for issues in relation to substance misuse, access to emergency contraception and sexual health advice and deliberate self-harm with a scenario provided to illustrate each of these. It will begin by briefly considering what makes adolescents different and the implications of this for the provision of health services.

Adolescence and health care

Adolescence is viewed in different ways. Freud saw adolescence as a period of recapitulation of the childhood oedipal complex and Erickson viewed it as a time of conflict between identity and role confusion. There have also been chronological definitions placed on the time of adolescence, the World Health Organization for example defining adolescence as the second decade of life, from 10–20 years. Rutter (1980) advocates a more general view on adolescence, in that it is merely a social construct, a rite of passage that is culturally and socially invented. As none of these definitions take into account the biological changes of puberty or the increasing central nervous system maturation and myelination, this chapter will view it as the period between the ages of 10 and 25 years of biopsychosocial maturation, leading to functional independence in adult life (Viner 2003).

This period between childhood and adulthood poses specific challenges for managing the health of this population group mainly due to the nature of adolescence. It is easy to be very generalist about the nature of adolescence but we should be mindful of the fact that adolescents are more different as individuals than they are similar. Health care professionals that work with young people are increasingly recognising the need for knowledge and understanding in respect of the specific needs of this client group. Young people between the ages of 10 and 20 years make up between 12 and 15% of the population in most developed countries (13% in the UK) and among minority ethnic communities the proportion is considerably higher. This is actually a client group as large as children under the age of 10 years in the UK (ONS 2000). They are, therefore, a significant number whose needs require specific attention and consideration.

It is also of note that young people have a distinct epidemiology of disease and health risk, which bring their own unique set of problems and symptoms not found in children or adults; these can be considered as either late onset childhood illnesses or early onset adult illnesses (Viner 2003). This, coupled with the physiological impact of puberty on common childhood illnesses such as diabetes, poses another set of adolescent specific complications. Further, the causes of mortality and morbidity in adolescents are distinct from those of both children and adults. For example accidents and suicide make up a larger proportion of total adolescent mortality than at any other age. Health care behaviours in early childhood are dominated by parental and family values. Adolescents in their quest for adulthood explore more 'adult' behaviours such as smoking, drinking alcohol, drug use, violence and sexual intimacy. Elkind's (1967) longstanding and often cited theory of adolescent egocentricism and the constructs of imaginary audience and personal fable could go some way to explain the somewhat risk taking behaviour of some young people. Elkind (1967) describes this imaginary audience behaviour as young people having a tendency to believe that others are always watching and evaluating them; the personal fable refers to the belief that the self is unique, invulnerable and omnipotent. The patterns of thinking reflected by both constructs seem to capture and explain feelings and behaviours typically associated with early adolescence, such as self-consciousness, conformity to peer group norms, and risk taking. However, Vartanian (2000) noted

in a theoretical and conceptual review of the imaginary audience and personal fable theory that this characterisation of adolescent social cognition was biased and faulty as it had not received adequate empirical testing largely because of the self report survey methodology used in previous studies. Yet despite these issues, the imaginary audience and personal fable constructs continue to be considered prototypical representations of social cognitive processes during adolescence (Vartanian 2000). Management of the health care of adolescents, therefore, needs to be specifically geared towards meeting their needs.

Surveys of this population group consistently provide evidence that young people want services that specifically meet their needs, especially in respect of confidentiality, privacy and being listened to. As noted above, adolescents sit between two camps with regard to emergency service provision. Neither the adult nor child services specifically respond to, or meet their needs. Reviews undertaken by the Commission for Health Improvement (CHI) indicate that even in hospitals that are found to provide otherwise high standards of care, a lack of dedicated adolescent facilities are highlighted. Although these hospitals have been commended for developing a 'child friendly' approach within their emergency departments, the lack of dedicated facilities which would provide privacy and dignity for adolescents are particularly of concern (CHI 2002). These concerns have also been raised by the Royal College of Paediatrics and Child Health in their report (RCPCH 2003) which outlines the health services that should be provided in order to meet the health care needs of young people. It highlights key issues which young people perceive as barriers to (their) effective use of both primary and secondary health care services, which include:

- Lack of information
- Difficulties in achieving low visibility access for confidential issues
- Services not seen as youth friendly because of concerns about confidentiality for those less than 16 years old

- Lack of expertise and continuity of care by professionals
- Failure to respect the validity of young people's views
- Young people in hospital having to be accommodated either in a children's area or with a population they regard as elderly.

N.B. Some groups of young people have particular difficulties accessing services, notably those who are disabled, socially excluded, living in poverty, or from a black or other ethnicity minority. Young people who are looked after and those who are unsure of their sexual orientation also face particular difficulties.

Acknowledging that adolescents have different needs during a time when they are required to make the transition to adulthood brings to light issues about decision making, rights and consent. Adolescents under the age of 16 years are categorised as children and fall under child and adolescent services, whereas adolescents over 16 years are generally provided for by adult services. Young people between the ages of 16 and 18 are regarded as having the same rights to consent to medical treatment as adults, this by virtue of the Family Reform Act 1969. However, for young people under the age of 16 years there is the added dimension of the concept of 'Gillick competence', and the 'Fraser' guidelines, which govern how decisions are made for young people who are not legally classified as an adult. (For a fuller consideration of how these apply, the reader is referred to Chapter 2 in this book.) The Sexual Offences Act 2003 allows for confidentiality in the discussion of under-age sex and advice on treatment, for this age group. The Act states that a person is not guilty of aiding, abetting or counselling a sexual offence against a child where they are acting with the intention to:

- Protect a child from pregnancy or sexually transmitted infection
- Protect the physical safety of a child
- Promote a child's emotional well-being by the giving of advice.

In all cases, the person must not be causing or encouraging the commission of an offence or a child's participation in it. Nor must the person be acting for the purpose of obtaining sexual gratification.

Substance misuse

Substance use amongst adolescents is increasing and is often regarded as being a 'normal' part of their lifestyle. There is evidence that some substance misuse is directly related to underlying psychopathology, and may be responsible for exacerbating mental health problems as well as other medical conditions.

Within the general population recreational substance use has reached epidemic proportions. It is estimated that 45 million European Union citizens have used cannabis at some time, with proportionately higher use among younger people (Ghuran *et al.* 2001). The consumption of 'hard' drugs such as cocaine and heroin is steadily increasing, with an estimated 1.5 million problem users in the EEC (Dixon 1998). A study conducted in the UK of almost 8000 15–16-year-olds indicated that 40% reported having tried illicit drugs at some time, with 30% reporting cannabis use in the 30 days prior to the interview (Miller & Plant 1996). Complications of drug use vary widely, but can result in serious medical conditions and premature death, as some recreational drugs have serious effects on the cardiovascular system. The management of young people who have accidentally ingested recreational drugs presenting for treatment can be challenging, especially as many will be unwilling or unable to provide an accurate history.

Scenario 1

Jake is a 15-year-old white English boy who has recently been admitted to the emergency department. He has been out for the evening with his friends and because he has become disorientated and incoherent they became concerned and have dropped him off at the department. Before leaving they reported that he started off the evening smoking some cannabis with his friends; later on they met some older guys who offered them amphetamines, which they believe he had taken for the first

> time. He has often smoked cannabis in the past;
> the first time he smoked he felt a little sick and
> was disorientated but subsequently seemed to
> have few side effects associated with its use. He is
> currently restless, agitated, disorientated, pacing
> around and talking a lot. The triage nurse is
> finding it difficult to gain his cooperation.

Immediate management

- Activated charcoal can be given within 1 hour
  of ingestion to reduce absorption (unless the
  patient is drowsy, fitting or vomiting).
- Base-line observations for at least 6 hours.
- Electrocardiogram (ECG) for approximately
  6 hours.
- Monitor fluid and electrolytes status.
- May need IV fluids and electrolytes (dextrose
  saline and potassium).
- Diazepam should be administered if convulsions occur.
- If the rectal temperature is >39°C, instigate
  cooling measures (fan, sponging, ice packs,
  cool IV fluids).

If Jake does not respond to this regime he will
need to be paralysed and ventilated. Caution
should be exercised when considering intravenous (IV) fluids as he may have ingested large
amounts of water prior to being admitted to
the emergency department if feeling hot, and
therefore water intoxication is a risk (Kerins *et al.*
2003).

Short-term management notes on amphetamine and ecstasy intoxication

Onset of symptoms from amphetamine consumption varies according to the route used. Transient nausea, increased muscle tone, muscle pain,
trismus (jaw-clenching), dilated pupils, blurred
vision, sweating, dry mouth, agitation, anxiety,
palpitations, vomiting, abdominal pain and diarrhoea are all possible symptoms of amphetamine
intoxication (Paton & Jenkins 2003). Hypertonia,
hyper-reflexia, hyperpyrexia, tachycardia, initial
hypertension then hypotension, tachypnoea and
visual hallucinations are also associated with
taking large amounts of amphetamines (Bobst
& Habraken 1997). Effects may be prolonged if a

patient has alkaline urine, which may be related
to a urinary tract infection, metabolic causes or to
a diet based mainly on vegetables.

In severe amphetamine or MDMA (ecstasy)
poisoning the following complications may occur:
delirium, coma, convulsions and cardiac dysrrhy-
thmias that may be fatal. A hyperthermic syndrome may develop with rigidity, hyper-reflexia
and hyperpyrexia (>39°C) leading to hypotension, rhabdomyolysis, metabolic acidosis, acute
renal failure, disseminated intravascular coagulation, hepatocellular necrosis, adult respiratory
distress syndrome and cardiovascular collapse.
Death from intracerebral haemorrhage has also
been reported in hyperthermic patients (Kalant
2001).

MDMA is also associated with hyponatraemia
and cerebral oedema. This can occur in patients
who have consumed excessive amounts of water
which may be related to an attempt to keep body
temperature under control. These patients present with mild hypothermia and confusion; they
may be unresponsive and have a staring appearance. It is more likely than not that young people
who present at an emergency department having
taken MDMA are also likely to have consumed
other substances such as alcohol or cannabis.
Staff need to be alert to this pattern of polysub-
stance use and to be prepared to assess patients
with this possibility in mind.

There is a range of substances that young people (and indeed adults) may consume. A summary of their effects and signs and symptoms
are provided below in Table 5.1.

Alcohol

In the period between the First and Second World
Wars in the UK, young people aged 18 to 24 years
old were the lightest drinkers in the population
and the group most likely to abstain from alcohol.
It was not until the 1960s that pubs and drinking
began to become an integral part of the youth
scene. By the 1980s, those aged 18 to 24 years had
become the heaviest drinkers in the population,
and the group least likely to abstain. Today, most
young people are drinking regularly, though not
frequently, by the age of 14 or 15 years (Ashley
2000). A national survey conducted in 1999 found

Table 5.1   Effects of commonly ingested substances encountered. Adapted from Mental Health Primary Health Care in Prison website: http://www.prisonmentalhealth.org/ (accessed 15 June 2005)

Substance	Syndrome	Vital signs	Mental state	Signs/symptoms
Atropine, phenothiazines, tricyclic antidepressants	anticholinergic	low BP, high HR	lethargy to coma	confusion, dilated pupils, dizziness, dry mouth, inability to urinate, flushed skin, convulsions
Metoclopramide, phenothiazines, some antipsychotics	extrapyramidal	low BP, high HR, high or low temperature	lethargy	dystonic movements, abrupt muscle contractions especially of the face and neck, torticollis, tongue protrusion, oculogyric crisis
Amphetamine, cocaine, ecstasy	hyperthermic	high BP, high HR, high temperature, high RR	fluctuating level of consciousness	rigidity, hyper-reflexia, disseminated intravascular coagulation, rhabdomyolysis, renal failure
Antipsychotics	neuroleptic malignant syndrome	high BP, high HR, high temperature, high RR	fluctuating level of consciousness	rigidity, hyper-reflexia, disseminated intravascular coagulation, rhabdomyolysis, renal failure
Codeine, heroin, methadone, morphine	opioid	low BP, low HR, low RR, low temperature	lethargy to coma	slurred speech, ataxia, pinpoint pupils
Barbiturates, ethanol, hypnotics	sedative	low BP, low RR, low temperature	lethargy to coma	slurred speech, ataxia, hyporeflexia
Aminophylline, amphetamine, caffeine, cocaine, phencyclidine, theophylline	sympathomimetic	high BP, high HR, high temperature, high RR	anxiety, agitation, delirium	dilated pupils, sweating, convulsions
Effect of withdrawal from opiates, e.g. heroin	withdrawal of opiates	high BP, high HR	normal	dilated pupils, sweating, nausea, vomiting, hyperactivity, piloerection, rhinorrhoea
Effect of withdrawal from alcohol and anxiolytics/sedatives	withdrawal of sedative hypnotics or ethanol/alcohol	high BP, high HR, high RR, high temperature	anxiety, restlessness, confusion	nausea, dilated pupils, tremor, convulsions, sweating

BP = blood pressure; HR = heart rate; RR = respiration rate.

approximately 28% of 14-year-olds had used alcohol at least once in the previous week. This figure rose to 48% for boys and 40% for girls at age 15 (Goddard 2000). In a survey of drug use, smoking and drinking among young teenagers in England in 2001, 54% of boys aged 15 had drunk alcohol in the last week, and 50% of girls of the same age had also drunk alcohol in the last week (National Centre for Social Research 2002).

Most studies concerned with young people and their alcohol use examines the 11 to 16 age group. Young people over the age of 16 years are often neglected from research, despite consumption patterns which have shown 16- to 24-year-olds are the age group most likely to consume more than the recommended weekly limits set by Government (Health Education Board for Scotland 2000). Boys *et al.* (2003), in their study of alcohol use amongst 15- to 17-year-olds in England, found that the normalisation of involvement with alcohol and other drugs appears to occur rapidly between 15 and 17 years. By 17 years, a fairly adult pattern of behaviour was established. This was due to a number of reasons which included easy access to alcohol in public situations, and acceptance (or reduction of conflict) among many parents of the adolescents' drinking behaviour. A substantial group in the study reported high levels of alcohol consumption and intoxication and negative consequences. Regular, heavy consumption of alcohol and binge drinking has been shown to have negative effects on both physical and mental health. This is exacerbated where alcohol is used to avoid or cope with difficult situations and relationships, which can impair psychological and emotional development.

Surveys suggest that there is a growing trend of drinking for effect and of drinking to intoxication. Teenagers aged 15 and 16 years in the United Kingdom have one of the highest rates in the international league of binge-drinking (consuming more than 5 drinks in a row), getting drunk and alcohol related problems (Hibell *et al.* 1997). Between 1995 and 1999 there was an 8% increase in those who binge drink more than three times a month (Hibell *et al.* 2001). Binge

drinking is common amongst adolescents who are still at school and who commonly drink alcohol at the weekend. Alcohol consumption is a common part of adult society in the UK: drinking has thus been recognised by young people as a part of the transition to adulthood; indeed drinking by adolescents often reflects both the attitudes and the practices of adult society, which, unlike drug use, is largely seen as a 'normal' and, for most people, an acceptable part of UK culture. Consequently, the way in which young people's alcohol usage is approached must be carefully considered in order that alcohol education and prevention is accepted, rather than treated by young people as being hypocritical. The WHO European Ministerial Conference on Young People and Alcohol advised 'alcohol policies directed at young people should be part of a broader societal response, since drinking among young people to a large extent reflects the attitudes and practices of wider adult society' (WHO 2001).

Alcohol use is inextricably intertwined with modern social living and is a visible part of everyday life. Most young people have seen adult drinkers before they reach their teenage years. The main difference between adults' social consumption of alcohol and young people's consumption is that young people do not always have sufficient experience or guidance to enable them to accurately evaluate potential risks such as the risks associated with the inappropriate consumption of alcohol (Commission of the European Communities 2000). Alcohol consumption amongst adolescents has been shown to have links with anti-social behaviour such as disorderly conduct, violence (including homicide) and criminal damage. The immediate effects of alcohol can, for some, result in lack of inhibitions, leading to other health consequences such as accidents (including alcohol related road traffic accidents), and unprotected consensual and non-consensual sex, which may in turn lead to unwanted pregnancies and sexually transmitted diseases.

Under-16-year-olds are governed by different laws with respect to alcohol and tobacco use and, as such, assessment of an adolescent under 16 years consuming high quantities of alcohol should trigger concerns for the health or social care worker around the adolescent's well-being. Under the 1989 Children Act (DoH 1989) a child is deemed in need if he or she is unlikely to achieve or maintain a reasonable standard of health or development.

Scenario 2

Ryan is a 14-year-old boy who has been in care since he was 9 years old. His father died of a heroin overdose when he was only 3 years old and his mother has a long history of serious mental illness. He has absconded from his care home on numerous occasions during the last year and has been mixing with older friends who are known drug users. The care staff are aware that Ryan has frequently been binge drinking and suspect that he has been shoplifting to finance his substance use. At 4 a.m. Ryan is brought into the department by the police. He has been picked up wandering the streets in an intoxicated state. He has admitted to the police that he has taken a mixture of drugs and has also consumed large amounts of cheap cider. He is unkempt, fluctuating between sleepiness and confusion. By the time Ryan is admitted he has become increasingly sleepy, has vomited all over the back seat of the police vehicle and appears to be shaky and tremorous.

Immediate management

- The patient should be positioned in prone position and endotracheal airway inserted. Vomiting may occur with the concomitant risk of inhalation.
- Continuous oxygen high flow needs to be administered to prevent fits and compensate for potential respiratory depression.
- Monitor blood oxygen levels.
- Monitor/assess for fits – intoxication with alcohol can cause epileptiform fits – this risk may be compounded by the drugs Ryan has taken.

- Assess hydration as he may need IV fluids – he has vomited at least once and alcohol causes increased diuresis.
- Monitor blood sugar – ingesting large amounts of alcohol depletes stored glycogen – combined with vomiting and dehydration hypoglycaemia can develop very rapidly.
- If Ryan becomes hypoglycaemic he will need glucose/dextrose IV.
- He may require diazepam per rectum or IV or if convulsions develop.
- Ventilation may be needed if respiratory depression is evident or severe hypoxia is evident.
- Regular, frequent base-line observation for least 4 hours but for longer if his condition is not improving significantly.
- Blood toxicology – determine blood ethanol (alcohol) level and to identify what drugs have been taken.
- Tailor the above regime depending on what drugs or other substances are identified by blood toxicology.

Short-term management

Ryan will need to be admitted overnight. Before discharge he should be assessed in accordance with the National Institute for Clinical Excellence (NICE) guidelines (NICE 2004). If there are concerns about Ryan's mental state then referral to Child and Adolescent Mental Health Services (CAMHS) should be arranged as soon as possible. Ryan needs to be educated about the dangers of excess alcohol and the risks of taking drugs and alcohol together. On-going drug/alcohol counselling is indicated if there is evidence that he uses alcohol or drugs on a regular basis. If this presentation is a recurrent one then CAMHS should be arranged even if his mental state appears stable, so that underlying emotional and psychological issues can be addressed.

The presentation of a young person who has consumed excessive amounts of alcohol will vary according to the amount. Table 5.2 below gives an outline of what behaviours can be expected based on the amount consumed, although this will vary according to an individual's alcohol tolerance level.

Table 5.2   The psychological and physical effects of alcohol. Adapted from Victory Over Alcohol Inc. website, *The Business of Alcohol*: http://www.voai.org/business_of_alcohol.htm (accessed 15 June 2005)

Drinking and blood alcohol levels

Number of drinks*	Resulting blood alcohol concentration (%)	Psychological/physical effects
1	0.02–0.03	no overt effects, slight mood elevation
2	0.05–0.06	feeling of relaxation, warmth; slight decrease in reaction time and in fine-muscle coordination
3	0.08–0.09	balance, speech, vision, hearing slightly impaired; feelings of euphoria, increased confidence; loss of motor coordination
	0.10% – Legal intoxication in most states; some have a limit of 0.08%	
4	0.11–0.12	coordination and balance becoming difficult; distinct impairment of mental faculties, judgment
5	0.14–0.15	major impairment of mental and physical control: slurred speech, blurred vision, lack of motor skills
7	0.20	loss of motor control – must have assistance moving about; mental confusion
10	0.30	severe intoxication; minimum conscious control of mind/body
14	0.40	unconsciousness, threshold of coma
17	0.50	deep coma
20	0.60	death from respiratory failure

Figures based on 150 pound male. For each hour elapsed since the last drink, subtract 0.015% blood alcohol concentration, or approximately one drink.

* Number of drinks based on the following equivalences, each containing approximately one half ounce of ethyl alcohol: 12 oz. (300 g) can of beer, 4% alcohol content; 4 oz. (100) glass of wine, 12% alcohol content.

Sexual health and emergency contraception

The UNICEF (2001) report on teenage pregnancy in industrialised countries listed the United Kingdom as having the highest teenage pregnancy rate in Europe and the second highest rate of all industrialised countries in the world after the USA (UNICEF 2001). The reasons for such high levels are complex and have been fully explored in the report by the Social Exclusion Unit (1999).

The amendment of the Prescription Only Medicines (Human Use) Order (DoH 2001a) enabled the purchase 'over the counter' of emergency contraception drugs to those over 16 years of age. The New Medicines Act legislation effective throughout the UK from August 2000 has paved the way for the supply and administration of prescription only medicines by designated health professionals under patient group directions (PGDs). A number of medicines including emergency hormonal contraception (EHC) have been made available under PGDs which has enabled a significant reduction in the waiting time from booking in to the emergency department and receiving treatment. A single hormone treatment levonorgestrel 0.75 mg is an effective method of preventing an unwanted pregnancy after unprotected intercourse or condom accident. This is given in two doses; the first must be given orally within 72 hours of the first act of unprotected intercourse and repeated 12 hours later. The efficacy of this treatment decreases markedly with time (95% of pregnancies prevented if given within the first 24 hours, falling to 58% by 72 hours – overall effectiveness 86%) (Mawhinney & Dornan 2004).

In 1999, a third of 18–19-year-olds had used emergency contraception at least once during the previous two years. By 2001/2002, 21% of 18–19-year-olds had used emergency contraception at least once during the previous year. However, 16–17-year-olds were the least likely to have heard of either hormonal or emergency contraception. In 1999, the use of emergency contraception at least once in the previous two years in this age group was 8% but by 2001/2002 the proportion in this age group that had used it at least once in the previous year had almost tripled (20%) (Graham *et al.* 1996). In addition to high conception rates, at least 10% of sexually active teenagers are estimated to have a sexually transmitted infection and chlamydia rates are increasing fastest among 16–19-year-old women. The *Sexual Health and HIV Strategy* (DoH 2001b) was published in an attempt to reduce these rates.

During out of hours periods the need for emergency contraception is a service which is frequently accessed by young people. Consequently increasing numbers of young girls access accident and emergency departments rather than primary health care facilities for advice on sexual health and particularly emergency contraception (Hogg 1997; Mawhinney & Dornan 2004), as they are seen as convenient and accessible. Moreover, if the young person is below the age of 16 years then they are more likely to attend an emergency department to obtain emergency contraception as over the counter sales usually only apply to those over 16 years. However, the exact extent of the use of emergency contraception amongst teenage girls is difficult to gauge, because specific data are not included in national contraception statistics (Fallon 2003). Lack of knowledge and understanding in respect of the use and effects of emergency contraception among young females could influence decisions about its use especially

if they do not fully understand the importance of timing for emergency contraception (Bullock 1997).

Research has shown that young people's access to emergency contraceptive services can be problematic with barriers apparent. Fallon (2003) reviewed the literature from a feminist perspective and highlights issues of power relationships, triage and law. Concerns around confidentiality and embarrassment have also been noted (Bullock 1997). Hadley (1995) examined attitudes of health care professionals and reported that the type of reception and help received by adolescents seemed to depend on the personality and moral viewpoint of staff members, whose attitudes varied from helpful to disapproving. Nurse (1993) further suggests that judgmental attitude and personal, moral, ethical and religious opinions all influence decisions in relation to the provision of emergency contraception in emergency departments. Mawhinney and Dornan (2004) recommend as a result of their study that a range of appropriate contraceptive services be available at the times of greatest demand (mainly weekends and evenings) if Government targets are to be realised in relation to reducing the high numbers of teenage pregnancies in the UK.

When considering issues in relation to the provision of emergency contraception for young women under the age of 16 years, issues of age, consent and confidentiality have to be considered. The 'best practice guidance' for doctors and other health professionals (DoH 2004) should guide practice. It is essential that these young people are assessed in line with the Fraser Guidelines to ensure that they are managed appropriately. The Fraser Guidelines specifically refer to contraception but the principles also apply to other treatments, including abortion. They refer to doctors but also apply equally to other health professionals in England and Wales. In relation to the issue of under-aged sex, the Sexual Offences Act 2003 does not affect the ability of health professionals and others working with young people to provide confidential advice or treatment on contraception, sexual or reproductive health to young people under 16.

Scenario 3

Ruth is a 15-year-old girl of Jamaican descent who attends an inner city college where she is doing GCSEs. She has had several boyfriends since the age of 13 years and met her current boyfriend, Leon, at college. Leon is two years older than her and is studying sports science. They see each other regularly and have developed an intimate sexual relationship over the last few months. Ruth and Leon have spent a lot of time with each other at weekends when Leon's parents are away socialising. Ruth was very worried that she might have been pregnant a month ago when they had unprotected intercourse but was relieved when her period arrived on time. Last night Ruth again had unprotected intercourse with Leon and is now very worried about becoming pregnant. She presents at the department alone late in the evening to request emergency contraception.

Immediate management

- Check whether Ruth is alone or accompanied by parents.
- Establish age and ability to consent to treatment (Fraser Guidelines).
- Clarify date and time of unprotected sexual intercourse.
- Establish whether any previous pregnancies.
- Assess risk of sexually transmitted infection.
- Establish whether the sexual intercourse was consensual.
- Dispense emergency contraceptive medication with full instructions on administration.

Short-term management

Ruth should receive information and instructions on the use of emergency contraception drugs. If Ruth is considered at risk of sexually transmitted infection she should be referred to the genito-urinary clinic and the local drop in centre where young people can get confidential advice on matters of sexual health. Advice on contraception should also be given. At all times Ruth should be assured of confidential treatment and management relevant to her cognitive ability in line with the best practice guidance (DoH 2004).

Young people who self harm

Attendance at emergency departments of young people who self-harm should not be confused with those who use substances for pleasure and entertainment. Deliberate self-harm (DSH) is also referred to as parasuicide, attempted suicide, suicidal behaviour or self-injurious behaviour, and is now recognised as a serious public health issue, with an increasing number of young people engaging in self-harming behaviours (Hawton *et al.* 2003). This is of significance, not least because an initial act of DSH renders the young person at an increased risk of subsequent self-harm which in turn increases their risk of suicide (Hickey *et al.* 2001). Suicidal behaviour has markedly increased over the last ten years and is reported to be among the highest in Europe especially in young males between the ages of 15 and 19 years (NICE 2002). Deliberate self-harm, especially in young females between the ages of 15 and 19 years, has also significantly increased in the UK. It is estimated that 1 in 10 teenagers self harm (Samaritans & Centre for Suicide 2002), although caution should be exercised in relation to these statistics as reported figures are not based on agreed definitions; further, the majority of young people who self harm do not seek medical advice or attend for hospital care (Hawton *et al.* 2002), but an estimated 25 000 young people are referred annually to general hospital services in England and Wales particularly with self-poisoning, frequently paracetamol overdose, or cutting themselves (Hawton *et al.* 2002).

Child Line, one of the UK's leading charities providing 24-hour telephone support for any child or young person with a problem, reported that they counselled around 120 000 children and young people during 2002–3. For 1122 (1%), concern about deliberate self-harming was the main reason for making the call. A further 2% (2223: 1998 girls, 225 boys) disclosed self-harm to the counsellor, though this was not the reason why they had called Child Line. In total 3345 (3032 girls, 313 boys) children and young people talked to Child Line in 2003 about self-harming. These statistics do not include children who had called Child Line about a friend they were concerned about.

Guidelines produced by the Royal College of Psychiatrists in respect of the management of young people who deliberately self harm have been available for at least 20 years and although they have recently been updated (Royal College of Psychiatrists 1998) are largely unchanged. However a study by Nadkarni *et al.* (2003), which considered young people up to the age of 17 years who presented over a one-year period with a (discharge) diagnosis of deliberate self-harm, found a disparity between recommendations and practice. Although it was acknowledged that only a small proportion of young people actually presented at the department with this diagnosis, one of the main concerns raised in this study was the lapse in the assessment process. Although 90% of the young people were physically examined and questioned about their social situation and the reason for self-harming, only about half of the young people were questioned about previous episodes of self-harm. This is of concern as several studies have shown that around 10–15% of children who self harm are likely to repeat within the following year (Hawton *et al.* 1996; Spirito *et al.* 1992). Moreover, previous episodes of self-harm along with affective disorder and hopelessness, is one of the primary risk factors associated with future self-harm (Stoelb & Chiriboga 1998). This, together with the fact that a person who has harmed themselves is at a hundred times greater risk of suicide than that of any other general population (NHS Centre for Reviews and Dissemination 1998), is a strong indicator of the need for referral to CAMHS. Contrary to the guidelines of the Royal College of Psychiatrists (1998), only one-third of the young people in Nadkarni *et al.*'s (2003) study were admitted to a suitable ward; one-third were seen by the CAMHS staff in the department prior to discharge, but a similar proportion were discharged without any input from the mental health services.

A study by Anderson *et al.* (2000) which examined nurses' and doctors' attitudes towards suicidal behaviour in young people found that nurses and doctors agreed that suicidal behaviour often represents a 'cry for help', but do not generally support the notion that suicidal behaviour reflects mental illness. This contrasts with previous studies which showed that physicians thought that suicide (in general) and mental illness were related (Domino & Perrone 1993). In a previous study by Platt and Salter (1987) it was found that nurses were more likely than psychiatrists to see suicidal behaviour as 'attention-seeking' behaviour. The term 'attention-seeking' is derogatory and earlier studies have suggested that seeing suicidal behaviour as 'attention-seeking' can lead to a less sympathetic approach among non-psychiatric professionals and can influence professionals' interaction with the suicidal patient (Hawton *et al.* 1981; Ramon *et al.* 1975). However a more recent study found more positive attitudes among nurses, with the most significant factor being length of experience (Anderson 1997), which also demonstrated more positive attitudes towards suicidal behaviour, a finding which mirrored that of McLaughlin (1994).

More recently the National Institute for Clinical Excellence (NICE 2004) have produced guidelines and made recommendations for the physical, psychological and social assessment and treatment of people in primary and secondary care in the first 48 hours after having self harmed. In relation to children and young people under the age of 16 years special recommendations are made that include overall assessment and management of care being undertaken by appropriately trained doctors and nurses, particularly in respect of mental health issues, and the need for full and detailed assessment being made prior to discharge. Issues in relation to age, developmental stage and consent, particularly Gillick competence, are addressed along with the importance of parental consent, child protection, the use of the Mental Health Act in young people and the Children Act (1989). The importance of liaison with the Child and Adolescent Mental Health Team for them to undertake appropriate assessment of the child and family and also liaison between social service and education staff if appropriate is recommended. In particular the involvement of child and adolescent mental health service practitioners in the assessment and treatment of children and young people who have self harmed is recommended who should:

- be trained specifically to work with children and young people, and their families, after self-harm
- be skilled in the assessment of risk
- have regular supervision
- have access to consultation with senior colleagues.

Scenario 4

Amanda is a 15-year-old girl and is currently studying for GCSEs in an inner city area. She is the eldest of three children and her parents are very eager for her to do well at school. Her mother is a successful business woman and her father is the headmaster of a local school. Her parents' wish is that she will go on to study Law and they are therefore eager for her to do well at her exams and have organised for her to have some private tuition. Amanda is a naturally gregarious person with lots of friends who are allowed to socialise more than her. Over the last few months Amanda has not been allowed to go out at weekends and evenings – the only outing she has at the weekends is to visit her private tutor. She is currently feeling very stressed and pressurised and has had several tearful episodes lately, but has been unable to express how she really feels to her parents as she is worried that she will not live up to their expectations. On a number of occasions she has cut her arms superficially but has managed to conceal these marks. However on this occasion she has become panicky as the bleeding seems quite severe. She used a ring-pull from a can of soft drink to cut herself and the wound is 'messy'. Her parents find her in tears in the bathroom attempting to stop her wrist from bleeding and take her immediately to the emergency department.

Immediate management in the emergency department

- Triage.
- Assess wound.
- Assess mental state.

- Ascertain whether this has happened before – have there been previous attendances for self-harm.
- Determine if there is a history of 'abuse' or other psychosocial problems.
- Assess blood loss.
- Clean.
- Suture or other closure.
- Antibiotics.
- Tetanus.
- Liaison with CAMH services.

Short-term management

- Admit overnight – parents may stay.
- Reassess next day – risk assessment of mental and physical health.
- Referral – on-going support from appropriate service – contact school and school nurse as this could be related to examination anxiety.

Notes on adolescents who self harm

People who deliberately harm themselves should always be taken seriously. Deliberate self-harm indicates that a child or young person may have an acute or chronic psychiatric disorder or have significant psychological problems. The young person may be experiencing depression, anger, anxiety or hopelessness, which they are unable to manage. Young people who have suffered a traumatic experience such as sexual abuse may experience guilt or shame which may become unbearable. Alternatively, they may try to convince themselves that the event or series of events never happened and so become more and more detached. For these people, self-injury is a way of dealing with their overwhelming feelings.

The appropriate procedure is thus to assess the predicament that the young persons find themselves in. Three factors are involved: the life stresses they are under; any internal distress they have arising from the experiences mentioned above; whether their emotionally supportive relationships are adequate. Treatment involves addressing any identified problems in these three areas. Some form of counselling may be required. This could be carried out by a mental health professional. Repetitive self-harm can have an addictive quality and, if it occurs often, a specific behavioural programme may be required which addresses the actions around self-harm and finds ways for the individual to directly express the concurrent feelings as an alternative.

Conclusion

In reviewing the services for young people who attend emergency departments in the UK it is clear that much work needs to be done in order to address the shortfall in provision of specific adolescent health care services. Difficulties in accessing the services and barriers experienced by young people have been highlighted as well as good practice in many areas. However it is important that practitioners acknowledge and appreciate the special and differing needs of this client group and strive to provide appropriate and desired services. It is anticipated that the successful implementation of the *National Service Framework for Children, Young People and Maternity Services* (DoH 2004a) will begin to address some of the major issues, particularly in relation to privacy, confidentiality, dignity and consent. In the interim period it is important that when dealing with adolescents in the emergency setting, procedures and guidelines are implemented to ensure that adolescents' health care needs are addressed in a manner specifically designed for them and are not a compromise between paediatric and adult services.

References

Anderson, M., Standen, P., Nazir, S. & Noon, J.P. (2000) Nurses and doctors attitudes towards suicidal behaviour in young people. *International Journal of Nursing Studies*, **37**, 1–11.

Anderson, M.P. (1997) Nurses' attitudes towards suicidal behaviour: a comparative study of community mental health nurses and nurses working in an accidents and emergency department. *Journal of Advanced Nursing*, **25**, 1283–1291.

Ashley, M.J. (2000) Balancing the risks and benefits of moderate drinking. In: *The Globe, Special Edition, Towards a Global Alcohol Policy*.

Bobst, M. & Habraken, P. (1997) *Substance Abuse, Clinical Nursing Series*. Western School Press, South Easton, MA.

Boys, A., John, M., Stillwell, G., Hutchings, K., Griffiths, P. & Farrell, M. (Alcohol and National Addiction Centre) (2003) *Teenage Drinkers: a follow-up study of alcohol use among 15–17-year-olds in England. Summary of main results*. Alcohol Concern, London.

Bullock, J. (1997) Raising awareness of emergency contraception. *Community Nurse*, **3**(7), 28–29.

Commission of The European Communities Brussels (2000) D/106330.

Commission for Health Improvement (2002) *Sheffield Children's NHS Trust and NHS Direct South Yorkshire and South Humber Report*.

Department of Health (1989) *An Introduction to The Children Act 1989*. HMSO, London.

Department of Health (2001a) *The Prescription Only Medicines (Human Use) Regulations*. HMSO, London.

Department of Health (2001b) *Sexual Health and HIV Strategy*. HMSO, London.

Department of Health (2004a) *National Service Framework for Children, Young People and Maternity Services*. The Stationery Office.

Department of Health (2004b) *Best practice guidance for doctors and other health professionals on the provision of advice and treatment to young people under 16 on contraception, sexual and reproductive health*. Gateway reference number 3382.

Dixon, P. (1998) *The Truth About Drugs*. Hodder & Stoughton, London.

Domino, G. & Perrone, L. (1993) Attitudes toward suicide: Italian and United States physicians. *Omega*, **27**(3), 195–206.

Elkind, D. (1967) Egocentrism in adolescence. *Child Development*, **38**(4), 1025–1034.

Fallon, D. (2003) Adolescent access to emergency contraception in accident & emergency departments: reviewing the literature from a feminist perspective. *Journal of Clinical Nursing*, **12**(1), 4–11.

Ghuran, A., Van der Wieken, L.R. & Nolan, J. (2001) Cardiovascular complications of recreational drugs. *British Medical Journal*, **323**, 464–466.

Goddard, E. (2000) *Drug Use, Smoking and Drinking Among Young Teenagers in 1999*, Report No. 189. Office for National Statistics, London.

Graham, A., Green, L. & Glasier, A.F. (1996) Teenagers' knowledge of emergency contraception: questionnaire survey in south-east Scotland. *British Medical Journal*, **312**, 1567–1569.

Hadley, A. (1995) Picking up the pieces. *Paediatric Nursing*, **10**(3), 169–174.

Hawton, K., Marsack, P. & Fagg, J. (1981) The attitudes of psychiatrists to deliberate self-poisoning:

comparison with physicians and nurses. *British Journal of Medical Psychology*, **54**, 341–348.

Hawton, K., Fagg, J. & Simkin, S. (1996) Deliberate self-poisoning and self-injury in children and adolescents under 16 years of age in Oxford, 1976–1993. *British Journal of Psychiatry*, **169**, 202–208.

Hawton, K., Rodham, K., Evans, E. & Weatherall, R. (2002) Deliberate self harm in adolescents: self report survey in schools in England. *British Medical Journal*, **325**, 1207–1211.

Hawton, K., Hall, S., Simkin, S. *et al.* (2003) Deliberate self-harm in adolescents: a study of characteristics and trends in Oxford, 1990–2000. *Journal of Child Psychology and Psychiatry*, **44**(8), 1191–1198.

Health Education Board for Scotland (2000) *Indicators for Health Education in Scotland. Summary of findings from the 1998 health education population survey.* Health Education Board for Scotland, Edinburgh.

Hibell, B., Andersson, B., Bjarnason, T., Kokkevi, A., Morgan, M. & Narusk, A. (1997) *The 1995 ESPAD Report: Alcohol and other Drug Use among Students in 26 European Countries.* Swedish Council for Information on Alcohol and other Drugs, Stockholm.

Hibell, B., Andersson, B., Ahlström, S., Balakireva, O., Bjarnasson, T., Kokkevi, A. & Morgan, M. (2001) *The ESPAD 1999 Report: Alcohol and Other Drug Use Among Students in 30 European Countries.* Swedish Council for Information on Alcohol and other Drugs, Stockholm.

Hickey, L., Hawton, K., Fagg, J. & Weitzel, H. (2001) Deliberate self-harm patients who leave the accident and emergency department without a psychiatric assessment: a neglected population at risk of suicide. *Journal of Psychosomatic Research*, **50**(2), 87–93.

Hogg, C. (1997) *Emergency health services for children and young people.* Action for Sick Children, London.

Kalant, H. (2001) The pharmacology and toxicology of 'ecstasy' (MDMA) and related drugs. *Canadian Medical Association Journal*, **165**(7), 917–928.

Kerins, M., Dargan, P.I. & Jones, A.L. (2003) Pitfalls in the management of the poisoned patient. *Journal Royal College of Physicians*, **33**, 90–110.

MacFoul, R. & Werneke, U. (2001) Recent trends in hospital use by children in England. *Archives of Disease in Children*, **85**, 203–207.

Masterson, A., Antrobus, S. & Smith, F. (2004) The Children's National Service Framework: from policy to practice. *Nursing Management*, **11**(6), 12–15.

Mawhinney, S. & Dornan, O. (2004) Requests for emergency contraception at an accident and emergency department – assessing the impact of a change in legislation. *Ulster Medical Journal*, **73**(1), 16–19.

McLaughlin, C. (1994) Casualty nurses' attitudes to attempted suicide. *Journal of Advanced Nursing*, **20**, 1111–1118.

Miller, P. & Plant, M. (1996) Drinking, smoking and illicit drug use among 15–16-year-olds in the United Kingdom. *British Medical Journal*, **313**, 394–397.

Nadkarni, A., Parkin, A., Dogra, N. & Evans, P.A. (2003) Management in Accident and Emergency (EMERGENCY) of Children and Adolescents Presenting with Deliberate Self-Harm (DSH). *Clinical Child Psychology & Psychiatry*, **8**(4), 513–520.

National Centre for Social Research and the National Foundation for Educational Research (2002) *Drug use, smoking and drinking among young people in England in 2001: preliminary results.* DoH, London.

National Institute for Clinical Excellence (NICE) (2002) *Self Harm Scope Document.* NICE, London.

National Institute for Clinical Excellence (NICE) (2004) *The short-term physical and psychological management and secondary prevention of self-harm in primary and secondary care.* Clinical Guideline 16. NHS. NICE, London.

NHS Centre for Reviews and Dissemination (1998) *Effective Health Care: Deliberate Self Harm.* University of York, York.

Nurse, N. (1993) Should we be turning them away? *Accident and Emergency Nursing*, **1**, 111–112.

Office for National Statistics (ONS) (2000) *Social Inequalities.* The Stationery Office, London.

Paton, J. & Jenkins, R. (eds) (2003) *Mental Health Primary Care in Prison.* Produced for HM Prison Service by the WHO Collaborating Centre, London.

Platt, S. & Salter, D. (1987) A comparison of health workers attitudes towards parasuicide. *Social Psychiatry*, **22**, 202–208.

Ramon, S., Bancroft, J. & Skrimshire, A.M. (1975) Attitudes towards self-poisoning among physicians and nurses in a General Hospital. *British Journal of Psychiatry*, **127**, 257–264.

Royal College of Paediatrics and Child Health (RCPCH) (1999) *Accident and emergency services for children: a report of a multidisciplinary working party.* RCPCH, London.

Royal College of Paediatrics and Child Health (RCPCH) (2003) *Bridging the Gaps – Health Care for Adolescents* (Council Report 114). RCPCH, London.

Royal College of Psychiatrists (1998) *Managing deliberate self-harm in young people* (Council Report CR64). RCP, London.

Rutter, M. (1980) *Changing youth in a changing society.* Harvard University Press, Cambridge, Mass.

Samaritans & Centre for Suicide (2002) *Youth and Self-Harm: Perspectives.* University of Oxford, Oxford.

Social Exclusion Unit (SEU) (1999) *The Teenage Pregnancy Strategy*. Cabinet Office, London.

Spirito, A., Plummer B., Gisbert, M., Levy, S., Kurkjian, J., Lewander, W., Hagbert, S. & Devost, L. (1992) Adolescent suicide attempts; Outcomes at follow-up. *American Journal of Orthopsychiatry*, **62**, 464–468.

Stoelb, M. & Chiriboga, J. (1998) A process model for assessing adolescent risk for suicide. *Journal of Adolescence*, **21**, 359–370.

World Health Organization (2001) *Declaration on Young People and Alcohol*. Available at http://www.youngalcohol.who.dk/PDFdoc?declarationE.pdf.

UNICEF (2001) A league table of teenage births in rich nations. *Innocenti Report Card*, 3 July, 43.

Vartanian, L.R. (2000) Revisiting the imaginary audience and personal fable constructs of adolescent egocentrism: A conceptual review. *Adolescence*, **35**, 639–661.

Viner, R. (2003) Adolescent medicine. In: *Forfar and Arneil's Textbook of Pediatrics*, 6th edn. N. McIntosh, P.J. Helms & R.L. Smyth (eds). Churchill Livingstone, Edinburgh.

Chapter 6 Treatment and Management of Minor Injuries

Lesley Wayne and Louise Bunn

Introduction

It is difficult to define what constitutes a 'minor injury'. The Department of Health (DoH 2003) defines a minor injury as one unlikely to require hospital admission. It is important to understand that the child's perception of their injury (and sometimes their family's perception) may differ greatly from that of practitioners. This may be illustrated by the child who complains of pain or injury from a relatively insignificant event, or one who frequently attends with parents requesting 'checks' for every minor scrape and bump. The important issue is never to be complacent about a child's attendance until a full assessment of their usual abilities as well as an assessment of the injury itself has been undertaken; only then can it be determined if the injury is minor.

With this in mind, this chapter will outline the main issues for assessment, management and treatment of minor injuries including minor head injuries, wounds, burns and scalds, foreign bodies, bites and stings, bruising and haematomas, and minor fractures, strains and sprains. Scenarios within the chapter illustrate actual clinical situations and their outcomes. They are examples arising from practice within a minor injury unit (MIU). Examples of patient group directives (PGDs) for the management of specific minor injuries are also given. These though of necessity vary from unit to unit (Cook *et al.* 2000; DoH 2003; NHS Executive 2000), so it is recommended that you familiarise yourself with those used in your own department.

The principles of assessing children with minor injuries

Assessment of the severity of the child's injury and the need for treatment is vital. However, as identified in Chapter 2, this needs doing simultaneously with an assessment of the child's developmental age and cognitive skills. The practitioner's skills in assessing these and in achieving a good relationship with the child and their family are essential to the assessment of the injury. Having established a rapport, you are subsequently able to proceed with your examination of the injury itself using strategies identified in Chapter 2. Remember that it is not only important to assess the presenting injury and its history but to document:

- The social context of the child, names of the person accompanying the child, who has parental responsibility, including details of whether they are present, need to be contacted and/or are aware that the child is attending the emergency department
- assessment of the child's pain using an appropriate pain assessment tool (please refer to Chapter 7)
- details of any medication, including analgesia already administered by parents
- known allergies.

Assessment and triage enables opportunity to check on immunisations, developmental progress and the feeding and sleeping patterns of the child. Whilst not always directly related to the minor injury itself, there may be implications for the overall welfare of the child. Additionally the ordered documentation of an injury assists the triage nurse in recognising injuries that are not consistent with the presenting history alerting child protection concerns, then managed in accordance with local and national policies, as discussed in Chapter 4 (HM Government 2006).

Alert: Assessing minor injuries in children can be challenging. There are many possible reasons why children may not cooperate with a physical examination/assessment as an adult would. These might include:

- Pain (see Chapter 7)
- Fear
- Shyness
- Lack of understanding due to age of development.

However, thorough assessment and adequate pain relief facilitates effective management of minor childhood injuries (Young *et al.* 2005).

Knowledge of anatomy is also essential in the assessment and management of injuries (see for example Field 1997; Tortora & Grabowski 2003; Waugh & Grant 2003). Treatments and local guidelines require regular review and should reflect national and local standards, policies and guidelines. The use of protocols and or PGDs is not a legal requirement, but strongly recommended as they provide a local tool for evidence-based information. The DoH (2003) also advocates the use of nationally agreed protocols dictating the recommended treatment and care. In our experience, PGDs aid the practitioner in assessing injuries. They should, however, be

- Evidence based (on nationally agreed protocols if available)
- Ratified and their use authorised by your employer
- Condition/patient specific, outlining treatment and referral
- Regularly revised, signed and dated.

Staff working in independent units, for example minor injury units, should work to the same guidelines as the parent department, using where possible the same documentation (Cook *et al.* 2000).

Specific injuries

Minor head injuries

The management of head injuries is complex, particularly when attempting to identify those that are 'minor'. NICE (2003) define a head injury as 'any trauma to the head other than superfi-

cial injuries to the face'. Primarily the modified Glasgow Coma Scale (NICE 2003) should guide the assessment and classification of children who have sustained a head injury.

However, where a rapid initial assessment of a child's conscious level is required, the AVPU method can be used (Resuscitation Council UK 2005):

A – **A**lert
V – Responds to **v**ocal stimuli
P – Responds only to **p**ainful stimuli
U – **U**nresponsive to all stimuli

Patients who score **P** or **U** have a Glasgow Coma Score (GCS) of 8 or less.

We would recommend that PGDs for the management of minor head injuries are based on the guidance provided by NICE (2003), who define infants as one year and under, and a child as 1–15 years of age. In certain circumstances, children aged 10 years or more can be treated as adults for the purposes of cervical spine imaging, but under the age of 10, there are increased risks associated with irradiation and a lower risk of significant spinal injury (NICE 2003). Our patient group directive also uses the evidence base of Young and South (2003), Resuscitation Council UK (2005), Currie (2000) and Glasgow and McGovern (2000).

Example patient group directive for the management of minor head injuries within a minor injuries unit

Assessment

- Determine whether the child has a treatable minor head injury or a more significant one potentially requiring referral. NICE (2003) guidelines recommend that all children presenting with a head injury are triaged by a trained member of staff within a maximum of 15 minutes of arrival. This assessment should establish whether they are high risk or low risk for clinically important brain injury and/or cervical spine injury using the guidance on patient selection and urgency for imaging (head and cervical spine). A suitably qualified practitioner should assess children identified as high risk within 10 minutes, and low risk children should be assessed within a further hour.

- Inform the child and parent of the role of the nurse practitioner and other professionals; obtain consent for treatment.
- Assess and document:
  — mechanism of injury to include assessment of c-spine
  — history of drug/alcohol intake
  — time of injury
  — relevant past medical history
  — loss of consciousness (LOC), amnesia, drowsiness
  — GCS, baseline observations including temperature, pulse, respiration, blood pressure, pupil size and reaction to light
  — motor function
  — visual disturbances
  — nausea/vomiting
  — headache/dizziness
  — size and position of any wound/presence of haematoma
  — palpate skull for presence of step/depression or bony tenderness
  — check ears and nose for blood/cerebrospinal fluid.

Alert: The most important sign is an alteration in the child's level of consciousness.

Exclusions
The presence of any of the following may indicate a more severe head injury:

- Mechanism of injury, including high velocity impact, i.e. a fall from a significant height. A risk fall is greater than one metre although a lower threshold should be used in infants and child under 5 years
- Loss of consciousness (LOC)
- Period of pre- or post-injury amnesia. **Alert**: Assessment of amnesia will not be possible in preverbal children and is unlikely to be possible in any child aged less than 5 years
- Severe headache

- Persistent vomiting. **Alert**: While vomiting is a high-risk variable, there remains some controversy regarding the number of episodes required to qualify as high risk (NICE 2003). This particularly applies to infants and children who have a tendency to vomiting, therefore limiting its predictive power. Sixteen per cent of infants and children aged 12 years or less vomit after a minor head injury with the cause of vomiting related to individual intrinsic factors such as a previous tendency to vomit rather than specific features of the head injury. Vomiting is, though, recognised as a sensitive, though not very specific, indicator of fracture risk in alert children after head injury and treatment therefore needs to be within the context of other aspects of assessment. However, to ignore this symptom risks overlooking a fracture of the skull vault, which substantially increases the risk of intracranial complications (Nee 2001). Thus, use clinical judgement regarding the cause of vomiting in children aged 12 years or less. This judgement should guide whether imaging is necessary (Barnard & Carley 2000; NICE 2003).
- Glasgow Coma Score (GCS) <13; <15 at any time since the injury; or equal to 13 or 14 at 2 hours after the injury. **Alert**: NICE (2003) highlight that a GCS of less than 13 was a significant predictor of an abnormal CT scan in children with head injury aged 14 years or younger. However, they also note that the prevalence of intracranial complications in infants and children is less than that in adults.
- Visual disturbance (blurred/double vision)
- Previously undiagnosed nystagmus
- Unequal pupils (remember to ask parent if pupils are normally unequal)
- History of fitting
- Abnormal neurological signs including: abnormal gait or balance, slurred or slow speech, limb weakness, drowsiness, floppiness, irritable cry, confused or inappropriate behaviour
- Abnormal baseline observations
- Pertinent medical conditions, e.g. haemophilia

- Lack of a responsible adult available to supervise the child on discharge
- **Alert**: Remember to consider other social factors in relation to safeguarding children (Humphries & Gully 2000)
- Inability to assess the child, e.g. special needs children, alcohol/drug intoxication.

Clinical signs suggestive of a skull fracture are:

- Soft and spongy scalp with localised swelling
- Depressed or open skull injury/severe wounds, e.g. wounds exposing a large expanse of periosteum or wounds bleeding excessively. Any visible trauma to the scalp or skull is of concern to the practitioner
- Blood or cerebrospinal fluid leaking from the ears and/or nose
- Battles sign (bruising in the mastoid area)
- Periorbital haematoma/raccoon eyes (bilateral periorbital bruising)
- Black eye with no associated damage around the eyes
- New deafness in one or more ear
- Any penetrating injury signs
- Children presenting with suspected c-spine injury (Glasgow & McGovern 2000; NICE 2003).

Alert: Head injury assessment/examination is an important opportunity to identify non-accidental injury. There is evidence of a distinct pattern of brain injuries associated with non-accidental head injury in children resulting from the different mechanisms of injury as opposed to those in accidental head injury. Non-accidental injuries are more likely to involve inertial forces such as shaking whereas injuries of an accidental nature are more likely to involve blunt trauma (NICE 2003).

It is recognised that the risk of abuse is highest in infancy reducing with increasing age (Sidebotham 2003). Infants under 12 months of age are more at risk of severe physical abuse. 'Shaken baby syndrome' is a condition referring to a young child who has been shaken violently resulting in subdural haemorrhage, which often coexists with retinal haemorrhages and little evidence of skull fractures (Sanders *et al.* 2003). These children commonly have associated extracranial injuries typical of physical child abuse (Jayawant *et al.* 1998). However, some children with subdural haemorrhages may present with relatively minor or non-specific symptoms (Sanders *et al.* 2003). Jayawant *et al.* (1998) argue certain clinical investigations should be mandatory in the assessment of all children under 2 years of age with subdural haemorrhage in order to minimise the number of abused children who might go undetected.

Where concerns about non-accidental injury exist, the clinical investigations advocated by NICE (2003) include:

- Skull x-rays as a part of a series of plain x-rays (skeletal survey)
- Other well-established examinations – e.g. opthalmoscopic examination for retinal haemorrhage; examination for pallor, anaemia, tense fontanelle
- Investigations such as CT and or MRI scans.

Management of a minor head injury

It is recommended that the management of a minor head injury is based on the NICE (2003) guidelines, who advise that National Health Service (NHS) minor injury clinics or community settings should refer patients who have sustained a head injury to a hospital emergency department if any of the exclusions identified above are present. Otherwise, the treatment of minor head injuries in the community, minor injury unit (MIU) or emergency department is as follows:

- Treat wounds in accordance with wound care policy – remembering to check tetanus status in relation to the child's age (Elliman & Bedford 2004) and against latest DoH guidelines regarding children's immunisation schedule. These are available online at: www.immunisation.nhs.uk.
- Give written and verbal head injury advice (NICE 2003). The NICE guidelines include discharge advice, which can be downloaded from the NICE website (www.nice.org. ukpdfheadinj) and adapted to suit local needs.

Box 6.1   Scenario utilising an example of a patient group directive for minor head injuries

Patient – A young mother presents at MIU with 9-month-old baby Jack.

Presenting complaint/history of presenting complaint – She is concerned, as when feeding Jack that morning she noticed that he had a significant swelling to the right side of his head. She has no explanation for this, despite protracted questioning.

Past medical history – There is no past medical history or history of congenital abnormalities to account for the swelling. Jack was born at full term, normal delivery, with normal development.

Medication/allergies – None.

Immunisations – Mum refused the MMR triple vaccine, opting to pay for individual vaccines. Jack had his mumps vaccine 5 days ago with no ill effect at all.

On examination – Jack was very happy, contented, looking around, verbalising normally and interacting with mother and staff. Mother was very attentive, caring, yet anxious. All baseline observations were normal: T 36.8°C tympanic, P 107, BP 80/50. There was no reported loss of consciousness, no vomiting, no abnormal drowsiness and no loss of motor function. It was, however, noted that he had a large swelling over the right parietal area, approximately 6 cm in diameter. On palpation, the swelling felt soft, spongy and fluctuant. There was no bony tenderness or indication of any other injuries to torso or limbs.

Diagnosis – A provisional diagnosis could not differentiate between the possibility of an underlying medical condition or a significant head injury with an underlying fracture (although this did not seem possible from the history given, despite the presence of significant scalp swelling).

Treatment/referral – A referral to the paediatrician for review and assessment with immediate transfer to the paediatric ward by ambulance was arranged. A routine referral to the Health Visitor Liaison Service was also completed.

Alert: Jack, admitted for observation, was subsequently found (some 24 hours later) to have sustained a skull fracture. His parents later recalled that he had pulled a stair gate onto himself two days prior to attendance. However, there is concern that the parents could not explain how the injury happened during the initial assessment and there was delay in seeking treatment. It is also likely that there would have been cuts/scratches around the injury site had he pulled the stair gate onto himself, as described by his parents. Conversely, Hobbs (1997) argues that if an infant presents with a cranial swelling a day or two after a minor head injury and has a hairline parietal single linear fracture, the cause is usually innocent. Therefore, a multidisciplinary assessment is required in accordance with national guidelines (HM Government 2006).

Wound management in the emergency department

Of the 2.3 million children attending emergency departments each year in the UK over 60% attend as a result of injuries including cuts/lacerations (which may be incised, puncture, penetrating or crush injury wounds), bites, stings and burns (Casey 1999). This section examines the assessment and initial management of some of the acute minor wounds and burns commonly seen in children. It is concerned with emergency/initial wound care and does not include advanced wound care such as delayed or secondary closure and tendon repair. It is, however, essential that you are familiar with the normal anatomy of the skin as wound healing itself is a complex sequence of cellular and molecular processes. Normal wound healing occurs in three stages: inflammation, proliferation, maturation, which can take two weeks or months depending on the wound's size, depth, position and general health of the child (Cole 2003). An informative source, which explores wound healing in depth, is Gould (2001).

Whilst treatment is usually straightforward, a thorough assessment of the wound or burn is vital to prevent short-term and long-term complications for the child (Cole 2003). Management depends on a number of factors:

- Mechanism and time of the injury
- Size and depth
- Site of the wound.

Additionally wounds caused by non-sterile agents increase the risk of infection.

Some general principles of wound assessment

Assessment should include the elements identified below (as evidenced by Cole 2003; Miller 1995; Miller & Collier 1996; O'Sullivan 2000; Rubin 1998; Small 2000) and in accordance with local wound care policy (Butcher & Reid 1997). Before initiating treatment to an emergency wound specific questions need to be asked to ensure an accurate wound assessment, the outcome of which is legibly documented in the child's record (Cole 2003).

- What
  — type of wound is it?
  — was the mechanism of the injury?
  — is the history?

Alert: If the history is not consistent with the type of wound – consider non-accidental injury.

- When
  — did it happen?

Alert: The time elapsed since injury is important as Moulton and Yates (1999) identify that wounds older than six hours are more prone to infection.

- Where
  — is the site of injury on the body? Is there an increased risk of infection because of the place where the wound has occurred? Could there be underlying damage? **Be aware of** unusual mechanisms, e.g. penetrating joint injuries. Is it the child's dominant hand?
- How
  — does it look? – Is it oozing blood suggesting a venous blood vessel or spurting blood suggesting an arterial bleed that needs to have pressure applied, elevation and expert help?
  — deep is the wound? Do the distal neurovascular and tendon functions need assessing? Could a foreign body be present? The presence of glass or metal suggests the need for an x-ray to locate or exclude this before dressing or closure.
  — wide is the wound?
  — does it feel to the child?

Alert: It is worth considering the use of a diagram with measurements documenting the length, depth and breadth of the wound; and wound grids and photographs to aid documentation. Clearly, document associated bruising, swelling, erythema and circulatory deficit, i.e. heat, tracking or pus may be indicative of infection. Also, wounds and burns can be very painful. Does the child need analgesia? Local anaesthetic/analgesia may be required to aid assessment.

Assessment should also include:

- Past medical and medication history to determine if there is anything that may affect wound healing such as immunosuppression
- Known allergies – which may be to drugs or dressings/dressing tapes such as elastoplast
- Tetanus and immunisation status
- Baseline set of observations of temperature, pulse and respiration
- Tissue viability, e.g. presence of slough, contaminants, contused wound margins and infection all affect healing and subsequent management.

Alert: Remember to exclude involvement of underlying structures, e.g. tendons, nerves, joints and fractures. X-ray suspected penetrating joint injuries as well as suspected fractures and remove rings or other items of jewellery if worn from the affected area.

Tetanus

The anaerobic bacterium *Clostridium tetani* found in soil and in human and animal excrement causes tetanus. Spores are introduced into the body through puncture wounds, burns or trivial unnoticed wounds. Immunisation programmes generally control the effects of tetanus in the UK, but if acquired the disease can prove fatal (Cassell 2002). The bacterial infection produces a toxin, which circulates in the body to cause severe and painful muscular contractions, and spasms, which can lead to death through respiratory problems and exhaustion. The incubation period is 4–21 days, commonly about 10 days.

Obvious contamination of wounds does not need to be evident for tetanus to develop in unvaccinated children or those with waning immunity. Even minor wounds can prove fatal (Thwaites and Farrar 2003).

The DoH (2002) lists tetanus prone wounds as:

- Any wound sustained more than 6 hours ago
- Any wound or burn at any interval after the injury that shows one or more of the following characteristics
  — a significant degree of devitalised tissue
  — puncture type wounds
- Any wound that had contact with soil or manure likely to harbour tetanus organisms
- Wounds with clinical evidence of sepsis.

Wound cleansing – some general principles

It is worth noting that the cleansing of wounds has been the subject of topical debate (Cole 2003), but most authors agree that emergency wounds are initially treated as contaminated therefore needing thorough cleansing. Additionally there is consensus that wounds need irrigating rather than swabbing or wiping clean. Notably avoid wiping with cotton wool and gauze swabs as fibres from the cotton wool can shed into the wound and gauze swabs can redistribute bacteria around the wound causing tissue damage (Gould 1999). Irrigation removes debris, reducing risk of infection. Both normal saline and 'drinking quality' tap water are the optimum agents therapeutically (Dealey 1999; Holt 2000; Riyat & Quniton 1997; Wardrope & Smith 1992). Antiseptic agents are not recommended for initial cleansing (Cole 2003).

Wound closure – some general principles

To improve wound healing, and sometimes cosmetic appearance, many emergency wounds need primary closure to bring the wound edges together. To hold the edges in place the following may be used: glue, hair ties, Steristrips, staples or sutures. The position of the wound, the nature of the wound and the age of the child influence the chosen technique. However, some wounds may not be suitable for primary closure and left to heal by secondary closure (inflammation, granulation and epithelialisation), for example abrasions, wounds with tissue loss or mammal bites, including human bites. Before any wound is closed, tendon and neurovascular damage must be excluded and the wound washed thoroughly (Cole 2003). Antibiotic therapy is prescribed for children where extensive contamination or tissue damage has occurred (Young *et al.* 2005).

Exclusions

- Extensive wounds needing general anaesthetic
- Deep wounds with tendon nerve or arterial damage – refer to surgical practitioners/ doctors
- Facial wounds needing referral to a plastic surgeon
- Large areas of skin loss or devitalised tissue – refer to a plastic surgeon.

Cuts and lacerations

A cut is defined as a breach in the skin caused by a sharp object leaving a straight, well-defined wound with little bruising. A laceration (Latin – lacerare – to tear) is a breach in the skin caused by blunt trauma, crushing or shearing forces, leaving a ragged, irregular wound (Small 2000).

Management should include:

- Written and/or verbal consent
- Selection of an appropriate local/topical anaesthetic/analgesia
- Thorough cleansing and exploration of the wound. Ensure the base of the wound is visualised and the extent determined. Use retractors and magnifying lights if necessary.
- Debridement of 'debris' (the removal of devitalised or infected tissue, fibrin or foreign material) to remove slough, contaminants and damaged tissue. The body can remove these by natural processes, but large quantities of debris can delay healing providing an environment for infection. This may be achieved by surgical debridement or use of topical treatments, for example hydrocolloid dressings; silver sulphadiazine ointment may

be of use when removing grit from wounds (Dearden 2001). Topical treatments should be used according to local protocols.

- Occasionally a tourniquet may be required to aid haemostasis when examining digits, but remember to remove it.
- Consider whether wound closure is indicated. Note that methods of closure vary, dependent on the type and nature of the wound and the age of the patient (Rubin 1998; Small 2000). Methods include:
  — Wound closure strips, useful for superficial/deep dermal wounds where haemostasis has been achieved, where friable skin is present and can assist where slight to moderate skin tension is required to appose wound edges.
  — Tissue glue for superficial/deep dermal wounds where haemostasis has been achieved. It can be used in conjunction with wound closure strips but should not be used on friable skin or where good skin apposition is not achievable. It should not be used on infected tissue.
  — Suturing (try to avoid using on children), necessary where closure using the above methods is unachievable, for example large subcutaneous wounds, wounds where haemostasis is difficult, wounds over highly mobile joints.
  — Staples, used as an alternative to suturing for linear scalp wounds. We would not advocate their use for young children.

Bites

It is worth noting here that bites by mammals whether superficial or deep have the potential for infection due to the oral bacteria that may be present. Dog, cat and human bites are the most prevalent seen in emergency departments (Medeiros and Saconato 2003). There is, however, debate in the literature over the use of prophylactic antibiotics. Whilst prophylactic co-amoxiclav is advocated by some for human and animal bites management may differ according to local policy, site and depth of the bite. Additionally the suturing of bite wounds remains a topic of

debate due to concerns about primary closure of a potentially infected wound. Therefore, the management of a bite by a mammal will also depend on local policy, the size, depth and position of the wound. For example, suturing and prophylactic antibiotics may be the choice of treatment for a facial wound where cosmetic appearance is a main concern (Chen *et al.* 2000). There is, though, agreement in the literature relating to the need for thorough cleansing of the bite itself and follow up to monitor healing.

Alert: Human bites in children may be indicative of child protection concerns. Therefore, act accordingly in line with local and national policy.

Dressings

The frequency of dressing changes, and acceptability for the child, influence the choice of wound dressing. Some wounds may be treated by gauze dressings kept moist and changed daily or more frequently, whilst others may be more appropriately treated using a modern dressing changed less frequently (Dearden *et al.* 2001). Dressings are largely a matter of practicality and individual preference based on clinical findings (Miller & Collier 1996; Owen *et al.* 2000; Small 2000) and a flexible, knowledgeable approach to wound management (Thomas 1997). They should of course:

- Be non-adherent (to avoid unnecessary pain and damage to delicate healing tissue on their removal)
- Be an effective barrier against infection
- Maintain wound temperature
- Provide an optimum environment for wound healing
- Allow absorption of exudates.

The fixation of the dressing is again largely a matter of practicality and individual preference. It may be necessary to bandage dressings in place, e.g. 'boxing gloves', but it is *never* necessary to tape the bandage onto skin. Stockinet placed over bandages maintains their position with tape applied over the stockinet. Flexible tape allows for easy movement, holds dressings in place and is easily removable with plaster remover solution. Children and/or their parents will require information about the type of dressing used and what to expect from that particular product. Whenever possible, give written advice in the form of an information leaflet. There is also an excellent web resource on wound healing and management initiated by Stanley Carson (MD FACS CWS), available online at www.woundhealer.com.

It is worth noting that if suitable for the wound, hydrocolloids are an ideal dressing for children. They allow the child to lead a full and normal life as many normal activities can still be undertaken, for example playing in sand, as the dressing protects the wound from urine, faeces and other matter such as sand and soil, as well as allowing the child to bathe and shower. An important feature for both children and their parents is that the dressing is removable without causing pain, the wound care is undertaken by the parent, so involving them in the care of their child (Forshaw 1993; Schmitt *et al.* 1996).

Box 6.2   Scenario concerning the management of a cut sustained by a 14-year-old

Patient – Emily is a 14-year-old girl who presents to MIU, accompanied by her aunt.
Presenting complaint – Emily has cut her left index finger using a knife one hour ago.
Past medical history – none.
Medication – none.
Allergies – none known.
Tetanus status – pre-school booster aged 5 years.
On examination – Emily is given a full verbal explanation of the intended examination (including an explanation of basic anatomy) and her verbal consent to proceed is sought having ascertained she is competent according to the Fraser Guidelines (as discussed previously in Chapter 3). Emily has a subcutaneous, 1 cm wound over the radial border of the proximal phalanx of her left index finger. The wound is bleeding profusely and difficult to assess. There is no obvious swelling or bruising to the joint. Circulation and sensation distal to the wound are normal. There is no specific bony tenderness apparent. She has full flexion and extension, abduction and adduction of the finger and pincer grip with the thumb indicates full power. Tendon function (flexor digitorum superficialis, flexor digitorum profundus, and extensor digitorum) appears normal.
Provisional diagnosis – Subcutaneous wound requiring further exploration under local anaesthetic (at this point Emily was asked for formal written consent, which she gave).
Plan – Using an aseptic technique explore the wound after achieving haemostasis. Consider the use of a tourniquet.
Treatment – Distraction techniques prior to treatment included the use of a medically orientated puzzle book specifically developed for adolescents. It depicts various emergencies and gives instructions in first aid treatment.

The wound and surrounding skin were cleaned with normal saline and the finger anaesthetised with 2 ml of 1% plain lignocaine via digital nerve block. The base of the wound (with the aid of skin retractors and magnifying light) was visualised. It was evident that while the joint capsule was intact, there was a small tear to the extensor tendon. In accordance to local protocols treatment proceeded as follows.

The wound was dressed with an anti-bacterial, non-adhesive pressure dressing and a high arm sling applied. Emily was prescribed 1 g oral paracetamol which she took.
Alert – A nurse practitioner should not treat wounds with visible or lacerated tendons.
Referral – A referral for medical review at the parent hospital's emergency department was completed.

Abrasions

These injuries present as the result of friction commonly sustained during a fall. Rubin (1998) defines abrasions as excoriations that remove the surface epithelium and may involve the dermis. Exposed nerve endings make these wounds particularly painful. Occasionally underlying structures are involved, with serious implications for treatment and cosmetic outcome. Assessment is the same as that for lacerations, paying particular attention to wound site, measurements, tissue viability and the involvement of tendons, joints etc. and pain. Where there is extensive tissue loss or other complication, urgent referral to plastic surgeons is required. Thorough assessment determines how the wound is managed, using local anaesthetic either topically applied or infiltrated. If the abrasion is too large to be adequately anaesthetised, or the amount of local anaesthetic required exceeds the therapeutic dose, for example when cleaning multiple abrasions, it may be appropriate to refer the child for admission and general anaesthesia (Young *et al.* 2005). Multidisciplinary assessment is therefore required.

Debris can be removed with sponges, surgical brushes, fine forceps and hypodermic needles.

Alert: As the sight of needles and other sharp metal implements often frightens children, we have found the use of distraction techniques invaluable in this situation. Syringing normal saline at high pressure using a large syringe (30–60 ml) via an 18 g needle (carefully removing the needle and using only the hub attached to the syringe produces a good result for 'needle phobic' children) will aid removal of contaminants (Rubin 1998).

Alert: Vigorous scrubbing of wound margins can cause further tissue devitalisation, therefore avoid.

It is though vitally important to remove debris. Clothing particles, road tar and sand are common contaminants that are difficult to remove and, if left, not only give rise to infection, but can also cause permanent tattooing. Flamazine or other silver-nitrate based dressings are extremely useful on these wounds as it emulsifies and lifts out contaminants (Dowsett 2004; Severn NHS Trust 2001; Thomas 2002). If Flamazine is used, the child should be reviewed the next day. Once the wound is debrided it should not be allowed to dry out. Facial abrasions benefit from the topical application of light liquid paraffin. Other areas may require the topical application of paraffin ointment, occlusive film or hydrocolloid dressings, or silver-based dressings. Again dressing choice is dependent on clinical presentation, site of wound etc (Heenan 1998). Large, deep abrasions may produce moderate to large amounts of exudates therefore dress accordingly.

Minor burns and scalds

Burns and scalds are one of the most common accidents in childhood, taking literally seconds to occur. In 2002 in the UK, approximately 42 000 children under 15 years of age sustained a burn or scald. The majority were under 5 years old (28 000) with scalds being the most common injury in children aged less than 3 years (Child Accident Prevention Trust 2002). Children are physiologically different from adults with a higher percentage of extracellular fluid that is more easily lost through thermal injury (Taylor 2001).

Thermal injury occurs when there is exposure to:

- Wet heat – steam, boiling water, hot fat
- Dry heat – contact with a hot surface (irons, radiators) or direct flames
- Radiation – sunburn
- Chemicals – many household items are caustic to skin, also consider systemic effects through inhalation, ingestion and skin absorption
- Electrical – there may be entry and exit wounds although cardiac assessment would be a priority. (Pape *et al.* 2001)

Alert: Note that burns affecting >5% body surface area (BSA), and those sustained from contact with chemical agents and electrical burns are significant thermal injuries requiring immediate referral for specialist management (National Burn Care Committee 2001).

Assessment

Your documented history should include:

- Time and duration of exposure
- Specific data relating to the causative agent and how it occurred
- Investigate the possibility of an inhalation injury
- Tetanus status
- An accurate estimation of the extent and severity of the burn/scald (essential)
- Use of a wound grid for burns affecting a small BSA to accurately assess their external dimensions.

Alert: It is important to establish the depth of the burn and pain associated with the burn, as this will alter your subsequent treatment and management. Areas of simple erythema should be ignored when estimating the severity of burns. The depth of burns should be described using the following terms in order to avoid confusion:

- Superficial epidermal (erythema only)
- Superficial dermal (erythema and blistering)
- Deep dermal (destruction of the epidermis and most of the dermis)
- Subdermal (full thickness). (Pape *et al.* 2001)

Superficial burns have normal capillary refill and sensation. Burns and scalds are more likely to be of mixed depth than uniform depth throughout. Remember the *deeper* the burn, the *less* painful it is likely to be. Burns that are more extensive are assessed using a Lund & Browder chart (Jenner *et al.* 2006). These estimate the percentage of BSA affected according to the age of child. The National Burn Care Committee (2001) has useful guidelines for children requiring admission or referral:

- Any burn exceeding 5% of total body surface area
- Children with small subdermal burns may benefit from early excision and grafting
- Burns or scalds to functionally important areas, e.g. face, hands, feet, perineum, joints or flexor surfaces
- Children with underlying medical conditions, e.g. diabetes
- Non-accidental injury concerns
- Burns with associated injuries, e.g. inhalation, electrical burns
- Infected burns or evidence of septicaemia
- Burns outside these guidelines may be treated in the emergency department/MIU, with careful monitoring and a review by a clinician within 24 hours.

Management of minor burns – some general principles

- The priority for any burn is to cool the area immediately (or in the case of a chemical burn, appropriate neutralisation of the contaminant) with plenty of cold water for a minimum of 15 minutes. However, be aware that

children lose body heat very rapidly due to their relatively increased BSA.
- Cooling reduces pain and swelling, therefore administer even if presentation to the department is initially delayed.
- Chemical burns may require longer irrigation dependent on their toxicity. Seek advice from a reliable source, i.e. Toxbase or National Poisons Centres.
- Clingfilm is an excellent first aid dressing as it is essentially sterile and minimises the risk of infection, reduces pain as air is not circulating next to the burn, is pliable, transparent for inspection and is non-adherent (Hudspith & Ryatt 2004).
- There is debate as to whether blisters should be left intact, aspirated with a needle or completely de-roofed (Cole 2003). Bosworth (1997) believes that leaving intact hinders the assessment process and joint movement may be restricted. Other authors (Flanagan & Graham 2001; Gower & Lawrence 1995) suggest blisters be left intact to maintain protection, being only aspirated if necessary to alleviate pressure. Our personal preference is to de-roof large blisters to aid patient comfort. Follow local policies and guidelines (Taylor 2001).

Dressings

The specific aims (and primary importance) of a burns dressing, in addition to those previously discussed, are to:

- Provide an aseptic environment for healing;
- Absorb exudates;
- Be easily removed without sticking;
- Allow freedom of movement. (Taylor 2001)

Topical applications

Many topical applications are available. The following are most frequently used in emergency departments/MIUs.

Flamazine cream

This is often the initial dressing of choice (it can be used for up to one week) and is widely accepted as the agent of choice for the prevention of gram-negative wound sepsis. It has the added benefit of being effective against pseudomonas and MRSA (World Wide Wounds 2002). Additionally to anti-bacterial properties, it soothes the burn, limiting blistering. Should slough occur, Flamazine aids removal. Added advantages are that hand and foot burns can be placed in a plastic bag with the cream applied, allowing joints to be exercised (Dowsett 2004).

Alert: Young children must not have bags applied; instead use boxing glove bandaging.

Limitations of use and disadvantages

- It should not be used on faces as it may cause temporary staining of skin (argyria may occur after prolonged application or if large areas are treated, but will eventually resolve).
- It should not be used on neonates, premature infants and infants younger than two years of age as it may cause haemolysis (destruction of erythrocytes), methaemoglobinaemia (inability of erythrocytes to transport oxygen) and leucopenia (elevated white cell count), although this has not been fully researched.
- It should not be used in near term pregnancy or breastfeeding (as sulphonamides are known to cause kernicterus). Dressings require changing at least every 24–48 hours depending on the exudates and frequent changing can impede tissue repair.
- The surrounding skin can become macerated, altering the burn's appearance, thereby making re-assessment difficult (Smith & Nephew 1997).

Despite limitations and disadvantages it is, however, generally agreed that Flamazine is a safe broad-spectrum agent (Klasen 2000).

Other topical treatments

- Facial burns should be treated with light liquid paraffin.
- Paraffin impregnated gauze may be used with caution. It has a tendency to dry out, causing adherence and 'gridding' may occur. This may be alleviated by the additional use of soft paraffin ointment next to the burn.

- Silicone dressings are very useful for their non-adherent properties.
- Polyurethane films are semi-permeable membranes excellent for use on superficial burns with low to moderate exudates. The exudates may facilitate wound healing since it contains immunoglobulins. Excessive exudates are aspirated through the dressing.
- Hydrocolloid dressings have their place in the management of small superficial burns. However, we would advocate caution in their use, as they can be particularly difficult to remove from the surrounding intact skin, thereby causing distress to the child.
- Secondary dressings provide thermal insulation, absorb exudates; when using, secure the primary dressing in place, protecting against further trauma. (Butcher & Reid 1997; Pudner 2001a,b; Taylor 2001; Thomas 1997)

Alert: Be aware of the possibility of toxic shock syndrome, even in children with very small burns. The symptoms include:

- Sudden onset of fever
- Vomiting
- Diarrhoea
- A diffuse, macular, erythematous rash
- Shock

Urgent treatment consists of fluid resuscitation and antibiotics (Pape *et al.* 2001).

Box 6.3 Scenario concerning the management of a burn

Patient – Helen is 10 years old and has attended with a teacher from her school.
Presenting complaint – Helen presented complaining of a burn to the dorsum of her right foot.
History of presenting complaint – Helen was reluctant to take part in PE. She stated that she had scalded herself with water from the kettle when she made a hot drink the previous night. Helen's mother had cooled her foot with water and applied some 'burn cream'. On looking at Helen's foot, the teacher had become concerned as she noticed that, 'fluid was oozing onto her sock'. School staff had left a telephone message at home for Helen's mother to contact them.

Box 6.3   (Continued)

Past medical history – Helen has attended the unit on three occasions for minor problems.
Medication – None.
Allergies – None known.
Tetanus status – Up to date.
On examination – Helen is shy, a little quiet, and although not withdrawn was reluctant to have her foot examined. The nurse practitioner spent time chatting to Helen generally about school and other activities she enjoyed. A few minutes later, Helen became more relaxed and was willing to have her foot examined. Her sock was stuck to her foot, so it was soaked off using lukewarm water. A 2 cm diameter, partially de-roofed blister was evident, situated over the navicular area of her right foot. It was oozing fluid+ and had fluff from her sock stuck to it. There was some localised erythema. A measuring grid was used to measure the wound, which was found to be 6 cm in diameter. Neither the wound nor the rest of the foot showed signs of infection (no heat, swelling, pus or tracking). Circulation and pulses were normal. The wound was tender+ on palpation. Helen had full range of movements in her ankle and toes with normal power and function. She said it was more painful when wearing shoes.
Provisional diagnosis – Superficial (dermal) burn, >12 hours old.
Plan – Clean and dress wound.
Treatment – Flamazine cream was the dressing of choice in the first 24 hours for its antibacterial properties, and patient comfort when applying, and later removing, the dressing. Helen was more than happy to have her foot dressed. Mother subsequently arrived in MIU and she was provided with the necessary information to continue her care.
Discharge and advice – It was arranged that Helen would be reviewed in the unit the next day. Her mother was instructed to give Helen regular paracetamol within the therapeutic dose for her age and to soak off her dressing at home in the bath prior to her attending for review the following morning. Although Flamazine is non-adherent, it tends to leave the skin macerated making re-assessment more difficult. Asking the patient to soak off the Flamazine and apply a temporary dry dressing (in this case a silicon dressing, gauze and tape were supplied to the patient) enables the skin to return to a more

normal appearance. This is particularly useful when re-assessing hand/foot burns treated with Flamazine in a polythene bag; older children can be given a dry bag that they can loosely tape on, having gently washed off the Flamazine at home.
On review – Helen re-attended the next day as planned. She had soaked off her Flamazine dressing and applied the temporary dressing herself. Plaster remover solution was used to remove the tape and the silicon and gauze came off without sticking. The blister had completely de-roofed itself leaving moist pink skin underneath. The dead skin from the blister had shrivelled and it removed easily when cleaned with normal saline. The wound bed was particularly tender. On re-assessment, the burn was superficial, 2 cm in diameter and the surrounding erythema had settled completely. The burn was re-dressed with a silicon dressing, gauze and bandage. Arrangements were made for 'follow up' with the practice nurse and Helen advised to stay off school for the remainder of the week. A burns advice card was given and a routine school nurse referral made.

Foreign bodies

Children present with foreign bodies (FB) for various reasons.

Common presentations include:

- Children who fall, sustaining cuts/abrasions on glass or stones
- Embedded earrings
- Objects that are swallowed (inhaled objects are a medical emergency and are therefore not dealt with in this chapter)
- All manner of objects inserted into ears and noses – Beware! It is extremely rare for children to insert objects into their anus or vagina. In 47 years combined accident and emergency experience only one child has presented with an FB in her vagina. This subsequently proved to be a child protection issue.

Assessment of a suspected FB with an overlying wound is similar as that outlined for cuts and lacerations. Other considerations are:

- The velocity involved in sustaining the injury, e.g. air gun pellets (Johnson 1998)

- X-raying for radio-opaque FBs, e.g. metal, ceramic and glass. There is no point in x-raying for most organic material, e.g. wood splinters. However some fish bones do show on x-ray (Raby *et al.* 1997)
- Visually checking for FBs.

To ascertain presence and location of an FB palpate and explore wounds carefully using needles, forceps or probes. Specialised removal techniques are required for removing some FBs, e.g. fish hooks, sheep ticks.

Alert: Remember glass does not always show on x-ray, this is dependent on the lead content of the glass. Therefore wounds that are suspected to contain glass should still undergo a thorough examination, despite a negative x-ray (Raby *et al.* 1997), as should wounds involving rose thorns, wooden splinters or other organic FBs, as also these do not show up on x-ray.

Some emergency departments use metal detectors to locate metal foreign bodies in wounds and those that have been swallowed, for example swallowed coins/metal objects. This avoids using x-rays during the initial assessment thereby not exposing children to unnecessary radiation. Follow local policies regarding this.

Removal of foreign bodies from wounds

Use appropriate local/topical anaesthetic in line with local protocols. Indeed, if topical analgesia is applied to the wound at triage or during initial assessment this can reduce treatment time, although sedation may still be required (Priestly *et al.* 2004). Pharmacy will advise on local anaesthesia options. Superficial foreign bodies can be removed using splinter forceps, needles, ring probes or wound brushes. Specific techniques may be required for the following:

- Fishhooks – The chosen method for fishhook removal depends on the type of fishhook embedded, its location and the depth of tissue penetration. Occasionally, more than one removal technique may be required. The retrograde technique is the simplest but least successful removal method, while the traditional advance and cut method is most effective for removing

fishhooks that are embedded close to the skin surface (Gammons & Jackson 2001). Using this method the fishhook needs to be pushed through the skin, cutting behind the barb with wire/ring cutters as it exits the new puncture wound. Do not attempt to pull them out. A simple dressing is applied. Prophylactic antibiotics are not normally required. There should be an assessment of tetanus status and toxoid administered if needed.

- Sheep ticks (a blood sucking insect, prevalent in moorland areas) can be removed applying an alcohol wipe to the tick then using forceps, grabbing the body and rotating several turns to free the head. Pulling directly leaves the head *in situ*, potentially giving rise to infection and abscesses. Give relevant advice regarding signs and symptoms of Lyme's disease.
- Embedded earrings commonly present in children who have recently had their ears pierced with studs. Studs can be manipulated through the pierced lobe, once the lobe is adequately anaesthetised with lignocaine and the back loosened. In our experience embedded 'butterfly' backs are usually more difficult to manoeuvre, fine skin hooks are ideal for this purpose. Very occasionally (as a last resort) an incision is made to the posterior lobe to aid removal. Advice given includes: using larger studs, flat studs, long posted earrings, 'button type' backs as opposed to 'butterflies', sleeper type small hoops (some schools will not allow this type due to an increased risk of catching the earring and lacerating the ear lobe) and general hygiene advice for newly pierced ears.
- Swallowed objects do not usually present a problem unless there is a possibility or evidence the object has become stuck in the gastrointestinal tract (retching, drooling, reluctance to drink/eat, nausea, vomiting, abdominal pain, altered bowel habit) or if it is known that the object is toxic, e.g. batteries. For those children seek urgent medical opinion. For the majority of children who swallow small objects, e.g. toy parts, buttons etc., little more than reassurance and safety advice for the parent is required.

Ears and noses

Some general principles of assessment

Assessing FBs in ears and noses is a relatively more straightforward procedure. Usually the child is less distressed as there has often been no associated trauma. They are therefore more compliant with you just 'having a look'. Play and distraction may assist you in simply looking, for example mobiles hanging from ceilings give the child something to look up at when trying to assess a nasal FB.

Whenever possible, attempt to identify the type of FB from the history or on visualisation, for example animal, vegetable or mineral, as removal techniques are dependent on its composition. Beans, paper and cotton buds (vegetable) swell and can even disintegrate in moist conditions making removal difficult. Toy parts and beads (mineral) are awkward shapes to get hold of and can become wedged in the orifice. Moths and other insects can cause extreme pain and agitation and need to be killed prior to removal (Davies & Benger 2000). Caustic foreign bodies, e.g. batteries require urgent removal or referral to Ear, Nose and Throat (ENT).

Essential equipment

- A good light source, e.g. auroscope, magnifying light/glass
- A ready assortment of probes (hooked/ring type), forceps
- Suction – useful for smaller objects
- A thudicum (a nostril retractor) may be required in older children
- The parent to help hold and position the child. This is not always necessary, some children are very happy to be examined without being held, ask the child what they prefer
- An extra pair of hands to help distract/hold the child as necessary.

Positioning the child

1   Sit the child on the parent's lap, sideways for ears and facing front for noses.
2   The parent places one arm across the shoulders, immobilising the child's arms in a firm 'cuddle'.

3   The other hand supports the child's head against the parent's chest.
4   Secure the child's legs between parent's crossed legs.
5   Another method is to lay the parent on the trolley with the child using the same holding technique.

Alert: It needs to be stressed that either technique should make the child feel secure but not bound or overly restrained.

When checking ears and nostrils:

- It is essential to visually check bilaterally, not just the reported side.
- Observe for signs of trauma, associated inflammation, infection etc.
- Identify the FB if possible, to aid removal.

Removal of foreign bodies from ears and nostrils

The type of object *in situ* guides removal strategies identified below (Reynolds 2004):

- Nasal FBs may be expelled by encouraging the child to blow their nose (even blowing bubbles with their affected nostril, while occluding the unaffected nostril, may have success).
- Suction providing 100–140 mmHg of pressure is safe to use both aurally and nasally (Davies & Benger 2000). Obtaining a solid seal on the object may be difficult. Some children find the noise and sensation very distressing despite opportunity to play with the equipment prior to the procedure.
- Tissue glue applied to the wooden end of a cotton bud, placed in contact with a *dry*, easily visualised FB and allowed to set, before gentle retraction is reportedly a highly effective method (Hanson & Stephens 1994; McLaughlin *et al.* 2002). **Alert**: Extreme care and skill is obviously required to avoid contact with mucous membranes or the auditory canal. Its use is, therefore, not advised in pre-school or younger school age children (Ansley & Cunningham 1999).
- Alligator or other forceps are useful for irregularly shaped objects that can be grasped.

Hooks, ring probes and curettes can be placed behind FBs to 'pop' them out using traction.

- Live insects in the ear canal can be killed initially with liquid paraffin and then may be gently irrigated out with warmed water/saline.

Alert: Difficulty arises in ensuring that foreign matter is not inhaled or pushed further into the orifice. It is therefore imperative that the child is willing to keep still and is not distressed. Being prepared with a wide assortment of the correct equipment enables expedience; often one attempt at removal is all even the most cooperative child will allow. Repeated tries are unlikely to be successful and may cause physical and emotional trauma, increasing the risk of perforation.

There is no point in attempting the procedure on a screaming, moving target! Conscious sedation with the use of topical anaesthetic or a general anaesthetic (and therefore referral to a medical practitioner) will be required if the child is significantly distressed.

After two or more unsuccessful attempts, refer the child to the ENT department. If successful, following removal examine the site to check that there is no trauma (Reynolds 2004).

Insect bites and stings

Venomous creatures in the UK are rare, the only poisonous snake being the adder (Bradley 2001). The treatment of bites and stings follows the same principles outlined above for wounds. There are however some pertinent factors to bear in mind regarding the assessment and subsequent management:

- History – how, where, when: elicit the exact history and time of injury in order to correctly identify and treat the potential pathogen, e.g. the immediate topical application of vinegar (acid) is the first aid treatment of wasp stings, conversely, bicarbonate of soda (alkaline) alleviates bee stings. Regular soaking in a bowl of water (as hot as the patient can comfortably tolerate) relieves weaver fish stings within the first 24 hours.
- Note and measure the extent of erythema and swelling (a good tip is to draw around the affected area, this helps in future assessment).

- Note tracking, exudates, pus or the presence of heat (particularly over joints).
- Pay particular attention to areas of demarcation, sensory deficit, reduced capillary refill and check local pulses.
- Palpate for tenderness checking joint movements above and below the injury site.
- Baseline observations of TPR and BP should be performed routinely.
- Carefully remove stings if appropriate; bees may leave a sting with a small sac attached, and wasps do not.
- Check for signs of lymphangitis palpating lymph nodes for lymphoedema.
- Consider antibiotics if there are signs of infection. As Richardson (2004) notes bacterial infection may be introduced at the time of the insect bite or as a result of scratching the bite or sting.

Alert: Be aware of the possibility of an anaphylactic reaction. Anaphylaxis from insect bites is less common than from insect stings (Prodigy 2004; Richardson 2004).

Special considerations
Refer to medical practitioner urgently, obtain baseline observations and monitor if the child presents with:

- Anaphylaxis
- History of previous severe reactions
- Excessive swelling/erythema
- Tachycardia (Prodigy 2003).

Anaphylaxis
The definitive body for guidance for the treatment of anaphylaxis is the European Resuscitation Council (of which the Resuscitation Council UK is a subsidiary). There are no generally accepted definitions of anaphylactic and anaphylactoid reactions (Resuscitation Council (UK) 2005). Signs and symptoms may include any of the following:

- Altered respirations, e.g. note rate (may range from tachypnoea to apnoea), colour (flushing/pallor/cyanosis) and effort (use of accessory muscles, diaphragmatic breathing

result in sternal recession, head bobbing and nasal flaring)
- Altered pulse rate and stroke volume (may be tachycardic or bradycardic)
- Lowered BP (a late pre-terminal sign in young children)
- May be febrile
- Altered GCS and/or pupil reaction
- Angioedema – swelling of mucous membranes around eyes, lips, tongue and larynx (may result in irreversible asthma)
- Urticaria
- Abdominal pain, vomiting, diarrhoea
- Rhinitis, conjunctivitis.

Management

Provide safe, supportive treatment, maintaining a low threshold for intervention by the following:

- Airway – ensure patent airway, give oxygen (high flow via a non-re-breathing mask).
- Breathing – observe and record respiratory rate, peak flow, oxygen saturation.
- Circulation – observe and record pulse, BP and blood glucose, consider cardiac monitoring and need for cannulation.
- Drugs – usually first line treatment will include adrenaline (IM), antihistamines (IM) and corticosteroids (IM/slow IV).
- Fluids may be required IV if no response to drugs.
- Urgent early transfer to an emergency medical facility will be required (Resuscitation Council (UK) 2005).

Box 6.4   Scenario involving an anaphylactic reaction

Patient – Emma, a 15-year-old girl, attends MIU accompanied by her parents.
Presenting complaint – She has sustained a wasp sting to her upper arm and feels unwell.
History of presenting complaint – Fifteen minutes ago, Emma was stung on her right upper arm by a? wasp. She feels faint and nauseous and

---

is complaining of 'tightness' in her chest. Her arm feels sore.
Past medical history – None reported.
Medications – None.
Allergies – None known.
Tetanus status – Last booster dose 6 months ago.
On examination – Weight 50 Kg (approximated weight).

Temperature 36.9, pulse 110, respirations 30, blood pressure 85/60. SPO_2 95% on air, PEFR 380 L/min, blood sugar 5.3 mmol, GCS 15.

Emma is anxious, looks flushed, has swelling ++ around her eyes and lips.

Her tongue is normal, with no difficulty swallowing, but she sounds wheezy and is short of breath.

She has no rash, no abdominal pain, diarrhoea or vomiting.

Right upper arm: there is some local erythema and non-fluctuant swelling ++. There is no lymphangitis, no axillary lymph nodes are palpable.

Sensation and circulation (pulses and capillary refill) are normal. The swollen area is itchy and tender + to touch and feels warm ++. Full range of movements is present in all joints on the affected arm.
Diagnosis – Anaphylactic reaction, secondary to insect sting.
Treatment

- Reassurance.
- Summon assistance.
- Emma was laid flat, and the trolley tilted to elevate her legs.
- Oxygen therapy was administered at a rate of 15 L/min via a non-rebreathing mask.
- She was given adrenaline 500 micrograms IM (0.5 ml epinephrine 1:1000 solution). NB this is repeated in 5 minutes if no improvement occurs.
- Antihistamine (chlorpheniramine) 10 mg IM was also administered (Resuscitation Council (UK) 2005, and given in accordance with local patient directives). Continuous 3 lead cardiac monitoring was performed. Respiratory rate was continuously observed. Pulse, respiratory rate and BP were recorded at 5-minute intervals.
- Ice packs were applied locally to her arm.
- Emma was transferred by '999' ambulance to the local emergency department accompanied by her parents.

Bruises and haematomas

Bruises occur from a direct blow to the skin. They are particularly common in children through normal play and sporting activity and usually cause little concern. The commonest sites of soft tissue bruising in children are the head and lower legs. As bruising generally occurs at or near the site of trauma the location assists the initial assessment/clinical examination, for example large bruising to the occiput makes it necessary to exclude intracranial trauma, similarly bruising to the fingers will raise suspicion of a fracture (Young *et al.* 2005). It is important to consider the pattern of the bruising to ensure it is consistent with the trauma. If the bruising is extensive, has a typical pattern or occurs in the absence of trauma or with only minor trauma the child may have a condition such as idiopathic thrombocytopenic purpura, Henoch Schonlein purpura or another bleeding disorder. However, small bruises require no treatment and, as Young *et al.* (2005) advise, a cool pack and oral analgesia might be helpful in the first few hours after bruising and early mobilisation assists a speedy recovery.

A **haematoma** is a large bruise, or collection of blood in the tissues. It is usually associated with swelling. Moderate bruising and haematomas require ice/cool packs and elevation where practicable. Pressure dressings help to avoid the formation of a haematoma, for example a bruised ear. Advise against the use of heat packs, hot baths, vigorous massage and exercise, as this will encourage further bleeding and can result in the following complications:

- Sepsis
- Skin necrosis
- Compartment syndrome – spontaneous bleeding into a compartment, characterised by excruciating pain
- Hypovolaemia
- Myositis ossificans – ossification of muscle tissue (Wardrope & English 1998).

After 48 hours encourage application of gentle warmth, and light mobilisation to aid reabsorption. Vigorous exercise is to be avoided for several days as this may lead to ossification of the haematoma, causing chronic pain. Occasionally these patients require physiotherapy and ultrasound to aid healing.

Specific injuries requiring urgent referral for aspiration or surgical intervention include:

- Large haematomas
- Any haematoma at risk of, or compromising nerves, muscles and circulation
- Septal haematomas
- Aural haematomas.

Subungual haematomas are collections of blood under the nail plate caused by a crush injury, for example when children trap their fingers in doors. They can be treated by trephining (making a hole in the nail) which releases the blood, subsequently relieving pressure and pain. Use a cautery tool specifically designed for this procedure. A dressing is then applied. X-ray a suspected fracture; if a fracture is present, trephining the nail has technically made the fracture compound. Prophylactic antibiotics are required to prevent infection thereby reducing the risk of osteomyelitis. Trephining is not suitable for all children, as success is dependent on their cooperation and keeping still is vital.

Alert – Bruises in unusual areas, of unusual pattern, or when the history given conflicts with the pattern of injury, raises suspicion of non-accidental injury. Children have accidents according to their age and stage of development. If you are concerned – ask the unthinkable and ask yourself could they have bruised themselves on that part of their body?

Clotting disorders as mentioned above also need to be ruled out.

Soft tissue injuries

Sprains

The term sprain refers to damaged ligaments. Denote the severity in grades or degrees. Any joint can be affected, most commonly ankles and wrists. For example, ankle sprains are graded 1–3 (see below), with grade 1 being the most common (yet least severe) type of injury.

Grade 1 (1st degree)

A partially torn ligament but no joint instability present on examination. Ligaments connecting the ankle bones are overstretched. Damage may be microscopic but the ligament is not actually torn. The lateral ligaments are those most commonly injured.

Grade 2 (2nd degree)

There is disruption (partial tear) of the ligament and there may be some (but not significant) laxity of the ankle but functional integrity is maintained.

Grade 3 (3rd degree)

There is complete disruption (a complete tear) of the ankle ligament and functional integrity is lost resulting in instability.

Strains

Over-stretching or irregular overloading at the muscle–tendon junction may result in partial or complete rupture of the muscle. Classify strains by degree of rupture:

- First-degree involve less than 5% of muscle fibres. There is no great loss of strength or restriction of movement. Pain on passive stretch or active movement is experienced.
- Second-degree strains involve a more significant number of muscle fibres; pain is aggravated by any attempt to contract the muscle.
- Third degree strains are complete ruptures resulting in deformity, pain and complete loss of function.

Localised tenderness, swelling, bruising and discolouration are symptoms that may be indicative of a strain (Peterson & Renstrom 2001).

Management and treatment of sprains and strains

Management depends on a number of factors and current trends. Consider the following factors:

- The age of the child
- The child's normal level of activity, e.g. are they athletic?

- Site of injury
- Severity of injury
- Need to immobilise e.g. severe swelling
- Need to remain mobile e.g. ankle sprain, may require physiotherapy.

Fractures should be ruled out, then initial treatment aimed at minimising haemorrhage, swelling, inflammation, cellular metabolism and pain to provide optimal healing conditions. For initial treatment rest, ice, compression and elevation (RICE) are advocated. However, avoid prolonging immobilisation to prevent atrophy of muscle and tendons. There is debate about the use of support and strapping in the literature and, generally, it is not the initial treatment in the emergency context (Wardrope & English 1998). Particularly the use of double tubigrip should be discouraged; it is not proven to have any beneficial therapeutic effect (Sexton 2002). Whatever the initial treatment, however, the consensus is that children should be encouraged to move the joint as early as possible within 24–72 hours as this helps remove some of the inflammatory biological debris that can build up after injury; pain relief should be used as necessary. Referral to physiotherapy may be considered.

Fractures

'A fracture occurs when there is loss of continuity in the substance of a bone. This may range from those that are highly comminuted to hairline and even microscopic fractures' (McRae 2002:4). Fractures may occur under excessive tension, torsion or compression, therefore frequently happen when playing or undertaking sporting activities. Thus, fractures of the upper extremities most commonly result from falls onto outstretched hands; fractures to lower limbs are more common in the older child. An accurate history of the mechanism of injury is therefore important to aid diagnosis. For example, pulling on a child's forearm is likely to cause a pulled elbow, conversely, a fall from a height onto an outstretched hand commonly results in a supracondylar fracture of the elbow.

Beware of the child who refuses to use a limb. Despite no obvious radiological abnormality, these children require review by a medical practitioner and subsequent follow up.

Common types of fractures in childhood include:

- Buckle or torus fracture
- Greenstick fracture
- Spiral fracture (beware of a spiral fracture of the tibia in a non-weight bearing child as this may be indicative of non-accidental injury)
- Radial head and supracondylar fractures
- Epiphyseal (Salter-Harris) fractures.

Supracondylar fractures

These often result from a fall backwards with the arm hyper-extended, elbow fractures commonly occurring in children aged 3–11 years. While some of these fractures may demonstrate little or no displacement and of the greenstick type, the clinician should be wary of a more significant injury, resulting in circulatory or neurological deficit. Always check sensation and circulation distal to the injury. Refer children with neurological or circulatory deficit to an orthopaedic surgeon immediately. Children severely compromised require immediate reduction to restore function and reduce the potential risk of them developing compartment syndrome.

Fractures of the elbow are difficult to see on x-ray. Be wary of a displaced anterior fat pad, which indicates an effusion (and therefore a fracture) particularly when associated with pain, swelling and decreased range of movement.

Epiphyseal (Salter-Harris) fractures

These fractures involve the growth plate of the long bones and are therefore peculiar to children. They fall into five categories ranging from type 1 (being the least severe where growth disturbance is uncommon) to type 5 (having poor functional prognosis). For further reading, refer to McRae (2002).

Assessment, examination and preliminary diagnosis

We recommend a look, move and feel method when examining children as a child may be reluctant to move a limb after palpating for tenderness. Note the point of maximum tenderness.

Look for clinical signs of a fracture:

- Swelling
- Bruising including non-specific bruising and pain
- Erythema
- Apparent deformity
- Effusion
- Site of wound.

Feel and palpate for:

- Bony tenderness, deformity or the maximum point of soft tissue tenderness (remember to include all joints proximal and distal to the site of the injury)
- Signs of effusion
- Crepitus – note if present
- Skin temperature, e.g. heat may indicate inflammation, coolness may indicate decreased circulation
- Sensation and circulation, e.g. capillary refill and pulses distal to the injury
- Arterial pulses (the presence of an arterial pulse distal to an injury DOES NOT exclude vascular injury or compartment syndrome).

Move the limb to assess function:

- Assess range of movement in comparison with unaffected limb, e.g. flexion/extension, inversion/eversion, adduction/abduction, internal/external rotation, where applicable.
- Check for crepitus on movement.
- Check joint stability.
- Note whether movements are passive or active and whether full power is achieved on testing resistance.
- Test specific tendon function, e.g. in finger injuries, each digit is isolated to test the two flexor tendons and the extensor tendon.
- Loss of function and or weight bearing ability, e.g. can the child walk, stand on tiptoes, take body weight on hands, grip, grasp toys?
- If lower limb – note gait.

Plus

- Time of injury; mechanism of injury; neurological deficit; dominant hand in upper limb injuries.

Management and treatment of fractures – general principles

- Assess the child for pain and administer appropriate analgesia. In MIUs children whose pain cannot be managed by the appropriate protocol will be transferred to an emergency department.
- Remove jewellery.
- Ensure examination of whole limb including joints above and below the area of injury.
- See all children who have a fracture in either fracture clinic or emergency clinic. Usually this is within one week. See suspected scaphoid fractures in clinic at 10–14 days. Fractures of the terminal phalanx of the fingers and toe fractures may be managed by the GP or in the community if:
  — there is no associated wound
  — there is no displacement or angulation
  — tendon function is intact
  — check tendon/nerve function, any patients with injuries to tendons/nerves must be referred to a district general hospital (DGH).

It is also important to consider:

- The child's age
- The child's normal level of activity, e.g. are they athletic?
- Site of injury
- Severity of injury
- Need to immobilise e.g. unstable fracture, severe swelling
- Need to remain mobile e.g. minor avulsion fracture may require physiotherapy.

X-ray

X-rays aid clinical diagnosis, but exercise caution when contemplating x-raying children. Radiological diagnosis can be difficult due to immaturity of the bones; it may therefore be necessary to x-ray the other limb for comparison (Raby *et al.* 1997).

Practitioners are to follow local x-ray protocols and patient group directives. It is however worth noting that the ability of nurses to request x-rays at triage accelerates the patient's overall stay in the emergency department (Larsen 2002). Take note of the following advice:

Exclusions

- Children in MIUs who may have sustained serious/multiple injuries that are best managed in the emergency department should not have their transfer delayed due to nurse requested x-rays.
- Children under 1 year of age.
- Grease gun and similar high-pressure injection injuries.
- Injuries suspected to have penetrated a joint.

Inclusions

Nurses may request x-rays for:

- The upper limb, below shoulder, and the clavicle
- The lower limb below knee.

The following details will assist the radiologist to interpret the films:

- History of injury
- Site of injury
- Suspected bony diagnosis
- If a fracture is suspected which requires special views, e.g. scaphoid, state this on the request form.

Evaluation following x-ray and radiological diagnosis

1 The radiographer using local policy performs initial x-ray interpretation.
2 If an obvious bony injury is immediately noted, practitioners in accordance with the appropriate protocol will instigate the approved treatment.

We recommend that x-ray protocols also state that no patient shall be discharged until either

- the appropriate treatment is instigated for bony injuries
- the appropriate investigation, diagnosis and treatment is completed for conditions that do not include a bony injury or

- all documentation is completed in accordance with documentation protocol PLUS completion of the department x-ray treatment form.

Treatment may include the following:

- Support bandages, slings, splints, casts, crutches, ice and elevation, etc.;
- Analgesia and instructions/advice sheets for mobilisation.

Alert: Key points in fractures and orthopaedic problems:

1 Children's injuries differ from those of adults. They are less likely to sprain a ligament and more likely to sustain a greenstick or avulsion fracture.
2 Injuries, which involve the growth plate, treat carefully as later growth disturbance may occur. However, a greater degree of angulation can be tolerated in children than in adults, as growth will remodel the bone. Any concerns refer to an orthopaedic specialist.
3 Thoroughly assess limps as there are several possible underlying causes, which may lead to problems if untreated.

Management of specific fractures

Hand injuries

- 1st metacarpal
  — dislocation and (or) fracture involving the joint: refer DGH
  — fracture not involving joint: Bennett's Plaster of Paris (PoP); check x-ray; fracture clinic
- 5th metacarpal
  — displaced/severely angulated >45°: (lateral x-ray to measure) *and* refer DGH
  — undisplaced or minor angulation: double Tubigrip (DTG)/crepe; finger exercise; consultant clinic
- Other metacarpals
  — displaced/multiple/angulated >30°: refer DGH
  — undisplaced or minor angulation: DTG/buddy strapping; finger exercise; consultant clinic

- Phalanx: check for rotation deformity and overlap.

Alert: Angulated transverse fractures of the proximal phalanx may be very disabling, if in doubt refer to a doctor for assessment.

- Displaced/angulated: refer DGH
- Undisplaced: buddy strapping; finger exercise; consultant clinic
- Mallet finger: always x-ray; mallet splint and instructions (inform patients splint will be in situ for 6 weeks); consultant clinic 7–10 days.

Wrist injuries

- No bony injury: treat according to severity of pain or swelling; supportive bandage with or without sling
- Undisplaced fracture: PoP backslab, sling; fracture clinic; instruction sheet regarding care of plaster
- Displaced fracture: splint/sling, PoP backslab; liaise with DGH re: transfer with documentation and X-rays, nil by mouth.

Scaphoid
Alert: The scaphoid bridges the two carpal rows and is at particular risk of breaking during a hyperextension injury. There are several clinical examinations that aid diagnosis but none are fool proof as other fractures to the wrist elicit pain on clinical examination of the scaphoid bone (Larsen 2002).

Clinical signs

- Specific tenderness and/or swelling in the anatomical snuffbox (The anatomical snuffbox is a depression found on the lateral aspect of the wrist when the thumb extends. On the floor of the snuffbox lies the radial styloid, the scaphoid, trapezium and the base of the first metacarpal. Direct pressure on the snuffbox will elicit tenderness on the injured scaphoid bone.)
- Pain on direct pressure over the scaphoid bone
- Specific tenderness over the scaphoid tubercle
- Pain on axial compression known as telescoping the thumb into the snuffbox

- Very poor grip
- Reduced wrist movement **Alert**: Fracture may not show on first x-ray
- History may be of a fall onto outstretched hand or a 'starting handle' type injury
- If the mechanism of injury or the clinical signs suggest a possible fracture of the scaphoid ALWAYS treat as for a fractured scaphoid
- Common in adolescents
- Uncommon in children under 12 years old.

Management

- Scaphoid PoP, sling 24 hours
- Fracture clinic
- Instruction sheet regarding care of plaster.

Radius and ulna

- No bony injury: supportive bandage, with or without sling; follow up at GP surgery if necessary
- Undisplaced fracture: PoP; sling; fracture clinic appointment
- Instructions regarding care of plaster
- Displaced fracture: full arm splint; liaise with DGH re: transfer with documentation and X-rays, nil by mouth.

Alert: An isolated midshaft fracture of one of forearm bones (except transverse midshaft ulna – defence fracture) with other intact suggests radio-ulnar joint dislocation.

It is essential that x-rays include joints above and below the injury: Monteggia, dislocation radial head with fracture ulna; Galeazzi, fracture radius with dislocation inferior radio-ulnar joint.

Elbow injuries

- Radial head/neck
  - undisplaced: collar and cuff; fracture clinic
  - severe/dislocated: refer DGH.

Alert: Effusion in elbow joint suggests fracture and should be referred to consultant clinic in 10–14 days.

- Supracondylar
  - displaced or dislocated: check radial pulse, if absent gentle traction may restore circulation; refer DGH
  - undisplaced: collar and cuff; fracture clinic
- Olecranon
  - displaced: refer DGH
  - undisplaced: long arm PoP and sling; next fracture clinic.

Alert: All elbow injuries are treated in collar and cuff not a broad arm sling.

Arm injuries

- Humerus
  - shaft – undisplaced: test radial nerve; collar and cuff; refer next fracture clinic
  - shaft – displaced: refer DGH
  - neck – undisplaced: collar and cuff; fracture clinic
  - neck – displaced, comminuted: refer DGH.

Shoulder injuries

- Clavicle
  - no bony injury: broad arm sling if necessary, early mobilisation
  - fracture: broad arm sling; fracture clinic
  - displaced: check pulse/nerve function – if normal broad arm sling and fracture clinic, if absent refer to DGH
- Dislocation of shoulder: refer DGH
- Dislocation/subluxation of acromioclavicular joint: broad arm sling; refer fracture clinic
- Complete disruption of acromioclavicular joint: refer DGH.

Leg injuries

- Fracture neck of femur: obtain chest x-ray; obtain ECG; requires orthopaedic admission; cannulate if practitioner has cannulation skills; refer DGH
- Fracture shaft of femur: refer DGH; analgesia in accordance with analgesia protocol; requires IV infusion, cannulate if possible; Donway splint (supplied by ambulance).

Ankle injuries

Assess the need to x-ray using the 'Ottawa ankle rules' below:

Ankle x-ray is required only if there is pain in the malleolar region and any of the following:

- Tenderness upon palpation of distal 6 cm of posterior edge and tip of lateral and/or medial malleolus
- Inability to weight bear both immediately after injury and in the department (4 steps).

Alert: Foot x-ray is required only if there is any pain in the midfoot area and any of the following:

- Tenderness upon palpation at the base of 5th MT and/or medial aspect of navicular
- Inability to weight bear, both immediately after injury and in the department (4 steps).

Injury:

- No bony injury: double Tubigrip or crepe if required; advice rest, ice and elevation; follow up GP/physiotherapy if required (unable to weight bear without crutches)
- Undisplaced fracture: below knee PoP, crutches non-weight bearing; fracture clinic; advice re: aftercare of PoP
- Displaced fracture: liaise with DGH.

Alert: A severely displaced fracture that poses a risk of neurovascular deficit or skin damage should be reduced immediately and prior to transfer to DGH.

Foot injuries

- Fracture calcaneum: wool and crepe; crutches; advice elevation; fracture clinic; may need admission for elevation of the affected limb.

Alert: If it involves subtalar joint/depressed fracture the child requires orthopaedic referral and admission.

- Bilateral fractures: orthopaedic referral and admission
- Fracture base 5th metatarsal: symptomatic treatment, usually crepe/DTG but if severe pain below knee PoP and crutches; refer fracture clinic

- Other fractured metatarsals
  — displaced or multiple fracture: may require admission and should be referred to DGH and orthopaedic specialist
  — undisplaced fracture: symptomatic treatment as above
- Fracture talus/subtalar/midtarsal: refer DGH
- Ruptured Achilles tendon
  — History of injury with pain in lower calf may be missed because of pain and swelling at the time of injury and foot can be plantar flexed by the long toe flexes
  — Signs of rupture include: gap in tendon; inability to stand on tiptoe on the affected foot; positive squeeze test (Simmonds test); therefore refer these children to DGH.

Toe injuries

- No bony injury: two-toe strapping if required; advise supportive sensible footwear
- Undisplaced fracture: two-toe strapping; advise supportive sensible footwear; refer GP
- Displaced fracture: liaise with DGH.

Box 6.5

For this scenario please refer to the protocol for fracture management given previously.

Patient – James is 18 months old and lives with his mother and her boyfriend. James' mother is present with James.

History of presenting complaint – James attended nursery yesterday and appeared to be fine. Today he has woken and will only intermittently weight-bear on his right leg. His mother is concerned he may have injured his leg at nursery or trapped it in the bars of his cot in his sleep. There is no reported witnessed injury.

Past medical history – James has had two hospital admissions; firstly, for a febrile convulsion aged 6 months and secondly a head injury (fall down stairs) aged 15 months. He was hospitalised for 24 hours on each occasion. He has had four further attendances at an emergency department within the last year; two minor head

Box 6.5   (Continued)

injuries, a pulled elbow and a scalded foot. He is up to date with his immunisations.

Medication – James does not take any medication routinely; his mother has given him paracetamol elixir this morning 2 hours ago.

Allergies – Elastoplast.

On examination – James is happy and smiling when carried by his mother into the examination cubicle. He appears clean and well nourished. He wants to sit on his mother's knee and appears to be interacting normally with her. He is spontaneously moving all limbs. He becomes very distressed, screaming, as his trousers, socks and shoes are removed, but he settles quickly afterwards. There are circular bruises to both shins of differing colours, with faint bluish bruising around his right ankle. The right foot appears to have some subtle swelling. Sensation and circulation appear to be normal. On palpation the foot and ankle are non-tender, however James does not like having his upper shin touched at all, pushing the nurse practitioner's hands away. His ankle, knee and hip appear to be fine with normal ranges of movement in each when examined passively. He will not stand on his right foot at all, despite being distracted.

Provisional diagnosis – ? Fracture right leg; ? Lower leg.

Plan – X-ray right leg (the whole leg).

The x-ray shows a possible spiral fracture to the proximal third of the tibia.

Diagnosis – Possible spiral fracture, ? cause (? risk of non-accidental injury).

Treatment – Analgesia as required. (N.B. As James had had paracetamol 2 hours before his attendance no further analgesia was available to the nurse practitioners in the MIU (see local protocol) and therefore this may have been an indication for urgent transfer to emergency department if pain relief was inadequate.) The application of a temporary, long leg, Plaster of Paris backslab aided pain relief. During this, distraction with bubbles maximised his cooperation.

Referral – A referral to the emergency department for consultant medical review was completed. The duty consultant paediatrician was also informed. Additionally there were referrals to the paediatric liaison health visitor and paediatric social services, outlining the concerns raised by the reported history of injury and subsequent findings (local policy dictates referral procedure).

The staff kept James' mother fully informed about the reasons for the referrals. She understood the concerns raised and was willing to co-operate. Subsequently James transferred to the emergency department. His mother took him in her car.

N.B. James' mother displayed no hostility and she appeared to be willing to cooperate. Staff were therefore able to voice their concerns openly and entrust her with his transfer. This may not always be the case and in order to ensure the child's safe transfer it may not be possible at this stage to inform parents fully of concerns and the reasons for a social services referral. It may also be necessary to transfer the child and his parents by ambulance.

Summary and conclusion

Minor injuries in children are extremely common. The younger the child, the less likely they are to recognise dangerous situations, and their willingness to robustly explore their environment means that children are more likely than adults to injure themselves (Young *et al.* 2005). The nature of the injury and therefore treatment will be influenced by their stage of physical and cognitive development. However, injury severity in children obviously forms a continuum, with no precise definition of what distinguishes a major from a minor injury. This chapter has therefore focused on injuries reasonably expected to heal with minimal medical intervention. Clearly, it is essential to recognise such injuries and exclude 'major' injuries.

Assessing minor injuries in children, however, can be challenging. As Young *et al.* (2005) note, children may not cooperate during an initial assessment or physical examination as an adult would. Reasons include pain, fear, shyness or a lack of understanding of what the examiner is requesting. Depending on the nature of the minor injury there will be specific areas that need to be focused on but this needs to be done within the context of the child's age and stage of development. Additionally, deal with pain early by using analgesics, splinting and distraction.

It is important to minimise the amount of additional pain by handling limbs slowly and sensitively, soaking dressings off wounds and avoiding unnecessary movement. Make only simple requests to the child – ask them to copy a movement demonstrated by you or the parent, and encourage them to reach or grasp toys. Ultimately, a creative and flexible technique with careful observation is crucial in examining children's injuries, especially in determining whether the injury has affected important structures, such as a nerve or tendon.

Initial treatment strategies should include:

- An assessment of the likelihood of the child being cooperative during a procedure
- Whether the child needs analgesia or sedation and the type of analgesia and sedation that may be necessary
- If they have a wound consider how the wound will be anaesthetised and how it will be closed
- Whether any treatment such as splinting is needed
- Finally, consider the child's vaccination status, allergies to antibiotics or dressings, and pre-existing medical conditions.

Any concerns should be referred and all interventions and management should follow evidence base protocols/patient group directives.

Remember that in order to deliver the care that is appropriate for the child and their family (and exclude the possibility of neglect or abuse) it is necessary at this point to assess the child's cognitive and physical abilities and decide whether these are conversant with their expected developmental stage. Be aware children are likely to regress in a strange environment and under stressful circumstances. The expert on the child is their main parent, so consult them, listen and document the parent/parents' assessment of or concerns about the injury. Useful *aides mémoires* on child development are available, for example the book *Accidents and Child Development* (CAPT 2000). We would recommend that a copy of these aides is kept readily available for quick and easy reference.

Remember that throughout the assessment and treatment period, the presence of a parent will reassure an anxious child and provide the practitioner with the opportunity to clarify details, obtain an in-depth history and give advice to the parent. Separation will only increase anxiety and cooperation might be lost.

Remember that confidentiality must be maintained according to local and national policies. Where there is an issue of child protection, you must act at all times in accordance with national and local policies.

References

Ansley, J. & Cunningham, M. (eds) (1999) Crazy Glue and Foreign Bodies. In Reply. *Paediatrics*, **103**(4), 857.

Barnard, J. & Carley, S. (2000) Vomiting and serious head injury in children. *Journal of Accident Emergency Medicine*, **17**(6), 400–402.

Bosworth, C. (1997) *Burns Trauma: Management and Nursing Care*. Bailliere Tindall, London.

Bradley, G. (2001) Reptiles. UK Safari Website. Available online at: www.uksafari.com/reptiles.

Butcher, M. & Reid, A. (1997) Policy for Wound Care in the local Community and Hospitals NHS Trusts. Unpublished policy document, compiled by the local Combined Trusts Tissue Viability Service.

Casey, G. (1999) Wound management in children: the physiological events in wound healing in children, and the importance of taking a holistic approach to wound management. *Emergency Nurse*, **7**(6), 33–38.

Cassell, O.C.S. (2002) Death from tetanus after a pretibial laceration. *British Medical Journal*, **324**(7351), 1442–1443.

Chen, E., Hornig, S., Shepherd, S.M. & Hollander, J.E. (2000) Primary closure of mammalian bites. *Academic Emergency Medicine*, **7**, 157–161.

Child Accident Prevention Trust (CAPT) (2000) *Accidents and Child Development, Guidelines for Practitioners*. CAPT, London.

Child Accident Prevention Trust (CAPT) (2002) *Factsheet: Burns and Scalds*. CAPT. Available online at: http://www.capt.org.uk.

Cole, E. (2003) Wound management in the A & E department. *Nursing Standard*, **17**(46), 45–52.

Cook, M.W., Higgins, J. & Bridge, P. (2000) *Minor Injury Services. The Present State*. Emergency Medicine Research Group, Universities of Warwick and Birmingham (Commissioned by the UK DoH). DoH, London.

Currie, D. (2000) *The Management of Head Injuries. A Practical Guide for the Emergency Room*, 2nd edn. Oxford University Press, Oxford.

Davies, P.H. & Benger, J.R. (2000) Foreign bodies in the nose and ear: a review of techniques for removal in the emergency department. *Journal of Emergency Medicine*, **17**, 91–94.

Dealey, C. (1999) *The Care of Wounds. A Guide for Nurses*, 2nd edn. Butterworth, London.

Dearden, C. *et al.* (2001) Traumatic wounds: local wound management. *Nursing Times Plus*, **97**(35), 55–57.

Department of Health (2002) *The Green Book: Immunisation Against Infectious Diseases (Tetanus)*. Available online at: www.doh.gov.uk/greenbook/greenbook-pdf/chapter30–layoutpdf.

Department of Health (2003) *Reforming Emergency Care – Practical Steps*. The Stationery Office, London. Available online at: www.doh.gov.uk/emergency-care/reformpracticalsteps.pdf.

Dowsett, C. (2004) The use of silver-based dressings in wound care. *Nursing Standard*, **19**(7), 56–60.

Elliman, D. & Bedford, H. (2004) The New Childhood Immunization Schedule. *Nursing Standard*, **19**(6), 37.

Field, D. (1997) *Anatomy, Palpation and Surface Markings*. Butterworth Heinemann, London.

Flanagan, M. & Graham, J. (2001) Should burn blisters be left intact or debrided. *Journal of Wound Care*, **10**(1), 41–45.

Forshaw, A. (1993) Hydrocolloid dressings in paediatric wound care. *Journal of Wound Care*, **2**(4), 209–212.

Gammons, M.G. & Jackson, F. (2001) Fishhook removal. *American Family Physician*, **65**(3), 384–386.

Glasgow, J.F.T. & McGovern, S.J. (2000) Imaging the less seriously injured child. *Archives of Diseases in Childhood*, **82**(4), 333–341.

Gould, D. (2001) Clean surgical wounds: prevention of infection. *Nursing Standard*, **15**(49), 41–45.

Gower, J. & Lawrence, J. (1995) The incidence, causes and treatment of minor burns. *Journal of Wound Care*, **4**(2), 71–74.

Guly, H.R. (1996) *History Taking, Examination and Record Keeping in Emergency Medicine*. Oxford University Press, Oxford.

Hanson, R.M. & Stephens, M. (1994) Cyanoacrylate assisted foreign body removal from the ear and nose in children. *Pediatric Child Health*, **30**, 77–78.

Heenan, A. (1998) Frequently Asked Questions: Hydrocolloid Dressings. Available online at: www.worldwidewounds.com/1998/april/Hydrocolloid-FAQhydrocolloid-questions.htm.

HM Government (2006) *Working Together to Safeguard Children: A guide to interagency working to safeguard and promote the welfare of children*. The Stationery Office, London. Available online at: http://www.nelincs.gov.uk/working together.

Hobbs, C. (1997) Fractures. In: *ABC of Child Abuse*, 3rd edn. R. Meadow (ed). BMJ: London.

Holt, L. (2000) *Accident and Emergency: Theory into Practice*. Bailliere Tindall: Edinburgh.

Hudspith, J. & Ryatt, S. (2004) First aid treatment of minor burns: clinical review. ABC of Burns. *British Medical Journal*, **328**, 1487–1489.

Humphries, L. & Gully, T. (2000) *Child Protection for Hospital Based Practitioners*. Whurr, London.

Jayawant, S., Rawlinson, A., Gibbon, F., Price, J., Schulte, J., Sharples, P., Sibert, J.R. & Kemp, A.M. (1998) Subdural haemorrhages in infants: population based study. *British Medical Journal*, **317**, 1558–1561.

Jenner, R., Potier de la Morandiere, K. & Mackway-Jones, K. (2006) Trauma and burns in children. *Paediatrics*, **7**(1), 11–15.

Johnson, A. (1998) Principles of wound ballistics. *Emergency Nurse*, **6**(8), 12–15.

Klasen, H.J. (2000) A historical review of the use of silver in the treatment of burns. II. Renewed interest for silver. *Burns*, **26**, 131–138.

Larsen, D. (2002) Assessment and management of hand and wrist fractures. *Nursing Standard*, **16**(36), 45–53.

McLaughlin, R., Ullah, R. & Heylings, D. (2002) Comparative prospective study of foreign body removal from external auditory canals of cadavers with right angle hook or cyanoacrylate glue. *Emergency Medicine Journal*, **19**, 43–45.

McRae, R. (2002) *Practical Fracture Treatment*, 4th edn. Churchill Livingstone, Edinburgh.

Medeiros, L. & Saconato, H. (2003) *Antibiotic Prophylaxis for Mammalian Bites*. (Cochrane Review). The Cochrane Library. Issue 2: Update Software: Oxford.

Miller, M. (1995) Principles of wound assessment. *Emergency Nurse*, **3**(1), 16–18.

Miller, M. & Collier, C. (1996) *Understanding Wounds*. Professional Nurse in association with Johnson & Johnson emap healthcare, London.

Moulton, C. & Yates, D. (1999) *Lecture Notes of Emergency Medicine*. Blackwell Science, Oxford.

National Burn Care Committee (2001) *Standards and Strategies for Burn Care*. British Association of Plastic Surgeons, London.

National Health Service (NHS) Executive (2000) *Patient Group Directions (England only)*. HSC 20001026. The Stationery Office, London.

National Institute for Clinical Excellence (NICE) (2003) *Head injury – Triage, assessment, investigation and early management of head injury in infants, children and adults*. NICE, London.

Nee, P. (2001) Why do children vomit after a head injury? *Journal of Accident and Emergency Medicine*, **18**(3), 234.

O'Sullivan, I. (2000) Wounds, *Pretibial Lacerations, Tetanus Prophylaxis*, United Bristol Healthcare NHS Trust website. Available online at: www.ubht.nhs.uk/edhandbook/wounds/wounds.htm.

Owen, A., O'Sullivan, I. & Arrowsmith, M. (2000) *Wound Dressings*, United Bristol Healthcare NHS Trust website. Available online at: www.ubht.nhs.uk/edhandbook/wounds/dressings.htm.

Pape, S., Judkins, K. & Settle, J. (2001) *Burns. The First Five Days*, 2nd edn. Smith and Nephew.

Peterson, L. & Renstrom, P. (2001) *Sports Injuries*. Martin Dunitz, London.

Priestly, S., Kelly, A.M., Chow, L. *et al.* (2004) Topical Anaesthetic Applied at Triage Reduced Treatment Time in Children Presenting to Emergency Department with Minor Lacerations. *Evidence-Based Nursing*, **7**, 9. Available online at: http://ebn.bmjjournals.com/cgi/content/full/7/1/9.

Prodigy (2004) *Prodigy Guidance – Insect Bites and Stings*. London: Prodigy. Available online at: http://www.prodigy.nhs.uk/guidance.asp?gt=Insect%20bites%20and %20stings.

Pudner, R. (2001a) Low/non-adherent dressings in wound management. *Journal of Community Nursing*, **15**(8), 2–17.

Pudner, R. (2001b) Hydrocolloid dressings in wound management. *Journal of Community Nursing*, **15**, 4. Available online at: www.jcn.co.uk.

Raby, N., Berman, L. & DeLacey, G. (1997) *Accident and Emergency Radiology – A Survival Guide*. W.B. Saunders, London.

Resuscitation Council (UK) (2005) *The Emergency Medical Treatment of Anaphylactic Reactions for Medical Responders and Community Nurses. A Project Team Report for the Resuscitation Council*. Available online at: http://www.resus.org.uk/pages/reaction.htm.

Reynolds, T. (2004) Ear Nose and Throat Problems in A & E. *Nursing Standard*, **18**(26), 47–53.

Richardson, M. (2004) Causes and effective management of insect bites in UK. *Nursing Times*, **100**(22), 63–65,67.

Riyat, M.S. & Quniton, D.N. (1997) Tap water as a cleansing agent in Accident and Emergency. *Journal of Accident and Emergency Medicine*, **14**(3), 165–166.

Rubin, A. (1998) Managing Abrasions and Lacerations. *The Physician and Sports Medicine*, **26**(55), 45–55. Available online at: www.physsportsmed.com/issues/1998/05may/rubin.htm.

Sanders, T., Cobley, C., Coles, L. & Kemp, A. (2003) Factors affecting clinical referral of young children with a subdural haemorrhage to child protection agencies. *Child Abuse Review*, **12**, 358–373.

Schmitt, M., Vergnes, P., Canarelli, J., Gaillard, S., Daoud, S., Dodat, H., Lascombes, P., Melin, Y., Morisson-Lacombe, G. & Revillon, Y. (1996) Evaluation of a hydrocolloid dressing. *Journal of Wound Care*, **5**(9), 396–399.

Severn NHS Trust (2001) *Patient Group Directions. Flamazine Cream for the Treatment of Burns and Grazes*. Last Modified July 2003. Available online at: http://129.11.239.213/protocols/DisplayProtocol.asp?ID=500.

Sexton, J. (2002) Managing soft tissue injuries. *Emergency Nurse*, **10**(1), 11–16.

Sidebotham, P. (2003) Protecting babies. *Child Abuse Review*, **12**, 353–357.

Small, V. (2000) Management of cuts, abrasions and lacerations. *Nursing Standard*, **15**(5), 41–44.

Smith and Nephew (2003) *Flamazine Cream*. Smith and Nephew. Available online at: http://wound.smith–nephew.com/uk/Category.asp?NodeId=2016.

Taylor, K. (2001) The management of minor burns and scalds in children. *Nursing Standard*, **16**(11), 45–51.

Thwaites, C.L. & Farrar, J.J. (2003) Preventing and treating tetanus. *British Medical Journal*, **326**(7381), 117–118.

Thomas, S. (1997) A Structured Approach to the Selection of Dressings. Available online at: www.smtl.co.uk/world-wide-wounds.

Thomas, S. (2002) *Surgical Materials Testing Lab Dressings Datacard – Flamazine*. Available online at: www.dressings.org/Dressings/flamazine.html.

Tortora, G.J. & Grabowski, S.R. (2003) *Principles of Anatomy and Physiology*, 10th edn. John Wiley and Sons, Hoboken, New Jersey.

Wardrope, J. & English, B. (1998) *Musculo-skeletal Problems in Emergency Medicine*. Oxford University Press, Oxford.

Wardrope, J. & Smith, J.A.R. (1992) *The Management of Wounds and Burns*. Oxford University Press, Oxford.

Waugh, A. & Grant, A. (2003) *Anatomy and Physiology in Health and Illness*, 9th edn. Churchill Livingstone, London.

World Wide Wounds (2002, updated 2003) Revision 1.2 *News Archive – July Wound Bed Preparation*. Available online at: www.worldwidewounds.com/News/News2002.html.

Young, S.J., Barnett, P.L. & Oakley, E.A. (2005) Bruising, abrasions and lacerations: minor injuries in children 1. *MJA Practice Essential Paediatrics*, **182**(11), 588–592.

Young, S. & South, M. (eds) (2003) *Major Paediatric Trauma – The Primary Survey*. Available online at: www.rch. unimelb.edu.au/clinicalguide/pages/trauma.php. Information regarding hard copies available from: Clinical Practice Guidelines of the Royal Children's Hospital, Melbourne, Australia. Child Health Information Centre, Royal Children's Hospital, Flemington Road Parkville Victoria 3052, Australia.

Chapter 7 The Principles of Assessment and Management of Pain in Children and Young People Attending an Emergency Department

Ann Rich

Introduction

Pain is a complex, subjective, elusive phenomenon. It is a unique human experience that is influenced by cultural learning, anxiety, and a multitude of cognitive, psychological and sociological factors. According to the Royal College of Paediatrics and Child Health (1997:1) 'uncontrolled pain has adverse effects on cardiovascular, respiratory, immunological and metabolic processes, as well as long term psychological effects that are not fully quantified but likely to be harmful'. Although there have been many advances in the assessment and management of children's pain since its emergence as an area of academic study 30 years ago, it remains a difficult area for staff to address in practice. It is a major area of concern within the emergency department as it is seen as a primary symptom that prompts people to seek medical attention and an integral part of the triage process (Manchester Triage Group 1997). This chapter will explore the nature of pain in children and young people and factors affecting its management. It will examine the physiological, psychological and socio-cultural elements of pain identified by Hayward (1975) in his seminal work on the study of pain. A review of pain assessment tools will be undertaken examining their appropriateness for children in the emergency setting. Pharmacological and non-pharmacological methods of pain management will be considered including the role of the emergency practitioner in this area of care.

Definitions of pain

Autton (1986) states that pain is 'a private personal experience common to all individuals, yet unique to each. It means significantly different things to different people, in terms of quality as well as quantity, and it is extremely difficult to define on account of its complex interactions'.

Many other early definitions of pain considered by Melzack and Wall (1996) rejected those that implied an exclusive relationship between pain and tissue damage, since this can occur in the absence of pain. Conversely pain can occur after tissue damage as in the case of sunburn, when it arrives too late to act as a warning. They favour the definition of pain proposed by The International Association for the Study of Pain (IASP) (1979) which defines pain as 'an unpleasant sensory and emotional experience associated with actual or potential tissue damage or described in terms of such damage'. This definition supports physical and psychological indicators of pain and fits in with the Gate Control Theory (Melzack & Wall 1996). One of the most popular definitions of pain is that by McCaffery and Beebe (1989, p. 15): 'Pain is whatever the experiencing person says it is, existing whenever he says it does.' This makes a statement about always believing the patient, but this presents difficulties when working with children, as they may not have either the verbal or cognitive ability to express their pain. The recent amendments to the IASP definition has acknowledged this aspect: 'The inability to communicate in no way negates the possibility that an individual is experiencing pain and is in need of appropriate pain relieving treatment' (IASP 2001: 2). It is essential therefore that pain is assessed objectively and managed effectively by emergency care practitioners.

What is pain?

Pain has physiological, psychological and sociological components, therefore an understanding of pain requires knowledge of all perspectives and how they interact.

Physiological aspects

Physiological responses are seen as good indicators of assessing pain, as they are objective and to some extent do not require the child or young person's cooperation. An elevation in vital signs is a visible physiological response, such as raised blood pressure, heart rate, respiratory rate, temperature; even sweating, vomiting, nausea and dilated pupils are all signs of pain being present. They are seen as less susceptible to a child's control and are therefore more objective, especially when trying to assess a child who has learned to control his or her facial expressions and crying after painful experiences. However they are similar to physiological signs of high anxiety levels and distress in children (Seyle 1976), so if used as pain assessment measures it is essential to ascertain whether the responses do actually reflect the child's pain experience.

Psychological aspects

The psychological aspect of pain can be a challenge especially in paediatric patients. Children with previous pain experience do not like to express their pain for fear of more treatment, such as unwanted medication or injections. Wallace (1989) sees temperament playing a part in the child's response to pain, and Warni (1990) describes pain as a complex 'cognitive developmental phenomenon', affected by such factors as anxiety, fear and separation. Children demonstrate a concept of pain that correlates with Piaget's stages of cognitive development and their pain experiences and perceptions of pain at different ages underline the importance of the individual stage of development and its influence on the physiological, psychological and experiential components of pain. Children learn to cope with pain through the diverse nature of their own pain experiences. Psychological factors such as situational and emotional factors that exist when children perceive pain may alter their pain perceptions so it is important that the practitioner should recognise this to enable them to manage pain in children and young people (McGrath 1990; Schechter 1989).

Sociological aspects

Just as there are physical and psychological components that influence our experience of pain there is also the sociological dimension. Gender, culture, religion, our society and our relationships will all contribute to our perception of pain (Zborowski 1952). The word pain is derived from the Latin word 'poena' that means punishment. It was once believed that pain was not due to physical injury but by offending the gods or being invaded by evil spirits. Within Western culture pain is often associated with punishment and wrongdoing and within other cultures pain may be inflicted at religious ceremonies (Melzack & Wall 1996). Children learn from their parents, society and their religion how to express and respond to pain and this may influence our behaviour in a painful situation. It is well documented that children observe and model themselves on their parents and modify fear, anxiety and distress accordingly (McGrath 1990). Alder (1990) gave an example of a boy who suppressed his pain experience in front of his father and then completely broke down when he was not present. This child was strongly influenced by what his father would think as he was raised in a society where 'men don't cry'. Within other cultures pain is expressed very differently with beliefs that it is natural to cry and moan when in pain, and this may lead an observer to believe that individuals have a low pain threshold. It is important for the practitioner to understand and acknowledge how different cultural backgrounds may impact on the perception and tolerance of pain.

Pain transmission

This can be discussed under three main headings: pain receptors, neuronal transmission and brain perception.

Pain receptors

Prior to a pain impulse being initiated the sensation of a harmful stimulus being applied is picked up by specialised pain receptors known as nociceptors, from the Greek word 'noci' meaning harmful. They consist of the nerve endings that represent the dendrites of sensory neurones whose cell bodies lie in the dorsal root ganglia of the spinal cord. They are present in the dermis, in muscles and joints, in the hollow parts of the gastrointestinal tract, in the walls of the arteries, and in the meninges. Once stimulated by trauma, chemicals such as substance P, bradykinin and the leukotrienes give rise to the sensation of pain (Carr & Mann 2000; McGrath 1990; Sofaer 1998).

Although the pain receptors respond to a number of different types of stimuli the perception does not depend on the strength of the stimulus but on the individual response to pain and also the psychological state. It is a not a rigid system that transfers a certain amount of pain from a constant stimulus; it has the capacity to respond differently to the same stimulus. For example, an injection will not produce the same amount of pain in all children. The system will also respond differently depending on the context in which the child receives the injection. In children who use a simple coping strategy such as squeezing a hand or helping to prepare the site it has been found they will generally experience less pain (Bernstein *et al.* 2000).

To cause pain a stimulus must reach threshold strength. The production of prostaglandins around the site of an inflamed area increases the sensitivity to pain. The sensation of pain is not lessened by prolonging the stimulus as is the case with other sensory receptors, in fact sensitisation may occur and an even smaller stimulus than the original one may elicit pain (McGrath 1990). Inhibiting the enzyme that produces prostaglandin through the use of anti-inflammatory drugs helps in the reduction of pain intensity, as does the use of opioids which are similar to the endogenous opioids produced by the body. These are morphine-like substances produced in response to painful stimuli, and the amount produced in each individual may vary, so this could also help to account for the fact that some individuals appear to have more pain than others following a similar injury.

Neuronal transmission

There are two main sensory nerves involved in relaying the pain stimulus back to the spinal cord and brain. For an individual to sense pain, a nerve impulse must be initiated in nerve endings, then pass along specific nerve fibres to the spinal cord where it travels to the area in the brain responsible for sensation of pain (Carr & Mann 2000). There are three types of nerve fibres, A delta (Ad) fibres and the smaller C fibres that carry pain sensation, and A beta (Ab) fibres that carry sensations that are not normally painful, for example warmth and touch.

Ad fibres are large (first pain) fibres that transmit quickly and result in an instant reflex response and a rapid withdrawal from the pain source, such as removing a hand quickly if it touches a hot iron. Pain is instant, sharp and localised and acts as a protective mechanism. From the dorsal horn in the spinal cord the fibres cross to the other side of the cord and travel to the thalamus and somato-sensory areas of the cortex. These fibres are also responsible for pin-prick sensation. There are no receptors on their surface, so the use of an opioid drug such as morphine has little value in providing pain relief, and the child may still jump with pain as the pain sensors remain intact. Morphine may help to make a person more comfortable but localised tenderness and pain sensation is present around the inflamed area, for example an appendix.

C fibres (second pain) are small diameter non-myelinated fibres that conduct pain impulses more slowly and are responsible for the dull, burning, aching, throbbing type of pain. They continue from the substantia gelatinosa of the spinal cord and terminate over a wide area within the brain stem carrying pain, thermal and pressure impulses. Pain sensation can be subdued by use of opioids so that it is on the C fibres that local anaesthetics work and block this type of pain (Nie & Hunter 1988). Prolonged stimulation of C fibres can lead to sensitisation.

A beta (Ab) fibres, concentrated in the skin, fast track to the brain on the same side. They are rapidly conducting and are activated by touch and sensation. Although not directly related to pain transmission, they are significant in our understanding of the gate control theory to be discussed later in this chapter.

The brain and pain perception

Once a pain impulse travels through, it is transmitted to the brain via the spinothalamic tract. The thalamus is an area of grey matter situated deep in the forebrain; it is capable of recognising pain but not interpreting it. At the level of the thalamus some of the second neurones synapse so impulses go to other regions of the cerebral cortex. It acts as a relay station sending impulses to the cerebral cortex where the pain is interpreted and its source is localised (Hinchliff & Montague 1988). It is possible that this may explain why it is possible to analyse the pain that is being experienced in the light of previous experience and to express an emotional response to it.

Theories of pain

There have been several theories to explain the process of pain and here we will consider three theories: specificity theory, pattern theory and gate control theory.

Specificity theory

This theory proposed by Descartes in 1664 suggests that there are special nerve pathways that carry pain impulses, received by specialised pain receptors to a nerve centre in the brain. It is further suggested that the pain is a specific response and that the intensity of pain relates to the severity of the damage. A minor injury will cause minimum pain and major trauma will cause maximum pain. This theory takes no account of the psychological influences on pain perception, but it is important to recognise that this theory provides the basis for surgery in cases of intractable pain (McGrath 1990).

Pattern theory

In this theory it is believed that pain is interpreted by the sensory cortex as a result of the particular patterns of pain impulses that are present. It is thought to be the quantity of the stimulation rather than the quality that accounts for the perception of different painful sensations. A small amount of stimulation (rubbing) may lead to the perception of warmth, whereas stronger stimulation of the same kind (friction) may result in pain.

Gate control

Melzack and Wall's (1996) gate control theory proposes that the transmission of pain impulses from primary afferent fibres to spinal cord transmission cells from which the impulses travel to the cerebral cortex, could be 'gated' to facilitate or inhibit such transmission. A beta fibres, activated by touch and sensation, are said to close the imaginary 'gate'. The gating mechanism is in the dorsal horn of the spinal cord through which peripheral information passes. The gating mechanism consists of two types of neurone: SC cell and T cell. T cells transmit information about pain whereas SC cells inhibit. Once a pain stimulus is initiated it brings about the release of a transmitter substance called substance P (SP) which is responsible for generating the pain impulse (Francis 1987). The two fibres carry the impulse to the substantia gelatinosa from where the impulse is transmitted to the thalamus unless the 'gate' is closed and impulses cannot get through. Touch impulses will normally act to close the 'gate' unless the volume of pain is so great that the gate is forced open.

Many factors may influence this gating system, which allows diminished or exaggerated effects of the nociceptive messages to pass to the brain, where they will eventually produce reaction, sensation and movement. A major part of the gate control theory is *central control*, referring to the influence that the higher centres of the brain have on pain perception. Activities such as anxiety, excitement, anticipation and previous experiences increase the perception of pain, while distraction, relaxation and sensory input close the gate preventing sensory transmission influencing how the individual perceives the pain impulse (Melzack & Wall 1999). This theory suggests that both physiological and psychological factors can affect pain perception and allows the possibility of alternative options such as guided imagery and distraction to address effective pain management. The gate control theory may help to explain why 'rubbing it better', a phrase frequently used by mothers to their children, is not simply an old wives' tale, as it may reduce the sensation of pain as the touch stimulus may close the gate (Carter 1994).

Scenario 1

Joshua, 3 years old, is playing on the bouncy castle with his older sister, Lauren, when he slips through the opening onto the concrete and hurts his leg. He cries and his father picks him up, cuddles him and rubs his sore leg gently but firmly. This stimulates the fast acting Ab fibres that synapse in the substantia gelatinosa and prevent the pain impulses getting through. By distracting Joshua with cuddles and attention it helps with the management of pain.

This theory is widely accepted as it takes account of both the physiological and psychological dimensions/aspects of pain. Despite increased knowledge of the physiology of pain leading to greater understanding of the process, and the analgesic effect of endogenous opiates, there is little evidence that the knowledge gained has been put into use in clinical practice. It is clear that although some physiological changes do occur in direct response to a painful stimulus, other changes may occur as a result of the child's stress.

Children in the emergency department

Most children attending emergency departments will be experiencing pain and for some it may be their first experience of pain and a strange environment, resulting in a great deal of anxiety and distress (Atherton 1995; Moorcombe 1998). Pain in children has been categorised into a number of areas and we will briefly examine these as they account for a number of children who attend the emergency department.

Acute pain

This follows on very quickly from the delivery of the stimulus, and although the strength of pain is generally proportional to the intensity of the stimulation, it can be altered by many other factors in addition to the nature and extent of the wound. Children experience two types of acute pain; the first caused by accidents as they go about their normal activities, and the second caused by invasive procedures during medical or dental treatments. Often children admitted to emergency departments have sustained acute trauma injuries and are then subject to painful procedures such as suturing, or cleansing of a wound.

Pain that occurs during normal play activities, generally does not create undue distress, but that experienced during medical treatments is viewed differently (McGrath 1990). Research by Eland and Anderson (1977), and Fowler-Kerry and Lander (1987) demonstrated that young children often described repeated invasive procedures as more distressing than any other aspect of treatment. Schechter (1989) found that children do not always understand the reason for procedures, especially if they do not feel ill and they may feel powerless in certain situations. These factors may lead to increased fear and anxiety for some children, so the practitioner needs to understand how children develop concepts relating to pain and give appropriate explanations and reassurance to the child and family.

Recurrent pain

This occurs in a large number of children who do not suffer from an underlying disease but have a history of unpredictable episodes of pain when they present in the emergency department. McGrath (1990) found that over 30% of otherwise healthy children experience headaches or abdominal pains. The children's episodes vary in frequency, sometimes daily on a regular basis then nothing for weeks. Others develop pains on a weekly or monthly basis and there appears to be no pattern. Early studies by Schechter (1984) have shown that for some children the onset may coincide with a major life trauma, death in the family, moving house, birth of a baby or starting a new school, but in most cases there are no precipitating factors.

Chronic pain

The third category, chronic pain, is long-lasting pain, persisting beyond the time for healing an injury, or it may be evoked by disease or psychological factors. It is by definition difficult and at times impossible to relieve. The most common chronic pains in children are those that are associated with disease, and when children are suffering pain they may either be treated and discharged or admitted to an acute area for further assessment and management (McGrath 1990).

Pain and its assessment

The National Service Framework for Children (DoH 2000) offers principles on which pain care should be based and emergency care departments are highlighted as an area which requires specific focus. While it is an essential element to assess and manage children's pain, it is one of the major difficulties facing the emergency practitioner. As indicated earlier, pain management always proved problematic, due to myths and misconceptions, the subjective nature of pain, and may be further complicated by the child's inability or unwillingness to express pain either through lack of cognition, physical or mental impairment, severity of illness, anxiety, culture or fear of painful procedures. Within the setting each child will be triaged, and ideally their pain is assessed; however no single approach would provide sufficient information on the level of pain and its subsequent management for children and young people due to the subjective and complex nature of the phenomenon (Franck *et al.* 2000).

Assessment

Assessment has been described as a judgement of worth or importance and assessment of pain as the understanding of the pain experience and working towards managing the child's pain (McCaffery & Beebe 1989; McGrath & Unruh 1987). Recognition of children's pain is not straightforward, although according to Carter (1994), and Craft and Denehy (1990), children will identify

the location and severity of their pain if they are given the right encouragement. They need to be asked about it, though, as they will not always volunteer the information (Franck *et al.* 2000). The Royal College of Nursing (RCN) (1999) Clinical Practice Guidelines on the recognition of acute pain in children urge health professionals to understand their own values and beliefs around pain, thereby reducing their influence on assessment.

The Manchester Triage Group (1997) examined the variety of ways emergency care was prioritised within all emergency departments in the United Kingdom, and presented algorithms as a triage decision making tool for the allocation of clinical priority in emergency settings and part of this process involves assessment of every patient's pain. Within the emergency setting, a child's pain may be assessed by an experienced practitioner with or without using a specific tool at triage, as even young children may be able to indicate levels of pain if the right techniques are used (Hammers *et al.* 1994; LaFleur & Raway 1999). A number of assessment tools could be used, from a visual analogue scale to others developed specifically for the young child, such as a simple descriptive scale, the faces scale and a numerical scale. As it is essential that the assessment accurately reflects the child's pain a specific research based tool that addresses all aspects of the pain experience should be sought. An examination of the literature on pain assessment tools indicates that they are based on the three major approaches to pain assessment, namely cognitive, behavioural, and physiological and we will review their usefulness in the next section (RCN 1990; RCN Institute 1999).

Pain assessment tools

Self-reports in the form of verbal responses and questionnaires can be described as cognitive techniques, and rely on the child's ability to communicate their feelings and the images they have of their pain. It can be argued that self-report is of the most value because it allows subjective reporting and provides important information about the quality, nature, duration and intensity of the pain, but by its nature it is descriptive and qualitative, not measuring the pain objectively (McGrath 1990). Verbal reports are often seen to be unreliable in the younger child due to limitations with language. A variety of faces scales have been developed to allow assessment of the younger pre-operational child who is unable to quantify, abstract or symbolise. These include a series of numbered cartoon faces with a range of expressions from smiling broadly to crying inconsolably, which could express mood/ happiness rather than pain (Wong & Baker 1988). An adapted cartoon version of the faces scale (Wong & Baker 1988) has proved to be the most popular of its type of self-report, and its simplicity of use and speed of result, could make it an ideal integral part of a multi-dimensional tool.

The Oucher (Beyer 1984) was a further development from the faces scale, using photographs of real faces with expressions ranging from obvious distress to neutral. Three different versions of this scale are available, using the photographs of European-American, Afro-American, and Hispanic children. The Oucher and faces tools demonstrate facial expressions of acute but not chronic pain. The ideal approach to using the Oucher is introducing it to the child when that child is neither anxious nor in pain, and this is obviously not a feasible proposition with the child arriving in acute pain in an emergency department, with all the accompanying fear and anxiety brought about by a strange environment.

The colour scale (Eland 1990) provides information on the level of a child's pain, as well as the location of the pain. A front and back body outline is provided, with eight coloured crayons for the child to select which colours signify their pain. It will capture a child's interest, and besides being fun to do, it will provide an opportunity for the child to report the nature of their pain. This tool might not be suitable within the paediatric accident and emergency department for children arriving in acute pain, because it is time consuming to do, and can be difficult to understand for the child who does not relate colour and pain.

The pre-pubescent or adolescent child is capable of using scales similar to those used by adults, and pain questionnaires can provide a wide range of data, not simply focusing on pain intensity. The Comprehensive Pain Questionnaire (CCPQ) (McGrath *et al.* 1985a) is a structured interview with quantitative pain scales, and consists of generated and supplied format questions with Visual Analogue Scale (VAS) and facial affective scales to assess the various dimensions of the child's pain experience. The CCPQ has evidence of satisfactory reliability and validity in the assessment of children with chronic or recurrent pain. Although these tools can provide a comprehensive view on which to base subsequent care, their use within an emergency department would be impractical, as they would incorporate individual interviews with each child, which would be too time-consuming (Rowley 2002).

Infants, children and young people fall into different categories in behavioural assessment due to their levels of maturation and cognition and various tools have been developed incorporating specific distress behaviours to define and describe pain in neonates and infants (Carter 1994). It is often difficult to differentiate pain-related behaviour from behaviour resulting from other forms of distress, and although the behaviours measured are suggestive of pain, they are not definitely indicative. Cry, facial expression, posture, rigidity of the torso and body movements are measured, though other behaviours such as poor sleep patterns, decreased activity, mood changes and lack of social interplay, may also be indications of distress, caused by pain (Carter 1994).

The Children's Hospital of Eastern Ontario Pain Scale (CHEOPS, McGrath *et al.* 1985a), among others, identified patterns of behaviour cry, facial expression, verbalising, movements of torso and legs, gives a systematic assessment structure, and provides documentation of pain. Its use within a busy clinical setting is restricted by the lengthy and cumbersome scoring system.

The faces, legs, activity, cry, consolability (FLACC) tool also provides a simple, consistent method for all members of the multi-professional team to identify, document and evaluate pain, and could be incorporated with ease into an existing pain assessment tool. Behavioural tools are practical, because they do not rely on the ability or desire of the child to communicate, although some may have a limited use because they have been developed from behaviours associated with specific situations (McGrath *et al.* 1985b).

Physiological signs can also be used to assess whether a child is in pain. These include assessment of heart rate, respiratory rate, blood pressure and oxygen saturation levels. Physiological assessment is particularly valuable in infants and young children or those unable to communicate verbally (Coffman *et al.* 1997). Care needs to be taken that the changes are not due to anxiety, or crying, so if possible should be used in conjunction with other tools when assessing pain.

The paediatric pain assessment tool developed by The Manchester Triage Group (1997) is a multi-dimensional tool, combining a verbal self-report, wide descriptors and visual analogue scales with a numerical scale (0–5) together with colours, red being immediate priority and excruciating pain to blue dictating minor injury with no pain which follows the triage criteria for prioritising the severity of pain (Manchester Triage Group 1997). These factors are blended into a pain ruler or ladder, presenting higher intensities of pain as higher rungs on the ladder, and can be used by a wide range of ages, including young people and adults. Beyer and Wells (1989) and Hester *et al.* (1990) examined the validity of a ladder scale, and found it applicable to a wide age range, but that it was not well validated in children. In practice, this tool has proven to be very effective in assessing children's pain and the addition of the cartoon faces, which increases its age rangeability, makes it a multi-dimensional pain assessment tool. It is quick and easy to administer and score, an essential requirement in an emergency department and based on a number of valid and reliable tools has the potential to become a useful tool for the emergency practitioner.

The challenge of managing pain with paediatric patients

Ascertaining the level of pain that a person may be experiencing is one of the most common and difficult tasks for practitioners to accomplish. Accurate and appropriate means of assessment are clearly a fundamental need in the management of infant pain (McCarthy *et al.* 2000). It is suggested in both medical and nursing literature that the reason behind inadequate pain relief in children is the beliefs of the staff (Collier 1997; Ely 2001; Gay 1992; McGrath & Unruh 1987; Moor 2001; Schechter 1989). These beliefs are often referred to as 'pain myths' and according to Schechter (1989) are at the core of under-treatment of pain in children. Eland (1985) identifies ten inconsistencies facing the nurse dealing with a child in pain, and Burr (1987, 1993) reports on 12 common misconceptions which inhibit good practice in paediatric pain management. Part of the problem arises from the way children react to pain at varying ages, dependent on their cognitive ability, thus an active child may be demonstrating a coping strategy to deal with pain, and a quiet, sleeping child may be exhausted, due to persistent pain. Schechter (1989) identifies that infants and toddlers do remember painful procedures, demonstrating changes in sleeping patterns and inability to feed, following a painful experience. Anand and Hickey (1987) dispel the notion that infants and children do not feel pain because they are neurologically immature, demonstrating that pain pathways and cortical centres are well developed late in gestation. There is also a need for individual assessment of pain, without the assumption of preconceived ideas of injury indicative of particular pain.

The focus often in emergency departments is stabilisation of a critically ill child or young person; therefore it may not be possible to medicate a child, due to their status. There are however other factors that are put forward for the under-treatment of pain in children, such as the many myths and misconceptions about paediatric pain, the most common myth being that children's experience of pain is not as severe as that of adults (Melzack & Wall 1999; Twycross 1997; Read 1994). One myth, that of the fear of respiratory depression if children are given opiates when the risk is no greater than that of adults (McCaffery & Beebe 1989), could lead to a child or young person not getting satisfactory pain relief and a violation of their human rights (Franck 1989; Rich 2000).

Non-pharmacological methods

Many non-pharmacological strategies can easily be used in the emergency setting without extra teaching; it is essential therefore that practitioners are cognisant with the benefits of the approach (Salentera *et al.* 1999). According to McCaffery and Beebe (1989), being active or playing may act as a distraction from pain for a child. Emergency care provision could include the use of a play specialist, and other members of staff who develop skills so play can be used as a form of therapy and distraction (Chen *et al.* 2000). Moorcombe (1998) believes this should be supplemented with child friendly surroundings, simple distraction techniques actively encouraging and supporting the families in the management of their child's pain. Eland (1990) found that parents seeing their child in pain found they were unable to assist in the management of their child's pain as they were dealing with their own stress and anxiety. However, many parents who were encouraged 'to cuddle and rub and kiss it better' found it helped them to be involved. It distracted the child so pain was put at the periphery of awareness with attention focused on the distracter and not the pain.

Children themselves have indicated that they found parental presence an excellent distracter from things that hurt, and found that they helped in the reduction of anxiety and pain levels (Polkki *et al.* 2003). The practitioner would need to ensure that parents are adequately prepared to support their child through a painful procedure otherwise it could be counterproductive. Children are usually distressed on admission to an emergency department particularly if they have seen a gaping wound or need sutures. They need calm emotional support as well as appropriate management of pain during treatment.

Children should be helped to feel in control of the situation as this reduces the anxiety and distress associated with the hospital visit (Bernstein *et al.* 2000). There should be no punitive measures imposed for non-cooperative behaviour, but cooperation rewarded with toys, prizes, stickers etc. Zeltzer *et al.* (1990), who undertook a study on children undergoing short medical procedures, found that children perceived coping with the procedure a challenge ending with a reward for achievement.

Scenario 2

Harry, aged 4, fell against the edge of the coffee table and sustained a laceration just above his right eyebrow. He was not knocked out when he fell. At triage following an assessment of pain, Harry told the practitioner he did not want any medicine, as it didn't hurt cause Mummy had 'kissed it better'. Harry and his Mum were told it would be cleaned and closed with Steri-strips and he was again offered pain relief. He refused and Mum said she usually just kissed scrapes and bruises better and he just carried on playing after a cuddle. While his face was cleaned Harry was held by his Mum who stroked and talked to him telling him his favourite story. When it was finished he went home with his Mum, happily clutching a bravery certificate.

When using distraction techniques a number of factors must be considered, the primary one being that it must be appealing to the child. It must also engage a child appropriate to her/his level of understanding, and be consistent with the child's energy level and ability to concentrate at that time (Hodges 1998). Muscle relaxation can be achieved through exercises, blowing bubbles, blowing up balloons and therapeutic touch. Keeping a supply of play equipment in the emergency setting should be regarded as essential equipment. Providing age appropriate information before a procedure has been shown to be effective in reducing behavioural stress. An understanding of child development is essential to develop specific communication skills. Encouraging relaxation should decrease anxiety and therefore lead to an increase in pain tolerance, a useful strategy for reducing anticipatory anxiety. Suggest using the child's past experience as a positive statement about the anticipated event asking them to repeat to themselves 'I've had this done before and it wasn't that bad'. The role of complementary therapies such as reflexology and aromatherapy could be used but it would require staff to undergo training (Carter 1994; Twycross 1998).

Pharmacological management of pain

Based on the pain assessment, appropriate analgesics should be given to control pain and it should be appropriate for the severity of the pain. According to Morton (1998) a multi-modal approach using local and regional analgesia, opiates, non-steroidal anti-inflammatory drugs (NSAIDs) and paracetamol is particularly useful with children, and with their range of actions and potencies, should be flexible and sensitive enough to meet a child's individual needs (Moriarty 1998). Drugs can be administered using several routes: orally, rectally, by patient controlled analgesia (PCA), intravenously, by epidural and subcutaneously (Howard 2003; Lloyd Thomas 1993; Morton 1998). Ideally, analgesia should be easy and painless to administer, have a rapid onset of action and predictable effective analgesic properties without side-effects. The choice of method and route will depend on many factors such as the intensity of pain, whether a child is vomiting, if venous access is a problem, the child's age and the views of the child and parent.

Route of administration can determine the rate of onset of action and the acceptability of the drug to child and family, an example of this being paracetamol given orally as it is familiar and less threatening to a child. Paracetamol is thought to inhibit prostaglandin synthesis, therefore, as explained earlier, pain intensity is decreased. Paracetamol does not have a strong effect at the peripheral level so does not produce gastric irritation nor affect platelet function. It is useful for non-inflammatory pain such as a headache. The disadvantage in oral administration is the delayed rate of pain relief and its variable absorption in comparison with the intravenous route (Paris 1987; Read 1994). The use of rectal administration, which has a higher absorption rate, could be more beneficial but this has become less acceptable to both parents and children as it is seen as invasive, and health professionals are in agreement. Selbst and Henritig (1989) describe paracetamol as an excellent analgesic for mild pain believing its efficacy in mild to moderate pain should not be underestimated. Parents may be content because they are used to seeing its therapeutic effects; on the other hand they may have greater expectations

in relation to pain relief and feel that something more potent should be administered.

The administration of an NSAID anti-inflammatory drug such as diclofenac, which can be used for mild to moderate pain, works by inhibiting the enzyme cyclo-oxygenase which is responsible for the production of prostaglandin. By inhibiting prostaglandin production, pain intensity is decreased. It does however block all the enzymes including those needed for the protection of the stomach and small intestine, as well as the chemicals that maintain renal function and platelet adhesion. They are very effective for mild to moderate pain and when given with an opioid they provide additional analgesia and reduce the need for large doses of analgesia. They are of particular benefit to those experiencing excessive prostaglandin release post surgery.

Opioids such as codeine or morphine with their origins in the opium poppy, have powerful effects on moderate to severe pain. They act by binding to the opioid receptors and activate them, behaving in much the same way as endogenous encephalins. Morphine is considered the so-called 'gold standard' by which all other pain relieving drugs are used. According to Carr and Mann (2000) a dose of oral morphine will produce rapid and adequate analgesia, with fewer side-effects than a larger dose of a weaker opioid, and it is particularly effective in children. According to Broadbent (2000) there is no evidence that the short-term administration of opiates to children can cause addiction but this is frequently used as a reason for withholding opioid analgesia (McCaffery & Robinson 2002; McGrath 1996).

Conclusion

The importance of pain assessment has been identified, and the responsibility for the assessment of pain could be said to lie with the multi-professional team, the child and the parents/carers. A child may become disempowered in the emergency department as a result of pain, fear, the strange environment, lack of understanding and behavioural changes in their parents. Parents may also be disempowered through loss of control, sudden onset of the illness and changes in the child's behaviour. Communicating with the child and their parents is an essential part of pain management. Managing pain effectively involves the whole multidisciplinary team who should ensure that health professionals provide a child-friendly environment and work in partnership with the parents to give the best possible care to the child with mutual respect and recognition of each other's contribution. Accurate assessment and management of the child's acute pain experience will empower the child to uphold their human rights, as managing a child's pain effectively is an ethical imperative. In order to manage paediatric pain effectively, the practitioner has to be able to communicate with the rest of the multiprofessional team, and a focus on the holistic approach to child and family by the whole team will lead to quality of care and effective pain relief.

References

Alder, S. (1990) Taking children at their word. *Professional Nurse*, **5**(8), 397–402.

Anand, K.J.S. & Hickey, P.R. (1987) Pain and its effects in the human neonate and fetus. *New England Journal of Medicine*, **317**, 1321–1329.

Atherton, T. (1995) Children's experiences of pain in an Accident and Emergency department. *Accident and Emergency Nursing*, **3**, 79–82.

Autton, N. (1986) *Pain on exploration*. Longman and Todd Dorton, London.

Bernstein, D.A. Clarke-Stewart, A. & Penner, L.A. (2000) *Psychology*. Houghton Mifflin, Boston, Mass.

Beyer, J.E. (1984) *The Oucher: a users' manual and technical report*. Judson Press, Evanston, Ill.

Beyer, J. & Wells, N. (1989) The assessment of pain in children. *Pediatric Clinics of North America*, **36**, 837–854.

Broadbent, C. (2000) The pharmacology of acute pain. *Nursing Times*, **96**(26), 39–41.

Burr, S. (1987) Pain in childhood. *Nursing*, **3**(24), 890–896.

Burr, S. (1993) Myths in practice. *Nursing Standard*, **7**(25), 4–5.

Carr, E.C.J. & Mann, E.M. (2000) *Pain: creative approaches to effective management*. Macmillan Press, Basingstoke.

Carter, B. (1994) *Child and Infant Pain: principles of nursing care and management*. Chapman and Hall, London.

Chen, E., Joseph, M. & Zeltzer, L. (2000) Behavioral and cognitive interventions in the treatment of pain in children. *Pediatric Clinics of North America*, **47**, 513–25.

Coffman, S., Alvarez, Y. & Pyngolil, M. (1997) Nursing assessment and management of pain in critically ill children. *Heart and Lung*, **26**(3), 221–228.

Collier, J. (1997) Attitudes to children's pain: exploding the 'Pain Myth'. *Paediatric Nursing*, **9**(15), 15–18.

Craft, M. & Denehy, J. (1990) *Nursing interventions for infants and children*. Saunders, Philadelphia.

Department of Health (2000) *The National Service Framework for Children*. DoH, London.

Eland, E. (1985) Myths about pain in children. *The Candlelighters*. Childhood Cancer Foundation V (1).

Eland, J. (1990) Pain in children. *Nursing Clinics of North America*, **25**(4), 871–884.

Eland, J.M. & Anderson, J.E. (1977) The experience of pain in children. In: A. Jacox (ed) *Pain: A Source Book for Nurses and Other Health Care Professionals*. Little Brown (Inc.), Boston, Mass.

Ely, B. (2001) Pediatric nurses' pain management: barriers to change. *Pediatric Nursing*, **27**(5), 273–280.

Fowler-Kerry, S. & Lander, J.S. (1987) Management of injection pain in children. *Pain*, **30**, 167–175.

Francis, I. (1987) The physiology of pain. In: J. Boore, R. Champlen & M. Ferguson (eds) *Nursing and the Physically Ill Adult*. Churchill Livingstone, London.

Franck, L.S. (1989) The ethical imperative to treat pain in infants: are we doing the best we can? *Neonatal Intensive Care*, **11**(5), 28–34.

Franck, L.S., Greenberg, C.S. & Stevens, B. (2000) Pain assessment in infants and young children. *Pediatric Clinics of North America*, **43**(3), 487–512.

Gay, J. (1992) A painful experience. *Nursing Times*, **88**(25), 32–35.

Hammers, J.P.H., Abu-Saad, H.H., Halfens, R.J.G. & Schumacher, J.N.M. (1994) Factors influencing nurses' pain assessment and interventions in children. *Journal of Advanced Nursing*, **20**, 853–860.

Hayward, J. (1975) *Information – a prescription against pain*. RCN, London.

Hester, N.O., Foster, R. & Kristensen, K. (1990) Measurement of pain in children: generalizability and validity of the pain ladder and the poker chip tool. In: D.C. Tyler & E.J. Krane (eds) *Pediatric Pain: Advances in pain research and therapy*, Vol. 15. Raven Press, New York. pp. 79–84.

Hinchliff, S. & Montague, S. (eds) (1988) *Physiology for Nursing Practice*. Bailliere Tindall, London.

Hodges, C. (1998) Easing children's pain. *Nursing Times*, **94**(10), 31–33.

Howard, R. (2003) Acute pain management in children. In: D. Rowbotham & P. MacIntyre (eds) *Clinical Pain Management: acute pain*. Arnold, London. pp. 437–62.

International Association for the Study of Pain (1979) Subcommittee on taxonomy. Pain Terms: A List of Definitions and Notes on Usage. *Pain*, **6**, 249–252.

International Association for the Study of Pain (2001) IASP definition of pain. *IASP Newsletter*, **2**, 2.

LaFleur, C. & Raway, B. (1999) School age child and adolescent perception of the pain intensity associated with three word descriptors. *Pediatric Nursing*, **25**(1), 45–55.

Lloyd Thomas, A.R. (1993) Postoperative pain control in children. *Current Paediatrics*, **3**, 234–237.

Manchester Triage Group (1997) *Emergency Triage*. BMJ Publishing Group, London.

McCaffery, M. & Beebe, A.B. (1989) *Pain: Clinical Manual for Nursing Practice*. Mosby, St Louis.

McCaffery, M. & Robinson, E.S. (2002) Your patient is in pain – here's how you respond. *Nursing*, **32**(10), 36–45.

McCarthy, C., Hewitt, S. & Choonara, I. (2000) Pain in young children attending an Accident and Emergency department. *Journal of Accident and Emergency Medicine*, **17**, 265–267.

McGrath, P.J. (1990) *Pain in Children*. Guildford Press, New York.

McGrath, P.J. (1996) Attitudes and beliefs about medication and pain management in children. *Journal of Palliative Care*, **12**(3), 46–50.

McGrath, P.J. & Unruh, A.M. (1987) *Pain in Children and Adolescents*. Elsevier, Amsterdam.

McGrath, P.J., Deveber, L.L. & Hearn, M.T. (1985a) Multi-dimensional pain assessment in children. *Advantages in Pain Research and Therapy*, **9**, 387–393.

McGrath, P.J., Johnson, G., Goodman, J.T., Schillinger, J., Dunn, J. & Chapman, J. (1985b) CHEOPS: A behavioural scale for rating postoperative pain in children. In: H.L. Fields *et al.* (eds) *Advances in Pain Research and Therapy*, Vol 9. Raven Press, New York.

Melzack, R. & Wall, P.D. (1996) *The Challenge of Pain*. Penguin, Harmondsworth.

Melzack, R. & Wall, P.D. (1999) *Textbook of Pain*, 4th edn. Churchill Livingstone, Edinburgh.

Moor, R. (2001) Pain Assessment in a Children's A&E: A Critical Analysis. *Paediatric Nursing*, **13**(2), 20–24.

Moorcombe, J. (1998) Reducing anxiety in children in A&E. *Emergency Nurse*, **6**(2), 10–13.

Moriarty, A. (1998) The pharmacological management of acute pain. In: Twycross, A., Moriarty, A. & Betts, T. (eds) *Paediatric Pain Management: a multidisciplinary approach*. Radcliffe Medical Press, Oxford.

Morton, N.S. (1998) Prevention and control of pain in children. *Pain Reviews*, **5**, 1–15.

Nie, V. & Hunter, M. (1988) The central nervous system. In: Hinchliff, S. & Montague, S. (eds) *Physiology for Nursing Practice*. Bailliere Tindall, London.

Paris, P.M. (1987) Pain Management of the Child. *Emergency Medicine Clinics of North America*, **5**, 699–706.

Polkki, T., Pietila, P. & Vehvilamen-Julkunem, K. (2003) Hospitalized Children's descriptions of their experiences with post surgical pain relieving methods. *International Journal of Nursing Studies*, **40**, 33–44.

Read, J.V. (1994) Perceptions of Nurses and Physicians Regarding Pain Management of Pediatric Emergency Room Patients. *Pediatric Nursing*, **20**(3), 314–318.

Rich, B.A. (2000) An ethical analysis of the barriers to effective pain management. *Cambridge Quarterly of Health Care Ethics*, **9**, 54–70.

Rowley, H. (2002) *Pain management in children attending A&E*. Unpublished BSc thesis, University of Greenwich, UK.

Royal College of Nursing (1999) *The Recognition and Assessment of Acute Pain in Children; Recommendations*. RCN Publishing, London.

Royal College of Nursing (1990) *Nursing Children in the Accident and Emergency Department*. RCN Publishing, London.

Royal College of Paediatrics and Child Health (RCPCH) (1997) *Prevention and Control of Pain in Children: a manual for health care professionals*. BMJ Publishing Group, London.

Salantera, S., Lauri, S., Salmi, T.T. & Helenius, H. (1999) Nurses' knowledge about pharmacological and non-pharmacological pain management in children. *Journal of Pain and Symptom Management*, **18**(4), 289–299.

Schechter, N.L. (1984) Recurrent pains in children: an overview and an approach. *Pediatric Clinics of North America*, **31**, 949–968.

Schechter, N.L. (1989) The under treatment of pain in children: an overview. *Pediatric Clinics of North America*, **36**(4), 781–794.

Selbst, S.M. & Henritig, F.M. (1989) Treatment of pain in the emergency room department. *Pediatric Clinics of North America*, **36**, 965–989.

Seyle, H. (1976) *The stress of life*. McGraw-Hill, New York.

Sofaer, B. (1998) *Pain: principles practice and patients*, 3rd edn. Stanley Thornes, London.

Twycross, A. (1997) Nurses' perceptions of pain in children. *Paediatric Nursing*, **9**(1), 16–17.

Twycross, A. (1998) Children's cognitive level and their perception of pain. *Paediatric Nursing*, **10**(3), 24–27.

Wallace, M. (1989) Temperament: a variable in children's pain management. *Pediatric Nursing*, **15**, 118–21.

Warni, J.W. (1990) Behavioral management of pain in children. In: D.C. Tyler & E.J. Krane (eds) *Advances in Pain Research and Therapy* Vol 15. Raven Press, New York. pp. 215–234.

Wong, D.L. & Baker, C.M. (1988) Pain in children: comparison of assessment scales. *Pediatric Nursing*, **14**, 9–17.

Zborowski, M. (1952) Cultural components in responses to pain. *Journal of Social Issues*, **8**, 16–30.

Zeltzer, L., Merson, C.M. & Schechter, N.L. (1990) Paediatric pain: current status and new directions. *Current Problems in Paediatrics*, **20**, 415–486.

Chapter 8 Emergency Care of the Critically Ill or Seriously Injured Child

Karen Chandler, Gill McEwing and Janet Kelsey

Introduction

A quarter of all patients attending emergency departments are children. Of these children 15–20% will be critically ill resulting from either an acute medical problem requiring urgent intervention or serious injury (DoH 2003; Royal College of Paediatrics and Child Health 1999; Salter & Maconchie 2004; Watson 2000). Children requiring emergency care have unique and special needs, and especially those with serious and life threatening emergencies. The functional survival of a critically ill and/or seriously injured child is influenced by timely and appropriate intervention. Effective management of paediatric emergencies may well prevent deterioration in respiratory and circulatory function regardless of the initiating event (European Resuscitation Council (ERC) 2005). Furthermore, whilst the safest way for a critically ill and injured child to travel to the emergency department is by ambulance, as Flaherty and Glasper (2006) note, only 6% travel this way. Children in critical conditions often arrive by private car, taxi or public transport. It is therefore important that emergency department staff are aware that critically ill and/or injured children are often carried into the department and in light of this should receive early triage and assessment of their condition (Flaherty and Glasper 2006; Royal College of Paediatrics and Child Health 2004; Royal College of Surgeons and the British Orthopaedic Association 2000).

This chapter is concerned with the child requiring urgent intervention in the emergency department. A definition of critical illness as applied to children will be given. Recognition of the deteriorating child will be discussed along with assessment and treatment decisions. The chapter will provide the evidence base for the assessment

required to ensure a critically ill child can be recognised quickly and the management required to prevent further deterioration. The chapter will initially discuss the intervention and management of the child with an acute illness and then consider the specific issues related to the seriously injured child.

Critical illness is characterised by acute loss of physiological reserve (Aylott 2006). It is defined as a derangement in physiology with the potential to result in significant morbidity and mortality without prompt and appropriate invasive and therapeutic intervention (Hazinski 1992). A wide variety of disease may lead to critical illness but the fundamental interventions required are limited. The course of illness may be prolonged and the underlying cause difficult to discern. However, the common pathway of deterioration in critical illness occurs as a result of progressive deterioration of respiratory and circulatory function with respiratory failure or shock as the pathological expression. The final denominator is cardiopulmonary failure (Advanced Life Support Group (ALSG) 2004; Aylott 2006).

Physiologically children are different from adults as they are more susceptible to illness because of their underdeveloped immune system. The onset of illness is often sudden and deterioration rapid and they do not tolerate extremes of heat, fluid and electrolyte loss, infection and tissue injury. Children tend to have secondary cardiorespiratory arrest, usually due to the body's immaturity and inability to cope with the underlying illness/injury. The primary cause of hypoxia in children is respiratory failure due to underlying respiratory disease. However, it can also be the result of fluid or blood loss, leading to hypovolaemic shock, and finally circulatory failure. Children will initially use compensatory mechanisms, such as tachycardia, tachypnoea and an increased vascular resistance, to provide the tissues and vital organs with oxygen. An increase in the secretion of antidiuretic hormone (ADH) will also compensate for fluid loss by reducing the body's urine output, and conserve water. Unless the child is assessed and managed correctly these compensatory mechanisms will begin to fail, and the child will enter into decompensatory shock, where bradycardia will occur as a result of tissue hypoxia, leading to myocardial dysfunction, and if not managed will lead to the preterminal rhythm asystole. Apnoea may occur, especially in the younger child, eventually the periods of apnoea will increase and the heart rate will fall further, which will lead to asystole or pulseless electrical activity. Vascular resistance, which maintains the body's blood pressure, will also fall and irreversible shock will result. This will subsequently lead to cardiac arrest and the potential death of the child (ALSG 2004; ERC 2005).

In addition to physiological differences, children are also psychologically, intellectually, emotionally and socially different to adults. A child's first experience of hospitalisation is usually as a result of illness or injury, which involves attendance at an accident and emergency department (DoH 2003; Flaherty and Glasper 2006). Therefore, it is vital that we consider the psychological impact of this experience for the child and their family, as well as ensuring their physiological needs are assessed and met. The outcome for the critically ill and or injured child is largely dependent upon accurate assessment and management. Early recognition and treatment of the seriously ill child should avoid progression to cardiopulmonary arrest, reducing related mortality and morbidity in the child.

A rapid structured assessment using the mnemonic ABCD (Airway (with cervical spine), Breathing, Circulation and Disability) assists the practitioner in an accurate assessment and management of the critically ill child (ERC 2005). Initially this will be an 'instant' assessment to determine any evidence of immediate life threatening symptoms which would require the implementation of BLS and or ALS. Having determined that

this is not immediately required, a rapid but more thorough assessment then follows. The following provides a guide, but in such situations, the child's condition can change rapidly thus requiring a flexible approach as the situation demands.

Rapid assessment of ABCD

A – Airway

- Open airway, Check patency and position of the airway.
  Patency of the airway is assessed observing for spontaneous ventilation and look, listen, feel. Remember – if the child is able to speak or is crying this indicates that the airway is patent.
- Is there any obvious obstruction e.g. secretions, foreign body?
- Is the head in the right position for the airway (neutral for the infant/sniffing for the child aged 1 year to puberty). If there is no evidence of air movement then chin lift or jaw thrust should be carried out and the basic life support algorithm commenced (Resuscitation Council (UK) (RC UK) 2006).

B – Breathing
In order to assess the adequacy of breathing the chest should be examined and the following assessed:

- The work of breathing.
- The effectiveness of breathing.
- The effects of inadequate respiration.

Respiratory rate, rhythm, effort and efficiency
Assess air entry – chest expansion, breath sounds, noisy breathing (e.g. stridor, wheeze, grunting).

Respiratory movements can be felt by placing each hand flat against the chest or back with thumbs in the midline along the lower costal margin. The hands move with the chest wall during respiration. The amount of respiratory excursion is evaluated and asymmetry is noted.

Palpation is also carried out for voice conduction (vocal fremitus). This is achieved by placing the palmar surface of the hand on the child's chest and feeling for vibrations as/if the child speaks, whilst moving the hand symmetrically on either side of the sternum and vertebral column. Vocal fremitus is usually most prominent at the apex and least prominent at the base of the lungs. Absent or diminished vocal fremitus in the upper airway may indicate asthma or foreign body obstruction. Increased vocal fremitus may indicate pneumonia or atelectasis. During palpation other abnormal vibrations that indicate pathological conditions are noted. These include pleural rub which is felt as a grating sensation and is synchronous with respiration and crepitation which can be felt as a coarse crackly sensation and is the result of air escaping from the lungs to the subcutaneous tissue. This may be caused by injury or surgical intervention. Both crepitation and pleural rub can often be heard as well as felt. Auscultation allows assessment of breath sounds for pitch, intensity, quality, location and duration. Fluid, air or solid masses in the pleural space all interfere with the conduction of breath sounds. Normal breath sounds are vesicular, soft and low pitched on inspiration followed by shorter sound on expiration (Kelsey & McEwing 2006).

Work of breathing

Observe use of accessory muscles, sternal, intercostal and subcostal recession, flaring of nostrils, head bobbing, tracheal tug, bilateral chest movement. Chest wall movement should be symmetric bilaterally and coordinated with breathing. Note any asymmetry of movement; decreased movement on one side may be the result of foreign body obstruction, pneumonia, pneumothorax or atelectasis. Intercostal, subcostal or sternal recession shows increased work of breathing. It is more easily seen in younger children whose chest wall is more compliant. In children over 6 or 7 years it suggests severe respiratory problems.

Alert: The degree of recession gives an indication of the severity of the breathing difficulty.

Nasal flaring is also an indication of increased work of breathing. The enlargement of the nostrils helps to reduce nasal resistance and maintain airway patency; it is usually described as either minimal or marked.

Alert: Respiratory rates should be measured over a full minute (Kelsey & McEwing 2006). It should be remembered that young children breathe diaphragmatically and therefore are observed by watching abdominal movement rather than the movement of the chest. A decreasing rate or rhythm may indicate deterioration rather than improvement in the child's condition (ERC & RC UK 2004; Mackway-Jones *et al.* 1997).

Effectiveness of breathing – skin colour, temperature, oxygen saturation monitoring

Further information about the severity of the child's illness may be gained by measurement of oxygen saturation levels with a pulse oximeter. A saturation of more than 92% should be aimed for (Advanced Life Support Group 2004). Although generally accurate if the pulse oximeter reading is above 80%, below this figure it tends to over-read, as it does in the presence of poor peripheral perfusion, oedema, hypothermia or jaundice, or in abnormal haemoglobins, such as methaemoglobin (an end product of inhalation of nitric oxide) or carboxyhaemoglobin. In these circumstances acute changes may not be detected, therefore one should be cautious of its accuracy (Davies & Hassell 2001). Rajesh *et al.* (2000) evaluated respiratory rate as an indicator of hypoxia in infants under 2 months of age and concluded that a respiratory rate of more than 60 per minute is a good predictor of hypoxia and that the infants should be treated with oxygen should the facility to measure SaO_2 not be available. If there is evidence of respiratory or circulatory failure then arterial blood gases are needed. Percussion or tapping of the lungs is carried out to determine the presence and location of air, liquid and solid material in the lung and to evaluate the densities, position and landmarks of the underlying organs. Normally the percussion note in a lung full of air is resonant. When there is fluid in the chest, for example pleural effusion or haemothorax, the note becomes flat. With pneumonia where there is an increased amount of fluid but not in the chest the note becomes dull. With excess air, for example in asthma, the note is hyper-resonant. It is normal to find dullness over the liver and heart (Kelsey & McEwing 2006).

Alert: The effects of inadequate respiration will affect the cardiovascular stability and level of consciousness of the child.

C – Circulation

The circulation is assessed by examining the cardiovascular status and effects of circulatory inadequacy on other organs (Mackway-Jones *et al.* 1997).

Vital signs

The child's vital signs should be appropriate for the child's age and clinical condition, but:

Alert: Normal vital signs are not always appropriate when a child is seriously ill, indeed a normal heart rate and respiratory rate may indicate cardiopulmonary arrest is imminent.

The trend in individual patients' vital signs should always be noted and considered when making diagnoses and decisions. The child normally has a faster heart rate and respiratory rate and a lower arterial pressure than an adult. The child's heart rate and pulse volume should be assessed by palpating both central and peripheral pulses. Absent peripheral and weak central pulses are signs of advanced shock and hypotension in children (Mackway-Jones *et al.* 1997).

Heart rate/pulse

Alert: An accurate pulse should be measured for a full minute. If measuring the heart rate of children less than 2 years of age, a stethoscope should be placed over the apex of the heart and the beats counted for a full minute. Sinus tachycardia is common in the unwell, anxious child and further assessment should be carried out to identify the cause. Hypoxia produces tachycardia in the older infant or child.

Alert: Severe or prolonged hypoxia leads to bradycardia which is a pre-terminal sign and indicates imminent cardiopulmonary arrest. The child's heart rate and pulse volume should be assessed by palpating both central and peripheral pulses. Absent peripheral and weak central pulses are signs of advanced shock and hypotension in children (Mackway-Jones *et al.* 1997).

Blood pressure

Children in early shock may initially have a normal blood pressure reading as hypotension is often a very late and pre-terminal sign of circulatory failure in the child. Therefore a rapid assessment will not usually include the assessment of blood pressure; it can however be used once the child has initially been stabilised and used to monitor a trend and manage accordingly. When taking the blood pressure, the size of the child's limb must be taken into consideration. Make sure the width of the cuff is about two-thirds the length of the child's upper arm. A cuff that is too large may produce a reading that is too low; a cuff that is too small may give a false high reading (ERC 2005; Thomas 1996).

Skin perfusion and body temperature

The skin colour and temperature should be consistent over the trunk and limbs. Clinical signs of poor perfusion include peripherally cool skin, pallor, mottling, peripheral cyanosis and capillary refill more than 2 seconds. By the time central cyanosis is visible in acute respiratory distress, respiratory arrest is very close. Ambient temperature should always be considered in the interpretation of capillary refill. The sternum can be used to obtain a capillary refill in the presence of cold peripheries. Normally the peripheral temperature should be between 1 and 2% of the core temperature (Kelsey & McEwing 2006).

It had been accepted that 37°C was the mean body temperature; however the normal circadian range of infants' temperatures over the 24-hour period has been described as ranging from 36°C at night to 37.8°C during active periods in the day. In addition there is now recognised to be a variable fluctuation between individuals of 0.5°C (Mackowiak *et al.* 1992). Therefore we should accept individual variations in normal body temperature recognising that time of day and age of child may affect expected normal values.

Perfusion of the key organs – the brain and kidneys – must be assessed and monitored. Level of consciousness will be a key indictor in respect of brain perfusion and is discussed below. With regard to renal perfusion, urine output must be measured and should be more than 1 ml/kg/hr.

D – Disability

The child's level of consciousness should be assessed using the AVPU scale, which is a quick accurate assessment of neurological response.

A – **A**LERT
V – Responds to **V**OICE
P – Responds to **P**AIN
U – UNRESPONSIVE

A child who responds only to pain (P) has a Glasgow Coma Scale equivalent to 8/15 and is unlikely to be able to protect their airway.

Parents are usually the first to recognise any changes in their child's level of consciousness, therefore it is important to listen to what they say. A hypoxic child may be irritable or agitated early on but increasingly lethargic later. They may fail to recognise or interact, for example to maintain eye contact with their parents, or they may not respond to stimuli such as unfamiliar nurses. A progressive drop in level of consciousness is a late sign of hypoxia and may be an indication of respiratory distress; other causes that need to be considered include shock, sepsis, ingestion of depressants, metabolic abnormalities, hypothermia and head injuries (Thomas 1996).

Glasgow coma scale, including pupil size and reaction

In addition the modified Glasgow Coma Scale may be used, with limb movement, pupil size and reaction noted as a baseline; the presence of convulsive movements should also be noted; any patient with decreased conscious level or convulsions should have a blood glucose carried out (ERC & RC UK 2004).

Alert: Any problem with ABC must be addressed before assuming that a decrease in conscious level is due to a primary neurological problem (Mackway-Jones *et al.* 1997).

In addition to the above assessment, further information needs to be obtained. An acronym that is suggested by the ERC & RC UK (2004) is **AMPLE:**

A – **A**LLERGY (to drugs/other known allergens)
M – **M**EDICATION
P – **P**AST MEDICAL HISTORY
L – **L**AST MEAL
E – **E**NVIRONMENT (history of injury/accident)

Two examples of assessment and management of the acutely ill child are demonstrated below:

Scenario 1   Respiratory arrest

A 10-day-old infant was brought to accident and emergency via the GP surgery, following a respiratory arrest. The infant had a 2-day history of not feeding and increased sleeping. The infant had received bag valve mask airway resuscitation by the paramedics and was assessed by the paediatric emergency nurse on arrival, using a structured assessment tool (ERC & RC UK 2004):
Airway – The infant's airway was obstructed with secretions; this was cleared with gentle visible oronaso-pharyngeal suction at 10 kPa of pressure, using a size 10 gauge suction catheter. This technique was used to prevent any trauma to the airway, and prevent stimulation of the vagal nerve, which can cause bradycardia. The airway was placed in the neutral position to enhance air entry.
Breathing – Signs of breathing were assessed using the look, listen and feel technique, which indicated the infant was breathing at a rate of 70 beats per minute (bpm). The infant's respiratory effort and efficacy were also assessed, which demonstrated an increased respiratory effort evidenced by sternal and diaphragmatic recession. The infant was displaying signs of compensatory shock, but was beginning to deteriorate into decompensatory shock, having regular episodes of apnoea requiring bag-valve-mask ventilation. In collaboration with the paediatrician the decision was made to electively intubate this infant, as it was not going to manage sustaining adequate ventilation with oxygen or via continuous positive airway pressure (CPAP). A size 3.5 cm

oral endotracheal tube (ETT) was inserted, using a straight blade laryngoscope to lift the epiglottis and visualise the cords. A bougie was inserted into the ETT to increase the rigidity of the tube, it was vital to ensure this rigid tube did not extend out of the bottom of the ETT as it can damage or perforate the trachea. The ETT was secured using a trouser leg technique and the skin was protected with a granuflex dressing. The chest was assessed for bilateral air entry as there is a great risk of displacement of the ETT tube and insertion into the stomach. This infant was bagged using 100% oxygen and bilateral air entry was evident. The infant was connected to a portable ventilator using pressure controlled ventilation, with pressure settings at peak 20 cm and positive end expiratory pressure (PEEP) set at 4 cm, and a rate of 40 breaths per minute. The infant required 30% oxygen to maintain their saturations above 95%. The blood glucose measurement was within normal limits. An arterial blood gas indicated a respiratory acidosis, with a below normal pH, low pO_2 and a high pCO_2. This was taken prior to intubation, so will require repeating to re-assess. A size 8 fg nasogastric tube was inserted as ventilation can increase the amount of air in the stomach, which may splint the diaphragm, reducing the lung air entry and reducing the tidal volume, which would reduce the infant's saturations.

Circulation – The infant was tachycardic with a heart rate of 180 beats per minute on admission. The infant was pink, and saturations were above 95% once the airway had been secured and respirations sustained at 20 breaths per minute. The infant's capillary refill time (CRT) was 3 seconds, indicating circulatory failure. An intravenous cannula was inserted; blood samples were taken to test for urea and electrolytes, blood glucose, blood gas and haemoglobin. A bolus infusion of 20 ml/kg of 0.9% normal saline was administered to correct the CRT. Electrolyte results were examined as the infant was at risk of hyponatraemia, due to dehydration, which could lead to convulsions. The sodium was within normal limits for this infant.

Disability – The infant was drowsy, with a AVPU of P for painful stimuli. The infant did not display any abnormal movements. He had equal reactive pupils.

Exposure – The skin was assessed for any spots, rash or bruising. There were no visible signs of any marks to the skin. The infant's skin was also assessed for colour perfusion and temperature. The infant had an axillary temperature of 38.4°C. Paracetamol 15 mg/kg was administered per rectum.

Re-assessment and stabilisation – The infant was regularly re-assessed. Airway and breathing were controlled by intubation and ventilation, observing for bilateral air entry and oxygen saturation, remembering the mnemonic DOPE in the intubated child – **D**isplacement, **O**bstruction of the ETT, **P**neumothorax or **E**quipment failure. This infant's airway was maintained with intubation; a respiratory rate of 40 breaths per minute sustained saturations within normal limits. Re-assessment of the circulation demonstrated an increased capillary refill time of 3 seconds, so a further 20 ml/kg bolus of 0.9% normal saline was administered. The child was assessed for signs of dehydration, using the Advanced Paediatric Life Support Group's (2004) assessment tool for dehydration, which indicated the infant to be 5–10% dehydrated.

Rehydration fluids were calculated, at 100 ml/kg for the first 10 kg. An approximate weight of 3.0 kg was calculated based on the birth weight of 3.5 kg, as at 10 days of age it was impossible to use the APLS recognised guesstimate and it was recognised that the infant was likely to have lost approximately 10% of body weight due to normal physiological weight loss in the first week of life and a reduction in fluid intake.

The infant was referred to the regional paediatric intensive care unit, which advised the team of interventions required whilst awaiting retrieval. Continuous monitoring of the heart rate, respiratory rate and oxygen saturations observed for any changes in the child. If changes occur re-assessment of the ABCDE should be performed. This infant remained stable, and was successfully retrieved to paediatric intensive care (PICU), where he remained ventilated until his condition, which was thought to have been bronchiolitis, improved. His parents were regularly kept informed of their infant's condition, were aware of the necessity to transfer to PICU and were given appropriate advice about their journey to PICU.

A 6-year-old child was brought to accident and emergency presenting with tonic/clonic movements of her arms and legs. The convulsion had begun at home and had lasted approximately 5 minutes. The paramedics had administered 5 mg rectal diazepam, with no effect. The child had a 1-day history of pyrexia, and was not a known epileptic. An approximate weight of the child was calculated at 20 kg, with an endotracheal internal diameter size of 4.5 cm.

On assessment:

Airway – The child is unable to maintain her own airway. There are copious clear secretions in the mouth and it is impossible to open the mouth due to the tonic/clonic rigid movements. A further dose of rectal diazepam is administered, as there is presently no intravenous access, this is the protocol for the child experiencing a fit (Resuscitation Council 2006). The airway is suctioned with a size 10 fg catheter as far as visible.

Breathing – There is currently no regular respirations. 15 Litres of oxygen is administered with bag valve mask ventilation (BVM). Oxygen saturations are 92%.

Circulation – The child is tachycardic with a heart rate at 120 bpm. Two large cannulas are inserted to administer a bolus dose of 1 mg of intravenous lorazepam. A maximum single dose of 4 mg can be administered, however with caution as apnoea can present as a potential side effect. 50–100 mcg/kg can be administered, with a maximum dose of 8 mg or 100 mcgs in 24 hours (Guys *et al.* 2005).

Disability – The child continued to convulse, despite two doses of rectal diazepam and one dose of 1 mg IV lorazepam. A second dose of 1 mg IV lorazepam was administered (ERC & RC UK 2004). The child was unresponsive on the AVPU scale, pupils were equal and reacting to light.

Exposure – No obvious signs of a rash/bruising or non-blanching spots were visible.

On re-assessment:

Airway – The child continued to fit, although it was possible to insert a guerdal airway into the mouth to protect the airway. This is measured by placing the guerdal airway from the edge of the mandible to the truncus of the ear (ERC & RC UK 2004). In children the airway is inserted the correct way up, not as in adults where it is inserted upside down and rotated. This is because it would cause significant trauma to the soft tissue of the child's airway. The purpose of using a guerdal airway is to protect the airway from obstruction mainly caused by the tongue. Equipment was prepared for intubation, a size 5.5 cm endotracheal tube was required, based on the estimate of age/4+4. 1–2 mg/kg of ketamine was administered over 1 minute prior to intubation.

Breathing – Respirations were irregular and the child was at risk of a respiratory arrest due to the anticonvulsants administered. Therefore BVM ventilation continued to maintain adequate oxygenation. Saturations remained at 96%.

Circulation – The child remained tachycardic and her capillary refill time was normal. A stat dose of atropine 20 mcg/kg was prepared in case of bradycardia at intubation. Intravenous antibiotics and antiviral therapy were commenced, in case of a diagnosis of encephalitis.

Disability – the child continued to have tonic/clonic convulsions, so a loading dose of phenytoin was administered. The child was unresponsive on the AVPU scale, pupils equal and reacting to light.

Exposure – unchanged.

On re-assessment:

Airway – An internal diameter size 4.5 cm endotracheal tube, cut at 12.5 cm to the lips, was successfully inserted into the trachea (ERC & RC UK 2004).

Breathing – Bilateral lung air entry was evident which indicated the ETT was in the correct position. Saturations were at 98%.

Circulation – Normal CRT and heart rate reduced to 100 bpm.

Disability – The child continued to have tonic/clonic fits, so paraldehyde 0.3–0.4 ml/kg was administered diluted to equivalent volume of olive oil or 1-in-10 sodium chloride given as a rectal enema. The child was unresponsive on the AVPU scale, pupils equal and reacting to light.

Exposure – unchanged.

On re-assessment:

Airway and breathing – The child's airway, breathing are maintained by ventilation via the ETT.

Circulation was unchanged and within normal limits.

Disability was affected as she continued to convulse and was unresponsive. A loading dose of 15 mg/kg phenobarbitone was administered as recommended by the Paediatric Formulary (Guys *et al.* 2005).

On re-assessment:
Airway and breathing – Maintained by ventilation via the ETT.
Circulation – Heart rate within normal limits.
Disability – The child continued to convulse. A midazolam infusion of 1 mcg/kg was advised by the retrieval team, if the previous drugs did not stop the fitting. Recommended dose for status epilepticus is 30–300 mcg/kg/hour or 0.5 mcg/kg/min, maximum of 20 mcg/kg/min (Guys *et al.* 2005). The child's level of consciousness was unchanged.

On re-assessment:
Airway and breathing – Maintained by ventilation via the ETT.
Circulation – Heart rate was within normal limits.
Disability – The fitting is no longer visible once the midazolam infusion is commenced.

The regional paediatric intensive care team (PICU) retrieved the child. A magnetic resonance image (MRI) was ordered to confirm a diagnosis of encephalitis. A continuous cerebral function analysing monitor (CFAM) was to be applied in PICU to monitor abnormal electrical activity, which would not be visible due to the midazolam infusion. The following day the child was extubated in PICU and transferred to the ward, although the MRI did not confirm encephalitis. Antibiotics and anti-viral therapy continued.

The seriously injured child in accident and emergency

Children are more susceptible to injury due their risk-taking behaviour, resulting in accidents. Furthermore, accidents are the main cause of death in children over 1 year of age. Four out of five accident and emergency contacts with children and young people are for injuries. Response to the care of the most seriously injured child must therefore be delivered speedily with a team approach to optimise survival (DoH 2003; Flaherty & Glasper 2006; Royal College of Surgeons and the British Orthopaedic Association 2003).

Trauma is the leading cause of death and disability over 1 year of age; blunt trauma is seen in 80% of paediatric cases, of which two-thirds are associated with brain injury (ERC & RC UK 2004). Furthermore 1.4 million people suffer head injury each year, of whom 150 000 will be admitted to hospital, some requiring specialist neurosurgical services. Children's cerebral tissue is thinner, softer and more flexible than that of adults, giving the brain less protection against impact. Toddlers and very young children are unstable on their feet and are prone to banging their head on hard surfaces, such as furniture (Woodrow 2000).

Alert: Whenever a young child presents with a head injury, practitioners must examine the history of the injury in an attempt to decide if the injury was caused by accident or by a deliberate action and consider this within the context of a holistic assessment and interaction with the immediate family and carers.

A neonate has two visible fontanelles; a raised fontanelle can indicate increased cerebral volume. However, palpation of the fontanelle places direct pressure on the brain tissue, which can cause damage. The front fontanelle closes in the first year of life, followed by fusion of the skull bones at approximately 18 months. This forms a rigid, inflexible container for the intracranial contents.

Intracranial pressure is the total pressure exerted by all contents within the skull. If intracranial volume increases as a result of intracranial haemorrhage, blocked drainage of cerebrospinal fluid or cerebral oedema, pressure increases. Normal intracranial pressure (ICP) is usually measured as a mean pressure, between 0 and 10 mmHg; in younger children it may be lower, 3–7 mmHg. Problems can occur with pressure above 15 mmHg (Woodrow 2000), and sustained high pressure can cause 'coning' (tentorial herniation), where the brainstem tissue is forced through the foramen magnum into the spinal cord. Vital signs are often depressed caused by cerebral compression. Respiratory failure often requires artificial ventilation and the gag reflex is often impaired, leading to aspiration. Ischaemic brain damage is often caused by hypoxia and/or hypotension, which can lead to death of tissue. The child may require transfer to PICU if the outcome is to be improved. Raised intracranial pressure is often recognised by three symptoms, hypertension, bradycardia and an abnormal respiratory pattern, collectively known as 'Cushing's triad'.

Some head injuries may result in basal skull fractures, which are not visually obvious, but can cause leakage of cerebrospinal fluid (CSF) from the nose or ear. CSF can be recognised by a yellowish ring surrounding a bloodstain. Any nasal tube (nasal airway or nasogastric tube) can enter through the basal skull fracture and infect the brain; insertion should therefore be avoided until such a time that a basal fracture can be excluded (Woodrow 2000).

The brain needs a constant supply of oxygen and glucose for aerobic metabolism; without this the cells will resort to the ineffective anaerobic metabolism, causing damage to the cell membranes, creating an acidotic environment, and cell death (Woodrow 2000). Cerebral perfusion pressure (CPP) is a priority and is determined as mean arterial blood pressure (MAP) minus intracranial pressure:

$$CPP = MAP - ICP$$

Patients with a CPP above 70 mmHg are more likely to survive and suffer fewer complications (Woodrow 2000). In health MAP significantly exceeds ICP, giving a normal CPP of 70–100 mmHg, but in head injury CPP is usually below 60 mmHg (Woodrow 2000). Once there is closure of the fontanelle, direct measurement of the cranial volume requires invasive monitoring, but this exposes the child to potential complications, including infection and meningitis. Consequently, the benefits of invasive monitoring must outweigh the risks.

Preventing raised ICP is vital when managing the care of children with head injury. Assessing the child and controlling the environment can make a significant difference to their outcome. Certain factors, such as pain, noise or a bright environment, can increase the pressure; body positioning, ventilation, knee flexion and pres-

sure on the skull can all increase ICP, thus actions taken to avoid or prevent the above will aid in maintaining a desirable ICP. An increase in intrathoracic pressure can reduce cerebral venous drainage, increasing ICP as can PEEP in artificial ventilation and suctioning of the airway. Coughing and constipation can also lead to transient increases in ICP; linctus can be administered if a gag reflex is present, and laxatives to prevent constipation (Woodrow 2000).

Children with head injury can suffer fits, which may be a result of compression of the brain tissue. This can occur when the Glasgow Coma Score is below 10: prophylactic anticonvulsants should be given in these circumstances. The airway and breathing must be maintained during the fit. Fits increase cerebral oxygen consumption, while reducing cerebral oxygen supply (Woodrow 2000). Dunning *et al.* (2004) cited that the NICE guidelines (2003) recommend that computed tomography should replace skull radiography, but, as Dunning *et al.* (2004) found in their study, this can vary depending upon available services and adherence to the guidelines.

The mnemonic AcBCDE (Airway (with cervical spine), Breathing, Circulation, Disability and Exposure to assess for other injuries) assists the practitioner in an accurate assessment and management of the critically ill child. The principles of resuscitation are similar to those of the critically ill child, yet there are a few important differences:

Airway and cervical spine stabilisation

Assessment and management of the airway involves a jaw thrust and the look, listen and feel approach to assess air entry. At the same time immobilisation of the cervical spine is essential to prevent damage to the cervical cord, which could result in quadriplegia or death.

Alert: Immobilise first.

A chin lift is never used if there is suspicion of cervical spine injury. The oropharynx is cleared of debris, blood, vomit or secretions by gentle suction under direct vision. Artificial airways may be required to maintain the airway, but if there is a gag reflex present this could lead to vomiting and aspiration into the lungs. If there is no gag reflex present, intubation to protect the airway is essential.

Alert: Nasal intubation should never be performed in a head injury, in case of a basal skull fracture.

Measurement of cervical collar

A cervical collar must be measured to fit exactly: if too large, the head may become flexed on the spine; if too small, the neck may be able to move and not be immobilised. In measuring the collar the accurate measurement is the distance between the angle of the jaw and the upper part of the trapezius while the child's head is in the neutral position. The number of fingers that comfortably fit in this space is compared to the markers on the cervical collar (ERC & RC UK 2004).

The collar should be slid under the hands of the person maintaining the in-line cervical spine immobilisation and airway and fastened anteriorly, in case access to the airway is required. It is essential that manual immobilisation of the cervical spine is performed if the collar is removed. Sand bags and adhesive tape must be applied to ensure immobilisation, and be secured to a fixable object, not one that will move. Prior to fastening the collar, inspection of the neck for tracheal deviation, dilation of the veins, or any wounds or swelling to the neck such as subcutaneous emphysema (air under the skin) should be undertaken. It is recommended that the collar should only be removed when a normal neurological examination is evident, as a normal cervical spine x-ray does not guarantee any cervical spine fracture (ERC & RC UK 2004).

Breathing

Once the cervical spine and airway have been managed breathing must be assessed, checking for bilateral air entry to exclude chest injuries such as tension pneumothorax, simple/open pneumothorax, massive haemothorax, flail chest or cardiac tamponade (ERC & RC UK 2004). If breathing is ineffective bag-valve-mask (BVM) ventilation

with 100% oxygen is required (Kinney *et al.* 1999). Tracheal intubation may be indicated if:

- Adequate oxygenation is not achieved by BVM.
- There is respiratory arrest/respiratory failure (hypoventilation and/or hypoxia despite 100% oxygen).
- There is a Glasgow Coma Score of less than 8 or the AVPU score is at P or below.
- There are signs of a flail chest or inhalation injury.
- Prolonged/controlled ventilation or broncho-alveolar lavage is required.

Intubation is a specialist skill and requires assistance to immobilise the spine during intubation as this must be performed without any extension of the neck. An orogastric tube should be inserted and cricoid pressure should be applied on intubation to remove contents of the stomach, to prevent aspiration. Hyperventilation should not be performed in head injury as cerebral vasoconstriction induces hypocapnia and aggravates brain ischaemic injuries. Arterial $PaCO_2$ should be maintained in normal ranges (4.6–6 kPa/ 35–45 mmHg).

Circulation

Assessment of the cardiovascular status and restoration of normal circulating volume is vital in the acutely injured child. Chest trauma can result in a pneumothorax, haemothorax, cardiac tamponade or flail chest. Assessment of the heart rate, respiratory rate, capillary refill time, pulse volume, skin temperature, level of consciousness, blood pressure and estimation of internal and external fluid loss is vital in the acutely injured child. Thoracic injuries must be managed appropriately, depending upon the clinical diagnosis. A chest drain is required if a pneumothorax or haemothorax is detected, but it is essential that intravenous/intraosseous access is obtained prior to the insertion of a chest drain if a haemothorax is detected, as there may be a large blood loss once the drain is inserted. A haemothorax or pneumothorax can be recognised by unequal air entry and reduced noise on auscultation of the chest. A cardiac tamponade can be identified by muffled heart sounds: the collection of blood needs relieving, as it will affect ventricular function, which will result in cardiac failure.

A large volume of blood can also be lost from open fractures, pelvic and long bone fractures. Re-alignment and splinting of a limb fracture can reduce the blood loss. Obvious blood loss from a vessel must be controlled using direct pressure with a thin layer of gauze. Tourniquets should only be used in exceptional cases of traumatic amputation. Haemorrhage may also be due to internal blood loss from an intrathoracic, retroperitoneal (usually associated with pelvic fractures), or intra-abdominal injury. Intra-abdominal bleeding may be due to rupture of an intra-abdominal organ, such as the spleen or liver. This can present with abdominal distension which does not decompress with a gastric tube, and signs of circulatory failure and shock. Blood or bile stained aspirate via a naso/orogastric tube are suggestive of abdominal bleeding (ERC & RC UK 2004).

Hypovolaemic shock can occur due to fluid/blood loss or displacement, and can be graded on a scale of I–V, I being the mildest, V the severest. Mild to moderate shock (grade I–II) is managed with a bolus of 20 ml/kg crystalloid or colloid. Re-assessment and further boluses should be administered if indicated. Packed red blood cells 15 ml/kg added to 10 ml/kg of crystalloid

should be administered if the child remains shocked. This should be reheated to body temperature to prevent hypothermia. Grade III–IV requires immediate infusion of 40 ml/kg of crystalloid or colloid followed by a bolus of 15 ml/kg blood added to 10 ml/kg crystalloid. If type specific is not available within 10 minutes, then O negative should be administered (ERC & RC UK 2004).

An experienced surgeon will need to decide if surgery is required, which may be indicated if response is poor after fluid bolus of 40 ml/kg or repeated blood transfusion is required to maintain normal physiological parameters.

Alert: Normal saline is the solution of first choice. It is ubiquitously available and carries mimimal risk. However, repeated administration of iso-oncotic crystalloid solution boluses can lead to extravasation of fluid from the intravascular to the interstitial space especially where there is increased capillary permeability such as in septic shock. Colloids may be useful as they have an important effect on the intravascular space. When infused, the osmotic colloid pressure on the intravascular space increases. As a result, fluid is drawn from the interstitial space into the intravascular space. Therefore, the blood is rehydrated by osmosis (Adelson *et al.* 2003; Docherty & McIntyre 2002).

Table 8.1 Clinical signs of grades of hypovolaemic shock (as percentage of ciculating blood volume) (ERC & RC UK 2004)

	Grade I–II	Grade III	Grade IV
Blood loss (% volume)	<25	25–40	>40
Heart rate	Mildly increased	Moderately increased	Tachycardia/bradycardia
Systolic blood pressure	Normal or increased	Normal or decreased	Decreased
Pulse volume	Normal/reduced	Moderately reduced	Severely reduced
Capillary refill time	Normal/increased	Moderately increased	Severely increased
Skin	Cool, pale	Cold, mottled	Cold, pale
Respiratory rate	Moderately increased	Severely increased	Sighing respiration Agonal breathing
Mental status	Mild agitation	Lethargic	Reacts only to pain/unconscious

Refer to Table 8.1 which shows the clinical signs of grades of hypovolaemic shock.

Two routes of vascular access are essential. If intravenous peripheral cannulation is not successful after three attempts over a maximum of 90 seconds or the child is shut down and it looks unlikely that intravenous access will be possible, then an intraosseous needle should be inserted (Evans *et al.* 1995; UK Resuscitation Council 2005).

To diminish the likelihood of raised intracranial pressure the ERC & RC UK (2004) recommend that the internal jugular veins should not be cannulated for central venous access, as it hinders venous drainage from the brain. The head and chest can be elevated to 45° to aid venous drainage from the brain, as long as there are no signs of hypotension. The $PaCO_2$ should be kept between 35 and 45 mmHg (4.6–6.6 kPa), hyperventilation should only be carried out under careful supervision if there is raised intracranial pressure. Mannitol 0.25 g/kg intravenous or intraosseous may be given if there is evidence of raised intracranial pressure. However, more recently 0.45% normal saline has been recommended for use in raised intracranial pressure instead of mannitol (Adelson *et al.* 2003). Fisher *et al.* (1992) compared the use of 3% saline to 0.9% saline in raised intracranial pressure, and found that 3% saline reduces the raised ICP after traumatic brain injury. Hyperglycaemia and hypoglycaemia must be avoided and seizures should be treated with benzodiazepines and antiepileptic medication.

The most common cause of death in trauma is hypovolaemic shock, which occurs before death from raised intracranial pressure (ERC & RC UK 2004). It is essential to treat the hypovolaemia with fluid resuscitation even if brain injury is present. Arterial blood pressure must be maintained to prevent secondary ischaemia damage to the brain which may arise from hypovolaemic shock. However, once the blood pressure has been stabilised fluids should be given cautiously to prevent fluid overload and worsening cerebral oedema.

Alert: Frequent re-assessment is essential in the management of circulatory shock to assess response to treatment and observe for the development of internal haemorrhage.

Disability

Assessment of the acutely injured child's level of consciousness is made using the AVPU scale, the pupil response to light and the child's posture. A reduced level of consciousness at P for pain is equivalent to a Glasgow Coma Score of 8 and intubation should be considered to protect the airway. Pupil size indicates cranial nerve III function. Pupil size and response to light should be equal; a unilateral pupil with head injury may indicate intracranial mass on the same side of the brain, which requires urgent neurosurgical opinion. Poorly restricted pupils may indicate opiate poisoning or a midbrain disorder (ERC & RC UK 2004); an oval shaped pupil can indicate coning (Woodrow 2000).

The child's posture must be assessed; decorticate posturing is where the arms are flexed towards the trunk, decerebrate posturing is where the arms are extended. Both signs are worrying and the underlying cause must be treated. Frequent re-assessment of disability is essential in the acutely injured child and any abnormal finding must be investigated.

Exposure

A log roll should be performed to examine the acutely injured child from head to toe (ERC & RC UK 2004). Clothes must be removed in an appropriate manner to assess for injuries, maintaining the child's dignity and ensuring that all procedures are explained, even if the child appears unconscious. Heat loss also needs to be considered as this can occur relatively quickly in the child as their body surface is larger than their body weight; warming devices should be used to keep the child warm.

Log rolling the acutely injured child

A secondary survey should be performed once the AcBCDE and resuscitation is complete. This is to examine for further injuries. The purpose of the log roll is to keep the child's spine in line with the rest of their body. Five people are required to safely perform a log roll on a child, and three

Table 8.2   Paediatric Trauma Score

Variables	+2	+1	−1
Airway	Normal	Maintainable	Unmaintainable
CNS	Awake	Obtunded	Coma
Body weight (kg)	>20	10–20	<10
Systolic blood pressure (mmHg)	>90	50–90	<50
Open wound	None	Minor	Major
Skeletal injury	None	Closed fracture	Open/multiple fractures

A score of +2, +1 or −1 is given to each variable then added to give a range of −6 to +12.

people for an infant. Each member must know their role; the team leader is responsible for controlling the c-spine and must give clear instructions before moving the child. The fifth person in the child or third person in the infant is responsible for examining the infant/child for injuries. This examination starts at the head, to thorax and abdomen, feeling along the spine, inspecting the anus and back of the legs. When the examination is complete the team leader must direct the remaining team in returning the child back to the supine position. All injuries must be documented clearly. The child must be told what is happening, the purpose of the examination and their dignity maintained, even if they appear unconscious. X-rays are carried out as part of the secondary survey. These should include lateral c-spine, thorax and pelvis (anterior and posterior views).

Alert: Any change in the child's condition requires primary assessment of AcBCDE.

As with the unwell child, further relevant history should be obtained, using the AMPLE acronym.

Paediatric trauma score

Although not entirely reliable in predicting outcome, the paediatric trauma score, which incorporates age, is used widely. A score of more than 8 indicates mild trauma, where a score of less than 0 indicates a high level of mortality (ERC & RC UK 2004). Please refer to Table 8.2.

Scenario 3   Road traffic accident

A 14-year-old boy was admitted to the accident and emergency department following a road traffic accident, where he was the passenger in a stolen car. He is brought to the department by ambulance, escorted by his 18-year-old brother, having sustained a head injury and a possible cervical spine injury.

On assessment:

Airway with cervical spine – He appeared to have a patent airway and had a cervical collar in place; however, he was not fixed to a firm object. One nurse manually secured his cervical spine while it was visually examined for further injuries or vein distension before re-securing the blocks to prevent him moving. His airway was assessed; there were no signs of debris, blood or vomit.

Breathing – His breathing was assessed; respiratory rate, rhythm, bilateral chest movement and auscultation of the chest did not indicate any chest injury. His respiratory rate was below normal limits at a rate of 12 bpm, his colour was pale and oxygen saturations was 92% in air. 100% oxygen was applied via facemask with reservoir bag attached.

Circulation – His circulation was assessed; his heart rate was 70 bpm, which is the lower of the normal limits for an acutely injured child. His capillary refill time was 3 seconds, above normal, indicating signs of circulatory failure. His skin was pale and cool to touch. Two intravenous lines were inserted and a 20 ml/kg bolus of 0.9% normal saline was administered.

Disability – An AVPU assessment was performed, which indicated a P, responding to painful

Scenario 3 (Continued)

stimuli. His pupils were of equal size, and responding to light. As his level of consciousness was reduced to an equivalent Glasgow Coma Score of 8, intubation was indicated. This was undertaken by a skilled anaesthetist as the head could not be extended due to cervical injury.

Exposure – He was log rolled using the five people technique to examine the body for other injuries. No other injuries were visible, which was documented.

Re-assessment:

Airway with cervical spine – The airway remained patent, with no visible occlusion. The cervical spine remained immobilised.

Breathing – The respiratory rate was reduced indicating possible raised intracranial pressure. He was intubated with a size 6 cm cuffed endotracheal tube, using a jaw thrust; visible suctioning of the airway was performed and an orogastric tube was inserted to relieve air from the stomach and prevent aspiration. Ventilation was performed by ambubag with 100% oxygen, there was bilateral air entry and the child's saturations were 98%. Intravenous thiopentone 4–6 mg/kg was reconstituted with 20 ml water for injection and administered over 10–15 seconds as recommended by the Paediatric Formulary (Guys *et al*. 2005). Alternatively, rocuronium 0.6 mg/kg can be used, but intubation is required within 60 seconds of administration.

Circulation – The heart rate increased to 100 beats per minute, capillary refill was within 2 seconds. The skin was pink and well perfused.

Disability – His level of consciousness remained at an AVPU of P. Pupils were equal and reacting to light. Full assessment of his motor response indicated flexion of the arms to pain.

Exposure – He was kept warm using blankets. Dignity was maintained and all procedures were explained. He was referred to the regional retrieval unit; frequent re-assessment of his condition was performed.

Re-assessment:

Airway with cervical spine – The airway remained patent, with no visible occlusion. The cervical spine remained immobilised.

Breathing – Ventilation was maintained at 20 breaths per minute via the ETT with 100% oxygen with the ambubag; there was bilateral air entry and his saturations were 96–98%.

Circulation – The heart rate remained between 80–100 beats per minute, capillary refill was within 2 seconds.

Disability – His level of consciousness remained at an AVPU of P. Pupils were equal and reacted to light. Full assessment of his motor response indicated flexion of the arms to pain.

He was retrieved to a paediatric intensive care unit, where a computed tomograph of the brain was performed.

Scenario 4   Chest injury from stabbing

A 16-year-old boy was brought to accident and emergency accompanied by friends following a fight. He has sustained a 3 cm-long injury to his upper abdomen, lower thoracic region. His mother had been contacted and was on her way to the hospital. His approximate weight was 40 kg.

Airway – On assessment the boy was sitting in an upright position, maintaining his own airway.

Breathing – He had an increased respiratory rate with unequal air entry. On examination he had reduced breath sounds and expansion on the right side of his chest. He was able to string two to three words together, but was in obvious respiratory distress. He was pale, with oxygen saturations of 89% in air: 100% facemask oxygen was provided. A clinical diagnosis of pneumothorax or haemothorax was made. He was prepared for insertion of a chest drain.

Circulation – On assessment he was tachycardic at 110 beats per minute. A large bore cannula was inserted in case of sudden blood loss on insertion of a chest drain. He had an increased capillary refill of 4 seconds. Twenty ml/kg of O negative blood was requested for immediate use. Twenty ml/kg of 0.9% normal saline was administered.

Disability – At that time he was alert and obviously anxious; he was reassured and his mother was on her way.

Re-assessment:

Airway – On assessment he was beginning to feel tired but was still maintaining his own airway.

Breathing – His respiratory rate was increased and air entry continued to be unequal. A chest drain was therefore inserted into the fifth midclavicular space (ALSG 2004). There was a blood loss of 50 ml into an underwater drainage bottle;

it was also bubbling, indicating a haemopneu-mothorax. Following insertion of the chest drain he had improved air entry to the right side of his chest. He continued to receive 100% oxygen via the face mask, and his oxygen saturations increased to 96%.

Circulation – His heart rate reduced to 90 beats per minute, although his capillary refill was still 3 seconds. A 20 ml/kg transfusion of blood was administered. His blood loss into the chest drain was now 100 ml, a total of 2.5 ml/kg fluid loss.

Disability – He was alert and in less discomfort. His mother arrived and he felt more reassured.

The boy was transferred to the paediatric high dependency area.

Stabilisation, retrieval and transfer

Referral to the specialist paediatric regional retrieval unit is essential once resuscitation has been achieved. If resuscitation or stabilisation is proving difficult an experienced practitioner should contact the paediatric intensive care unit (PICU) for further advice. Where acutely injured or ill children are cared for depends upon the level of care they require. Level 1 is where the child requires closer observation/monitoring in a high dependency care bed/cot (HDC) as recommended in *Bridge to the Future* (BTTF) (NHS Executive 1997a, 1997b). Children requiring level 2 or 3 paediatric intensive care should be cared for in a PICU because they are suffering one or more organ failure (NHS Executive 1997a). Specialist PICUs are allocated to provide level 3 paediatric intensive care and the regional PICU is responsible for making a telephone assessment of the child and finding a bed in an appropriate level high dependency unit (HDU) or PICU. Based on the retrieval unit's assessment of the child the specialist centre will provide advice, support and an estimated time of arrival at the referring hospital (ERC & RC UK 2004). On arrival at the referring hospital the retrieval team will make a structured assessment of the acutely injured or ill child. The referring hospital will make a formal handover to the retrieval team. It is advisable if the referring hospital continues to support the retrieval team, as although they bring all equipment with them, it is an unfamiliar environment. On occasions referring hospitals may be asked to transfer the child to the HDU or PICU, it is essential that the most competent practitioner undertakes this role, has the appropriate equipment to do so and can intubate or resuscitate the child if required (DoH 2004). It is essential that all ambulance services work with hospitals to ensure that all inter-hospital transfer procedures and arrangements for neonates and children are jointly agreed, and that key items of equipment are compatible and familiar to ambulance and hospital staff and should have child-friendly features in the interior design of vehicles (DoH 2004). The family and, wherever possible, the child, should be involved in decision making. The child may be under a specific hospital, which may influence the PICU/HDU that the child is referred to. It is also an anxious time for the child and family, and procedures should be explained to them to reduce this anxiety.

Summary

An acutely unwell child can deteriorate quickly and requires urgent assessment using AcBCDE. This chapter has considered the assessment and interventions required for the child presenting with either a critical illness or serious injury. It is vital that accident and emergency practitioners are able to recognise the deteriorating child in order to put interventions in place to help improve outcomes and long-term prognosis. The key issues have been addressed and the specialist skills required in this context identified.

References

Adelson, P.D., Bratton, S., Carney, N. *et al.* (2003) Guidelines for the acute medical management of severe traumatic brain injury in infants, children and adolescents. Use of hyperosmolar therapy in the management of severe pediatric traumatic brain injury. *Pediatric Critical Care Medicine*, **4**, S40–S44.

Advanced Life Support Group (ALSG) (2004) *Advanced Paediatric Life Support: The Practical Approach*, 4th edn. BMJ Publishing Group, London.

Aylott, M. (2006) Caring for Children with Critical Illness. In: E.A. Glasper & J. Richardson (eds) (2006) *A Textbook of Children's and Young People's Nursing*. Churchill Livingstone Elsevier, London.

Davies, J.H. & Hassell, L. (2001) *Children in Intensive Care: A Nurse's Survival Guide*. Churchill Livingstone, London.

Department of Health (DoH) (2003) *Getting the Right Start. NSF for Children Young People and Maternity Services: Standard for Hospital Services*. Available at: http://www.doh.gov.uk/nsf/children/gettingtherightstart.htm.

Department of Health (DoH) (2004) *The National Service Framework for Children, Young People and Maternity Services*. The Stationery Office, London. Available at: http://www.dh.gov.uk.

Docherty, B. & McIntyre, L. (2002) Nursing considerations for fluid management in hypovolaemia. *Professional Nurse*, **17**(9), 545–549.

Dunning, J., Daly., J.P., Malhotra, R., Stratford-Smith, P., Lomas, J.P., Lecky, F., Batchelor, J. & Mackway-Jones, K. (2004) The implications of NICE guidelines on the management of children presenting with head injury. *Archives of Disease in Childhood*, **89**(8), 763–767.

European Resuscitation Council (2005) *European Resuscitation Council Guidelines for Resuscitation 2005. Section 6 Paediatric Life Support*. Elsevier. Online at: www.elsevier.com/locate/resuscitation.

European Resuscitation Council and Resuscitation Council UK (ERC & RC UK) (2004) *European Life Support Course: Provider Manual for use in the UK*. Resuscitation Council (UK), London.

Evans, R.J., Jewkes, F., Owen, G., McCabe, M. & Palmer, D. (1995) Intraosseous infusion, a technique available for intravascular administration of drugs and fluids in the child with burns. *Burns*, **21**(7), 552–553.

Fisher, B., Thomas, D. & Peterson, B. (1992) Hypertonic saline lowers raised intracranial pressure in children after head trauma. *Journal of Neurosurgical Anesthesiology*, **4**(1), 4–10.

Flaherty, J. & Glasper, E.A. (2006) Emergency Department Management of Children. In: E.A. Glasper & J. Richardson (eds) (2006) *A Textbook of Children's and Young People's Nursing*. Churchill Livingstone Elsevier.

Guys and St Thomas', King's College and University Lewisham Hospitals (2005) *Paediatric Formulary*, 7th edn. London.

Hazinski, M.F. (1992) *Manual of Pediatric Critical Care*. Mosby, New York.

Kelsey, J. & McEwing, G. (2006) Respiratory Illness in Children. In: E.A. Glasper & J. Richardson (eds) (2006) *A Textbook of Children's and Young People's Nursing*. Churchill Livingstone Elsevier.

Kinney, S.B. & Tibballs, J. (1999) An analysis of the efficacy of bag-valve-mask ventilation and chest compression. *Resuscitation*, **43**, 115–120.

Mackowiak, P., Wasserman, S.S. & Levine, M.M. (1992) A critical appraisal of the upper limit of the normal body temperature and other legacies of Carl Reinhold August Wunderlich. *Journal of the American Medical Association*, **268**, 1578–1580.

Mackway-Jones, K., Molyneux, E., Phillips, B. & Wieteska, S. (1997) *Advanced Paediatric Life Support. The Practical Approach*, 2nd edn. BMJ Publishing Group, London.

National Institute for Clinical Excellence (NICE) (2003) *Head Injury Guidelines*. Available online at: http://www.NICE.org.uk.

NHS Executive (1997a) *Paediatric Intensive Care: a framework for the future. Report from the National Co-ordinating Group on PIC*. NHS Executive, Leeds.

NHS Executive (1997b) *Paediatric Intensive Care: a bridge to the future. Report of the Chief Nursing Officer's Taskforce to the Chief Executive*. NHSE, London.

Rajesh, V.T., Singh, S. & Kataria, S. (2000) Tachypnoea is a good predictor of hypoxia in acutely ill infants under 2 months. *Archives of Disease in Childhood*, **82**, 46–49.

Resuscitation Council (UK) (2006) *Resuscitation Guidelines 2005*. Resuscitation Council (UK), London. Available at: http://www.resus.org.uk/pages/guide.htm.

Royal College of Paediatrics and Child Health (1999) *Accident and Emergency Services for Children: A Report of a Multi-Disciplinary Working Party*. RCPCH, London.

Royal College of Paediatrics and Child Health (2004) A Joint Inter-Collegiate Working Party on A & E Services for Children. *General Paediatrician with Responsibilities for the Child in A & E: The Designated Liaison Paediatrician*. RCPCH, London.

Royal College of Surgeons (RCS) and the British Orthopaedic Association (BOA) (2000) *Better Care for the Seriously Injured*. RCS, London.

Salter, R. & Maconchie, I.K. (2004) *Implementation of Recommendations for the Care of Children in UK Emergency Departments. National Postal Questionaire Survey*. BMJ. Available online at: doi:10.1136/bmj.38313.580324.F7.

Thomas, D.O. (1996) *Assessing Children – it's different*. RN, **59**(4), 33–44 (quiz 45).

Watson, S. (2000) Children's nurses in accident and emergency department: literature review. *Accident and Emergency Nursing*, **8**, 92–97.

Woodrow, P. (2000) Head injuries: acute care. *Nursing Standard*, **14**(35), 37–44.

Chapter 9 **Paediatric Resuscitation**

Rebecca Hoskins and Karen Chandler

Introduction

Paediatric cardiac arrest is a rare event. However, most occur or are managed in the emergency department (Castle 2002). The aim of this chapter is to discuss issues related to paediatric resuscitation and advanced life support (ALS) within the emergency setting. It presents the principles of basic and advanced life support in the context of resuscitating an infant and a child. Basic life support (BLS) is the foundation for successful advanced life support. Additionally basic life support is not simply the scaled-down version of the techniques and skills required for adult resuscitation. Specific techniques are required and employed according to the needs of the child (Advanced Paediatric Life Support (APLS) 2004; Resuscitation Council UK 2005). Furthermore, the aetiology of cardiorespiratory arrest in children is different from that of adults, largely due to anatomical, physiological and pathological differences (European Resuscitation Council and Resuscitation Council UK (ERC & RC UK) 2005). Thus, the BLS algorithm will be presented before describing the ALS algorithm and identifying common paediatric resuscitation drugs, strategies for estimating drug dosages and the appropriate equipment for paediatric resuscitation. Firstly, implications for assessment and intervention will be addressed in relation to the causes of paediatric arrest and the anatomical, physiological and pathological differences between children and adults.

Definitions

For the purposes of resuscitation the ERC (2005) and the RC UK (2005) provides the following definitions:

- An **infant** is a child under the age of 1 year.
- A **child** is aged between 1 year and puberty.

Why are children different?

Cardiopulmonary (CPR) arrest is uncommon and usually unpredictable in children (Byrne & Phillips 2003). It is rarely due to primary cardiac disease such as in adults where the primary arrest is often cardiac and is usually due to cardiac arrhythmia, such as ventricular fibrillation (VF) or pulseless ventricular tachycardia, requiring immediate treatment, as every minute's delay to defibrillation decreases the chance of returning to spontaneous circulation by 10% (ERC & RC UK 2005). In adults cardio-respiratory function may remain normal until the moment of arrest.

Alert: Automated external defibrillators (AED) may be used in children over 1 year of age (over approximately 25 kg). AEDs can accurately detect VF in all ages but may be inaccurate in the detection of tachyarrhythmias in infants. The ERC (2005) recommend purpose made paediatric pads, or programmes, which attenuate the energy output of an AED for children over 1 year. If it is the only machine available then an unmodified adult AED may be used for children older than 1 year who require defibrillation in cardiac arrest. Currently there is insufficient evidence to support or refute the use of AEDs in children aged less than 1 year (ERC 2005). Facilities that care for children under this age must provide defibrillators capable of appropriate energy adjustment.

In children most cardiac arrests are secondary to hypoxia. Hypoxia is the most common cause of cardiac arrest in children, followed by fluid loss, the underlying causes being respiratory disease and/or fluid loss. Respiratory arrest also occurs secondary to neurological dysfunction resulting from poisoning or convulsions, raised intracranial

Table 9.1 Anatomical differences of a child's airway and the implications for practice

Anatomical difference	Clinical application
Narrow airways	Greater risk of obstruction due to obstruction or swelling At greater risk of airway compromise
Large head and short neck	Tends to cause the neck to flex in the unconscious child and therefore contribute to airway obstruction
Relatively large tongue	May fall backwards in the unconscious child obstructing the airway
Infants less than 6 months old are obligate nasal breathers	A baby with a cold and therefore a 'blocked' nose is at far greater risk of respiratory compromise and failure
In children aged 3–8 years old, the tonsils and adenoids may be enlarged (hypertrophy)	May cause airway obstruction in the unconscious child and make airway management more problematic
Trachea is short and soft	Overextension of the neck can result in an obstructed airway
The cricoid ring is the narrowest part of the airway in a child as opposed to the larynx in adults	The cricoid ring acts as a physiological cuff and is susceptible to oedema and because of this, uncuffed ET tubes are used in children before puberty

pressure due to head injury or acute encephalo-pathy. Most other cardiac arrests are secondary to circulatory failure (shock). The worst outcome is in children who have had an out-of-hospital arrest and who arrive apnoeic and pulseless (APLS 2004). Thus it is argued that earlier recognition of seriously ill children and paediatric cardiopul-monary training for the public as well as health care professionals could potentially improve the outcome for this group of children (APLS 2004).

As highlighted within this book, children are not simply small adults. It is important to remember that children will have important physical and psychological differences as well as physio-logical responses to illness and trauma that change with age. Understanding these differences will ensure a modified approach to resuscitation in accordance with the age of the child.

Anatomy and physiology of the respiratory tract

The changes and differences in the anatomy and physiology of the respiratory and cardiovascular systems of children influence the emergency care given to them. These are summarised in the chap-ter concerned with respiratory emergencies. It is, however, important to remember that differences in the anatomy and physiology of the respiratory and cardiovascular systems of children influence emergency care (Hazinski 1992; Mackway-Jones *et al.* 1997). Therefore the important differences and their implications for resuscitation are high-lighted below and shown in Table 9.1.

Airway

The anatomical features outside and inside the airway have relevance to care and resuscitation techniques:

- Large head and short neck causing neck flexion
- Small face and mandible
- Loose teeth or orthodontic appliances
- Large tongue with the potential to obstruct the airway in an unconscious child, but may also impede the view during a laryngoscopy
- Compressible floor of the mouth with implica-tions for holding the jaw for airway positioning
- Narrow nasal passages easily obstructed by mucus secretions
- Adenotonsillar hypertrophy in 3–8-year-olds potentially causing obstruction and difficulty when the nasal route is used to pass pharyn-geal, gastric, or tracheal tubes
- Horseshoe shaped epiglottis – which when projecting posteriorly at 45 degrees makes tracheal intubation more difficult

- High anterior larynx – making it easier to intubate an infant using a straight blade laryngoscope
- Short soft trachea therefore overextension of the neck causes tracheal compression.

Breathing

- Immature lungs with a small total surface area in the infant with a tenfold increase in the number of small airways from birth to adulthood.
- Notably the upper and lower airways are relatively small and consequently more easily obstructed and when they are this has significant effects on air entry in children.

- Horizontal ribs reduce air expansion.
- Flail chest is tolerated badly.

The child's respiratory system does not reach full maturity until approximately 8 years of age (Seidal *et al.* 2003). See Table 9.2 which shows the implications of this.

Circulation

- Small cardiac ventricles
- Circulating blood volume is higher per kilogram body weight (70–80 ml/kg) than that of an adult thus in infants and small children relatively small absolute amounts of blood loss can be critically important. See Table 9.3 which makes reference to this.

Table 9.2 The implications for breathing of children's respiratory anatomy

Anatomical difference	Clinical application
Infants rely mainly on diaphragmatic breathing The muscles have fewer type 1 fibres than adults	These muscles are likely to fatigue more quickly and as a result small children are more at risk of respiratory failure
The chest wall of a younger child is relatively thin	Increased work of breathing and respiratory distress can be identified by the increased work of breathing of a child, seen as intercostal/subcostal and suprasternal recession
The chest wall is more cartilaginous and compliant	Large forces are required to fracture ribs and underlying damage to the lung parenchyma may be present without evidence of rib fractures
The ribs lie more horizontally in infants	The ribs contribute less to chest expansion

Table 9.3 Implications of cardiovascular physiology

Anatomical difference	Clinical application
At birth the right and left ventricles are of similar size and weight	In a 12-lead ECG, right ventricular dominance is apparent until approx. 6 months old
	As the heart develops, the P wave and QRS complexes increase in size and the P-R interval and QRS duration become longer
The child's circulating volume is higher per kg, but the actual circulating volume is small	A child's circulating blood volume is 70–80 ml/kg; this means a 10 kg child (aged 1 year) has a total circulating volume of just 700–800 ml
The stroke volume is small and relatively fixed in infants, thus cardiac output is directly related to heart rate	A 'normal' resting heart rate for an infant is much faster than in a larger child <1 year normal heart rate = 110–160 bpm >12 years normal heart rate = 60–100 bpm

Pathways leading to cardiac arrest in children

In the adult experiencing cardiac arrest, cardio-respiratory function may be nearly normal until the moment of arrest (APLS 2004). However, in children the aetiology of cardiac arrest differs considerably from those in adults (Kuisma *et al.* 1995). The origin of the cardiac arrest is most likely to be hypoxia secondary to respiratory failure originating from a respiratory problem or disease (Morton & Phillips 1992; Thompson 1990). It can also be the result of fluid or blood loss, leading to hypovolaemic shock, and finally circulatory failure. By the time the child suffers a cardiac arrest there will usually have been a history of respiratory failure that will have caused hypoxia and respiratory acidosis; this in turn will have caused cell damage in vital organs such as the brain, liver and kidney. Cardiac arrests caused by a primary circulation problem leading to circulatory failure will also have contributed to tissue hypoxia and acidosis (Phillips *et al.* 2000). Two-thirds of paediatric cardiac arrests occur during the first 18 months of life (Kuisma *et al.* 1995). It is also worth highlighting that children who survive out-of-hospital cardiopulmonary arrest (3–15%) usually have a devastating neurological outcome, although a neurologically intact survival of over 50% has been reported in children with respiratory arrest alone (Zaritsky *et al.* 1987).

Byrne and Phillips (2003) point out that the most common causes of out-of-hospital paediatric cardiopulmonary arrest are:

- Drowning
- Trauma
- Sudden infant death syndrome
- Poisoning
- Choking
- Sepsis
- Severe asthma.

Inpatient cardiac arrests tend to be caused by:

- Sepsis
- Respiratory failure
- Drug toxicity
- Metabolic disorders
- Arrhythmias.

These in-hospital causes often complicate an underlying condition (American Heart Association 2000).

It is rare for a child to suffer a cardiac arrest from a primary cardiac problem, although children born with congenital cardiac problems may do so (Castle 2002). Children with sudden collapse may have a prolonged QT syndrome, hypertrophic cardiomyopathy, or drug-induced cardiac arrest (Richman & Nashed 1999).

It is more likely that children have a secondary cardiorespiratory arrest, due to the body's immaturity and inability to cope with the underlying illness/injury. Children will initially use compensatory mechanisms, such as tachycardia, tachypnoeas and increased vascular resistance, to provide the tissues and vital organs with oxygen. An increase in the secretion of antidiuretic hormone (ADH) will also compensate for fluid loss by reducing the body's urine output and conserve water. Unless the child is assessed and managed correctly these compensatory mechanisms will begin to fail, and the child will enter into decompensatory shock, where bradycardia will occur as a result of tissue hypoxia, leading to myocardial dysfunction and if not managed will lead to the pre-terminal rhythm asystole. Apnoea may occur, especially in the younger child, eventually the periods of apnoea will increase and the heart rate will fall further, which will lead to asystole or pulseless electrical activity. Vascular resistance, which maintains the body's blood pressure, will also fall and irreversible shock will result. This will subsequently lead to cardiac arrest and the potential death of the child. Causes of death of a child vary according to age and gender. The most common cause of death in the child under 5 years of age is from congenital abnormalities, followed closely by respiratory disease (WHO 2005). From the age of one year this changes and trauma becomes one of the most common causes of death in children, rising significantly between the ages of 15 and 24 years.

The outcome of resuscitation from secondary cardiorespiratory arrest is poor, especially if prolonged (ERC and RC UK 2005). Resuscitating a child in respiratory arrest has a long-term survival of 50–70%, but the child in cardiorespiratory arrest (without a heartbeat) will only have a survival rate 5% (ERC and RC UK 2005). Children who survive cardiorespiratory arrest may suffer organ failure, including an increased long-term neurological morbidity. Hypoxia and acidosis causes cell damage and death before myocardial damage is severe enough to cause cardiac arrest. When circulatory failure is the primary cause, the organs are also deprived of essential nutrients and oxygen as shock progresses to cardiac arrest and circulatory failure, and causes tissue hypoxia and acidosis. Thus a child might survive initially but die later from multi-organ failure. Organs particularly at risk are the brain, liver and kidney (APLS 2004).

Asystole is seen as the most common cardiac arrest rhythm in children followed by pulseless electrical activity (PEA). Asystole is thought to be the most common arrest rhythm in children because the response of a young heart to prolonged severe hypoxia and acidosis is progressive bradycardia leading to asystole (APLS 2004). Ventricular fibrillation is a less common rhythm seen in collapsed children. It is thought that the development of VF is related to cardiac mass and the developing autonomic nervous system and therefore VF is less likely to occur in children with a small heart (Walsh & Krongrad 1983). The likelihood of VF appears to increase with age based on a study of out-of-hospital data. In children with non-traumatic arrest, VF was only reported in 3% of children aged 0–8 years but was seen in 17% of people aged 8–30 years (Appleton *et al.* 1995).

The outcome of resuscitation interventions is largely dependent upon accurate assessment and management and effective BLS.

Basic life support

Although the principles of paediatric basic life support are similar to the adult guidelines, paediatric basic life support is not simply a scaled down version. As the underlying pathology of cardiac arrest differs in children the priorities are different. The techniques of resuscitation for health care professionals in children need to be modified in order to take the child's age and size into account.

Remember – for the purpose of resuscitation children are divided into two groups:

- Infant below 1 year of age
- Child between 1 year and puberty.

When approaching a collapsed child, a safe approach is of paramount importance. It is essential that the rescuer does not become a second casualty and that help is summoned quickly. A useful mnemonic is the SAFE approach:

- Shout for help.
- Approach with care.
- Free from danger.
- Evaluate ABC (APLS 2004).

See Figure 9.1.

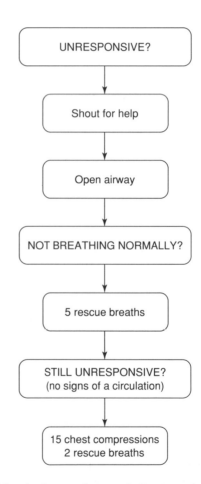

After 1 minute call resuscitation team then continue CPR

Figure 9.1 Paediatric basic life support (healthcare professionals with a duty to respond) (RC UK 2005).

Checking for responsiveness

The first priority is to ascertain whether the child is responsive to voice or stimulation. In an infant it is important not to shake the child and cause further injury. An approach of putting a hand on the child's forehead and using the other hand to gently shake the hands or feet of the child while asking them if they are all right is safe.

While a young child may not be able to answer the question, signs of life may be ascertained such as crying or opening of their eyes.

If the child responds then:

- They should be left in the position in which they were found unless they are in danger.
- They should be checked regularly and help contacted if required.
- The child should be reassessed regularly.

If the child does not respond then:

- The rescuer should shout for help.
- The child's airway should be opened using a chin lift, head tilt manoeuvre or a jaw thrust manoeuvre if trauma to the neck is suspected.

In an infant the head should be placed in the neutral position in order to open up the airway and in a child the head is placed in the sniffing position.

Opening up the airway of the collapsed child may be all that is required to relieve the obstruction of the tongue or soft tissues to allow the child to breathe spontaneously.

Look, listen and feel for breathing

The rescuer should then assess whether the child is breathing spontaneously for up to ten seconds by:

- LOOKING for chest/abdominal movement
- LISTENING for breath sounds
- FEELING for air movement.

If the child is breathing they can be put into the left lateral position, help sent for and regular reassessment carried out.

Breathing

If the child is apnoeic or making only occasional gasps then the rescuer should:

- Remove any obvious airway obstruction, under direct vision only. A blind finger sweep should never be used in children.
- Give five initial rescue breaths, the volume used should be adequate to make the chest rise and fall only. If the chest does not rise with each breath then the airway may be obstructed and the following actions should be instituted: removing any visible obstruction from the child's mouth under direct vision, ensuring that there is adequate head tilt and chin lift without over-extending the child's neck. If this is still not successful, then the jaw thrust method should be attempted. If after five attempts to achieve effective breaths despite the above actions the chest does not rise then the rescuer should move onto chest compressions.

In an infant the rescuer should cover the mouth and nose, ensuring a good seal with their mouth. In a child the rescuer should cover the mouth ensuring a good seal and pinch the child's nose.

The rescuer should blow for about 1–1.5 seconds.

Alert: If after five attempts an effective breath is not achieved then the rescuer should move on to chest compressions (RC UK 2005).

Assess for signs of circulation

Having given five rescue breaths, the rescuer should assess the child for signs of circulation.

- The rescuer should assess for any signs of circulation such as swallowing or coughing while simultaneously checking a pulse for 10 seconds (for trained health care providers only).
- In infants the brachial pulse is felt; because the necks of infants are short, the carotid pulse is difficult to palpate.
- In a child over a year old, the carotid pulse is felt.

If a pulse (of a rate above 60 beats per minute) is felt, then continue with ventilation, checking for a pulse every minute.

Delivering chest compression

If the child has no signs of circulation then external chest compressions should be commenced. There is no evidence to indicate the definitive rate at which cardiac output is insufficient, but the ERC (2005) and RC UK (2005) recommend that chest compressions are commenced in children up to puberty who have a bradycardia of less than 60 beats per minute and signs of poor perfusion, or if the rescuer is not sure whether a cardiac output is present.

In all children the landmark for chest compressions is the lower third of the sternum. In order to avoid compressing the upper abdomen, the chest compressions should be delivered one fingerbreadth above the xiphisternum. In infants two fingers are used to deliver chest compressions. An alternative method is to encircle the infant's chest and deliver the chest compressions with the rescuer's thumbs in the same position. This method has been found to be more effective in increasing coronary perfusion (Kinney & Tibballs 1999).

In children the landmarks for chest compressions are one fingerbreadth above the xiphisternum using the heel of one hand to depress the sternum. In larger children or if the rescuer is small then a two-hand technique with interlocked fingers can be used.

In all ranges, chest compressions should be delivered at a rate of 100/minute and the chest depressed to a third of the depth of the chest. Chest compressions and ventilations should be delivered at a rate of 15 compressions to 2 ventilations irrespective of the age of the child. Lone rescuers may use a ratio of 30:2.

When to go for help

Phone fast or phone first?

In general, paediatric out-of-hospital cardiac arrest is characterised by a progression from hypoxia and hypercarbia to respiratory arrest and bradycardia and then to asystolic cardiac arrest (Young & Siedal 1999). It would therefore seem more appropriate to prioritise immediate ventilation and compressions rather than phoning first as in adult resuscitation, the rationale being that the primary cause of the cardiac arrest, usually respiratory in origin, may be reversed by these manoeuvres. After 1 minute of resuscitation the lone rescuer is advised to phone for help even if this means leaving the child. If more than one rescuer is present then one should start resuscitation while another goes for help.

The exception to this rule is if the child has a witnessed, sudden collapse when the rescuer is alone, as a cardiac arrhythmia is more likely to be the cause of the collapse. In this case the lone rescuer should phone first in order to gain access to defibrillation as quickly as possible.

Foreign body obstruction sequence

The majority of deaths from foreign body aspiration occur in pre-school children (APLS 2004). Children in whom airway obstruction has occurred because of infection such as croup or epiglottitis should be taken to hospital as soon as possible. The foreign body obstruction sequence should NOT be used in these children.

This sequence should be used in children in whom: there is a definite history of foreign body aspiration; if the onset of signs and symptoms was very sudden; and there are no other signs of illness (ERC 2005; RC UK 2005).

Effective and ineffective coughing

The assessment of whether the child is able to cough effectively is key in the treatment of the choking child. If the child is:

- Crying or able to answer questions
- Has a loud cough
- Is able to take a breath before coughing
- Is fully responsive
- Then the child is able to cough effectively and should be monitored closely for signs of deterioration and encouraged to cough while help is summoned.

See Figure 9.2.

If the child is still conscious but has absent or ineffective coughing then back blows and thrusts (either chest thrusts for an infant or abdominal thrusts for children over the age of 1 year) should be given until the object is removed.

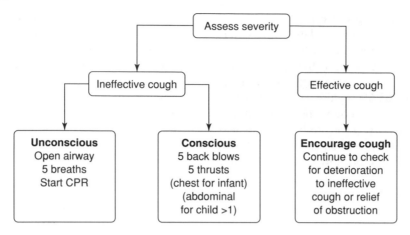

Figure 9.2 Paediatric foreign body airway obstruction treatment (RC UK 2005).

Obstruction sequence in conscious infant/child with ineffective cough

- Perform up to five back blows, try to position the head lower than the chest with the airway open. The blows should be delivered between the scapulae. If the foreign body is not dislodged go on to the next step.
- In infants perform up to five chest thrusts. Again the head should be lower than the chest. Give up to five chest thrusts to the sternum. The landmarks are the same as for chest compressions, but the chest thrusts are sharper and more vigorous than compressions and carried out at a slower rate.
- In the child if back blows have not successfully removed the foreign body then abdominal thrusts can be attempted in the conscious child. Standing behind the child a fist is placed in the child's epigastrium and the other hand pulls inwards and upwards sharply. This can be repeated five times.

Following chest or abdominal thrusts the child/infant should be reassessed; if the foreign body has not been removed and the child/infant is still conscious then the chest/abdominal thrusts can be repeated. Help should be sent for.

Alert: Abdominal thrusts should not be carried out in infants because of the risk of intra-abdominal injury.

If the child or infant becomes unconscious then:

- They should be placed on a flat surface, and help called for, although you should not leave the child at this point.
- Open the mouth looking for a foreign body which can be removed under direct vision.
- The airway should be opened and five rescue breaths attempted. If the chest does not rise between each breath then the head should be repositioned before each attempt.
- If there is no response to rescue breaths, chest compressions should be commenced, the sequence should be repeated until the foreign body is removed (RC UK 2005).

Advanced life support

The current paediatric universal algorithm is based upon the best available scientific evidence and particular emphasis has been placed on identifying and treating the causes of cardiac arrest as this is vital during paediatric resuscitation (Castle 2002). There has been a strong emphasis on the simplification of the guidelines based on the fact that many children do not receive any resuscitation at all because of the fear of rescuers that they will cause harm to the child because they have not been taught paediatric guidelines or cannot remember them. There is still a separate paediatric algorithm for health care professionals because of the physiological differences leading to arrest in children (RC UK 2005).

The priority in advanced life support is to ensure that adequate basic life support is instituted and ongoing since this is the foundation upon which adequate advanced life support measures are built. Once basic life support has been established with effective ventilation and supplementary oxygen, the child is attached to a cardiac monitor. The next phase is to then treat the presenting rhythm. As Castle (2002) identifies, paediatric resuscitation rhythms are divided into ventricular fibrillation/ ventricular tachycardia (VF/VT) and non VF/VT. Ventricular fibrillation is rare in children, seen in less than 15% of paediatric arrests in children under 10 years (Hampson-Evans & Bingham 1998). Note that VF can be caused by electrocution and poisoning, and therefore may be seen in children under 10 years of age.

Ventilate/oxygenate

Self-inflating bag-valve-mask ventilation allows the team to successfully ventilate the apnoeic child. Self-inflating bags are made commercially in three different sizes, neonatal, paediatric (500 ml) and adult (1600 ml). The smallest bag should not be used in resuscitation since it may be inadequate to support effective tidal volume and the longer inspiratory times required (American Heart Association 2000).

The mask should be an appropriate size, so as not to put any pressure on the child's eyes as it can produce a vagal response. The mask is sized from the cleft of the chin to the bridge of the nose. An airway adjunct such as an oropharangeal (sized from the middle of the mouth to the angle of the jaw and inserted the 'right way up') or a nasopharangeal airway (sized from the tragus of the ear to the tip of the nose and no wider than the child's external nares) may assist in preventing airway obstruction. More effective bag-mask ventilation can be achieved with two people, and this technique may be necessary when there is significant airway obstruction or poor lung compliance (Jesudian *et al.* 1985). High flow oxygen should be used at all times at 12–15 litres/minute. Tracheal intubation should only be attempted if an experienced anaesthetist is present.

Alert: Uncuffed or cuffed endotracheal tubes may be used in infants and children in the hospital setting only (ERC 2005; ERC & RC UK 2005).

Internal diameter for ETT (in mm) = age/4 + 4

Oral length for ETT (in cm) = age/2 + 12

A size above and below the calculated ETT size should be readily available. For example if a 4.5 mm ETT is calculated then a size 4.0 mm and 5.0 mm would also be required.

A straight blade laryngoscope is used for young children in order that the anaesthetist can sweep the epiglottis out of the way rather than place the curved blade in the vallecula.

Once a child has been intubated then asynchronous ventilations and compressions may be carried out.

Assess rhythm

Asystole/pulseless electric activity

Non-VT/VF is the most common presenting rhythm in children in cardiac arrest (Castle 2002). The treatment of asystole and pulseless electric activity is effective ventilation, using high concentration oxygen and 3-minute cycles of CPR. The 3 minutes of CPR aids circulation of drugs and the correction of hypoxia and acidosis. Adrenaline at a dose of 0.1 ml/kg of 1:10 000 (10 mcg/kg) is given at 3–5-minute intervals in order to increase coronary perfusion pressure (Saunders *et al.* 1984). Subsequent doses of adrenaline should remain at this dose. It is imperative to gain as much history prior to the child's collapse in order to try and ascertain the underlying cause of the arrest.

As in adults the potentially reversible causes should be sought and treated. If a circulatory cause is discovered such as sepsis, then fluid boluses of 20 ml/kg of crystalloid or colloid should be given.

Ventricular fibrillation/pulseless ventricular tachycardia

If the rhythm is found to be ventricular fibrillation or pulseless ventricular tachycardia then the child will require asynchronous DC shocks at

4 J/kg, followed immediately (without checking for the presence of a pulse) by 2 minutes of CPR 4 J/kg then a brief pause is taken to check the cardiac monitor, if the rhythm is still VF/VT then another shock at 4 J/kg is given followed immediately by 2 minutes of CPR and so on.

A simple and accurate way of calculating a child's weight is to use the formula:

$$(Age + 4) \times 2 = child's\ weight\ in\ kg$$

This formula can be used in children aged 1 year to puberty.

If after the first three shocks and 1 minute of CPR the rhythm is still VF/VT then subsequent shocks are given at 4 J/kg (RC UK 2005).

Paediatric paddles should only be used in children who weigh less than 10 kg (children under 1 year old) (ALSG 2004), otherwise transthoracic impedance will be higher and will contribute to an unsuccessful outcome.

Adrenaline should be administered every 3 minutes in the doses discussed above. In refractory VF/VT then amiodarone should be considered at a dose of 5 mg/kg with defibrillation following within 60 seconds of administration (ALSG 2004).

Biphasic defibrillation

At present there is no evidence to support or refute the use of biphasic defibrillators in children. The current recommendations are that if a biphasic defibrillator is to be used in a child, then the energy should be set as recommended for current monophasic shock energies: 4 J/kg, 4 J/kg and 4 J/kg (ERC 2005).

Additional drugs considered

The use of sodium bicarbonate at a dose of 1 mmol/kg should only be considered in prolonged cardiac arrest once effective ventilation is instigated and adrenaline and chest compressions are provided to maximise circulation (American Heart Association 2000).

Alert: 4.2% is used as 8.4% can cause alkalosis (EPLS 2005).

Glucose

Children, especially infants, have high glucose requirements and low glycogen stores. During periods of increased energy requirements, the child may very quickly become hypoglycaemic (American Heart Association 2000). It is essential as soon as vascular access is secured that a bedside glucose is measured. If the child is found to be hypoglycaemic (<3 mmol/l) then 10% glucose at a dose of 5 ml/kg should be administered (ALSG 2004).

Intra-osseous access

Vascular access can be difficult and time consuming to gain in children (Jewkes 1998). The current recommendations from the Resuscitation Council (UK) (2005) are that intra-osseous access should be the first line of vascular access in the child who presents in cardiac arrest without any vascular access.

Physiology

Drugs or fluids infused via the intra-osseous route enter the network of venous sinusoids within the medullary cavity, drain into central venous channels and enter the venous circulation via nutrient or emissary veins (Evans *et al.* 1995). Intraosseous injection of adrenaline has been shown to reach similar blood levels when compared with the central and peripheral venous infusion during cardiac arrest (Orlowski 1990).

Intra-osseous cannulation has a high success rate and infrequent complications.

Correct placement of the IO needle is verified by aspiration of bone marrow, by the IO needle 'standing proud' and by careful evaluation of the site when fluid is infused (Evans *et al.* 1995). Marrow aspirate can be used to estimate blood chemistry and a bedside glucose can be carried out using aspirated bone marrow.

Potential complications include:

- Local cellulitis
- Abscess formation
- Skin necrosis
- Fractures
- Compartment syndrome
- Microemboli
- Osteomyelitis
- Extravasation of drugs.

It is, however, important to put these potential complications into context, as this is a fast and relatively easy technique carried out in life threatening situations in order to allow access to the central circulation and complications have been reported in <1% of patients (American Heart Association 2000).

Sites for cannulation:

- Proximal tibia, the most commonly used site
- Distal femur
- Iliac crest
- Calcaneum (McCarthy & Buss 1998).

Any drug or fluid can be infused via an IO needle (with the exception of bretylium) (ALSG 2004). Thus resuscitation drugs, anaesthetic drugs and anticonvulsant drugs can all be administered effectively using this route. Blood and fluids can also be given via this route. In order to overcome the resistance of emissary veins, it is important to remember that fluids and drugs will have to be given under pressure.

Heat loss

As Castle (2002) notes, the management of a child's temperature is vital during resuscitation. It is acknowledged that this can be difficult but ideally the child should be covered at all times, fluids should be warmed, an overhead heater should be available and the area should be warm and free from drafts.

Post-resuscitation care

The post-resuscitation phase begins after return of spontaneous circulation in the child who was in cardiac arrest. Children are at risk of reperfusion injury following cardiac arrest, which may contribute to death hours or days later from multiple organ failure (ALSG 2004). Reperfusion injury means that cellular damage continues after circulation has been restored. This is due to depletion of adenosine triphosphate (ATP), entry of calcium into cells, free fatty acid metabolism activation and free-radical oxygen production (ALSG 2004).

The aim of post-resuscitation care is to preserve brain function, to avoid secondary organ injury by achieving and maintaining homeostasis, and to seek and correct the cause of the illness.

Another consideration to be taken into account is that the child will probably have to be trans-ferred either from the emergency department or ward to a paediatric intensive care unit (PICU). This may entail an interhospital transfer to a tertiary centre. A policy framework for providing critical care to children has been developed (NHS Executive 1997). This guidance describes how services should be regionalised around large paediatric tertiary referral centres, where expertise and resources are concentrated in caring for critically ill children. The outcome should be a reduction in mortality and morbidity for critically ill children (Maybloom *et al.* 2002).

Post-resuscitation stabilisation continues assessment and support of the child's airway, breathing and circulation with the addition of preservation of neurological function and the avoidance of multiple organ failure.

Airway and breathing

- All children should receive high flow oxygen.
- The majority of patients will require intubation and ventilation due to a decreased level of consciousness and a depressed gag reflex.
- The aim should be to keep the oxygen saturation above 95%.
- Other ventilation parameters are adjusted in response to arterial blood gas measurements.
- Capnography should be measured to ensure the ET tube remains in the correct place.

Circulation

Persistent circulatory dysfunction is observed frequently after resuscitation from cardiac arrest (Kern *et al.* 1997). This may be due to underlying cardiac abnormality, the effects of hypoxia and acidosis on the myocardium, continuing acid-base or electrolyte disturbance or hypovolaemia. Frequent reassessment is important:

- Support ventilation.
- Assess blood pH and oxygenation through blood gas measurement.
- Identify and correct metabolic disturbances.
- If indicated a bolus of fluid at 20 ml/kg may be required with further reassessment.
- Inotropic drugs may be required to support the circulation.

- Appropriate vascular access should be in place; this might also include an arterial line for blood pressure measurement as well as blood gas measurement. A central venous pressure line may also be necessary in order to measure systemic venous pressure. Continuous ECG monitoring will also be required.
- An appropriate urinary output will demonstrate adequate renal perfusion. In infants this should be 2 ml/kg/hour. In children 1 ml/kg/hour is adequate.
- Baseline blood tests should be carried out, such as urea and electrolyte measurement, full blood count, glucose, and a coagulation screen as clotting factors may be depleted following the cardiac arrest.

Disability (neurological assessment)

Secondary brain injury can be minimised by ensuring that homeostasis is achieved as far as possible. Ensuring that airway, breathing and circulation are assessed and corrected will contribute to minimising damage to the brain. Normalisation of blood sugar and body temperature will also minimise damage. Recent data suggest that post-arrest hypothermia (core temperatures of 33–36°C) may have beneficial effects on neurological function (Bernard *et al.* 1997). There is insufficient evidence at present to recommend hypothermia routinely in the post-arrest phase.

The child may also require analgesia and sedation and control of any seizures that may occur in the post-resuscitation phase.

Exposure

Assess the child from head to toe. Assess the skin for spots, rash or bruising. However, consider heat loss as well as maintaining the child's dignity. Heat loss can occur relatively quickly in the child as their body surface is larger than their body weight.

Care of the family

It is essential that the family are kept informed of their child's progress and the plan of care and transfer. Ideally a nurse should be allocated to the care of the family in order to answer questions, clarify information and act as the family's advocate.

The presence of family during resuscitation has been debated in recent years. It is however argued that wherever possible parents should be present during the resuscitation of their child. As Castle (2002) states, it is, however, paramount that a senior member of staff supports them through this experience.

When to terminate resuscitation

It is well documented that the outcome of arrest is poor although more successful for an isolated respiratory arrest. It is important that both parents and more junior members of staff are prepared for a poor outcome.

It is suggested that resuscitation efforts are discontinued if there is no return of spontaneous circulation at any time up to 30 minutes of cumulative life support and in the absence of recurring or refractory VF/VT. Exceptions are patients with a history of poisoning or a primary hypothermic insult in whom prolonged attempts may occasionally be successful. Seek expert help from a toxicologist or paediatric intensivist. Decisions should be made according to the individual case.

Following an unsuccessful outcome the parents need time to come to terms with the death of their child. This may be a time consuming process but is a vital element of the grieving process. These issues are further discussed at the end of this chapter.

It is also important to debrief the staff involved as this provides important opportunity to discuss feelings and reflect on practice in order to develop practice in the future and possibly helps to improve outcomes for children and their families (Castle 2002).

Equipment

It is advocated that a separate area is set up to deal with the seriously ill child and/or the child requiring resuscitation, although ideally all areas in a resuscitation room should be able to cope with a paediatric or adult emergency in case of multi-emergencies (Castle 2002). Whilst some children arrive by ambulance many will arrive by car as in an emergency parents are likely to pick their child up and rush to hospital. The department should be prepared for this and equipment should be set up using the ABCD+E approach.

There should be airway equipment, circulation equipment with IV/IO cannulae easily accessible. The RC UK (2005) advocate that all items be LATEX FREE. Also all IV equipment should be Luer locking. Common drugs should be available in an unlocked cupboard in the emergency department. An exhaustive list of equipment required can be found at: http://www.resus.org.uk/pages/PCAequip.htm.

Newborn resuscitation

There is the chance that an unplanned delivery may take place in accident and emergency thus there is the potential that a neonate might require resuscitation in the accident and emergency department. Newborn resuscitation has some differences from the resuscitation of a child. Most neonates need little resuscitation other than stimulation but should they require CPR the main difference is that the compressions are performed as 3:1 as opposed to 15:2 at a compression rate of 120 beats per minute (Bingham 2001). Drugs are only needed if there is **no significant cardiac output** despite effective lung inflation and effective chest compression (ERC 2005). See Figure 9.3.

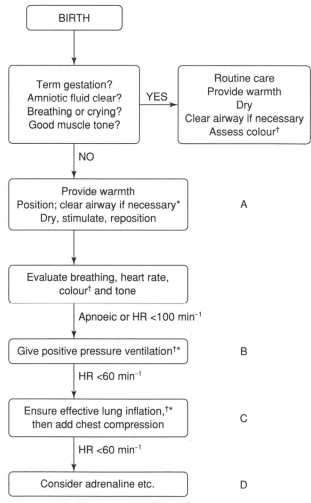

Figure 9.3   Newborn life support (RC UK 2005).

* Tracheal intubation may be considered at several steps.
† Consider supplemental oxygen at any stage if cyanosis persists.

Box 9.1	Review of learning – PBLS	
	Infant	**Child**
Airway opening head-tilt position	Neutral	Sniffing
Breathing initial slow breaths	5 rescue breaths	5 rescue breaths
Circulation pulse check	Brachial or femoral	Carotid
Chest compression landmarks	One finger breadth above xiphisternum	One finger breadth above xiphisternum
Chest compression technique	Two fingers or encircling with thumbs	One hand or two hands in larger children
CPR ratio of compressions to ventilations	15:2	15:2
Compression rate	100/min	100/min
Removal of foreign body	Back blows/chest thrusts	Back blows/abdominal thrusts

Box 9.2   Review of learning – PALS

- There are important anatomical and physiological differences to be taken into consideration when assessing, treating and resuscitating children
- For the purposes of resuscitation guidelines children are divided into 2 groups:
  — Infant – below 1 year old
  — Child – above 1 yr old up to puberty
- Formulae can be used in the calculation of weight and appropriate equipment depending on the age of the child
- Appropriate drug dosages are calculated taking into consideration the child's weight.

Useful guesstimates

1 Weight in kg = (age + 4) × 2
2 Adrenaline: 1st dose = weight divided by 10 – > no. ml 1:10 000 (i.e. minijet) 0.1 ml/kg of 1:10 000
3 Fluid resuscitation = 20 ml/kg bolus 0.9% Normal Saline (NaSal)
4 Glucose = 5 ml/kg of 10% solution (or a 5 ml syringe per kg)
5 Size (internal diameter) of endotracheal tube in mm = (age/4) + 4
6 Length of oral endotracheal tube in cm = (age/2) + 12
7 Length of nasal endotracheal tube in cm = (age/2) + 15
8 Total blood volume in infants = approx. 80 ml/kg
9 Urine output = 1–2 ml/kg/hr

Pre-terminal signs

- Bradycardia
- A silent chest
- Central cyanosis
- Hypotension
- Exhaustion

Four H's and Four T's

Hypoxia
Hypothermia
Hypovolamia
Hypo/hypercalcaemia/kalemia
Tamponade
Tension pneumothorax
Toxins
Thromboembolic events

Key points

- The most common cause of cardiac arrest in children is respiratory failure.
- Circulatory failure can result in cardiac arrest, usually caused by fluid or blood loss.
- Cardiac arrests of cardiac origin are uncommon.
- Maintaining a clear airway and oxygenation are essential.

Bereavement

Unfortunately not all resuscitation interventions have a successful outcome. It is therefore important to consider bereavement within the context of this chapter. The death of a child is undoubtedly one of the most painful and heartbreaking experiences a parent will ever endure. The death of a child caused by traumatic or unexpected circumstances can be such an intense loss that the resources of bereaved parents may be profoundly overwhelmed and one could almost expect the grieving process to be complicated.

McKissock and McKissock (1991) described bereavement as a 'natural disaster'. The death of a child contradicts our belief that children will outlive their parents and parents grieve both for the loss of the child and a loss of self. Parents could feel a huge sense of guilt for failing to protect their child (Murphy *et al.* 1998). Consequently a traumatic or sudden death for which there is little or no time for preparation can result in a very abrupt and difficult grieving process due to the sudden shock of loss and a sense of being overwhelmed.

It is, therefore, extremely important that parents and families are afforded appropriate emotional and educational support immediately after a sudden or traumatic death of a child. Coping with such a loss can be very laborious and draining for the entire family, children, adolescents and adults alike, the grief response being intense and prolonged. It must also be recognised that each member of the family will respond to the situation in their individual way and will need to deal with such a loss in their own individual way (Rubel 2004).

Murphy *et al.* (1998) found that the sudden death of a child could interfere with emotional expression and cognitive performance. Without support and intervention parents could experience increased mental distress, trauma symptoms, delayed loss accommodation, declining physical health and marital problems. For example many parents blame each other and stop communicating which could result in marital breakdown.

Those families touched by such tragedies as the sudden death of an infant or the death of a child through traumatic circumstances need to respond to their loss in some way. The way the family are supported and communicated with during the first few hours after hearing the news is critical. The way health care professionals respond to their needs at this time of crisis could have an effect on their whole grieving process.

Whilst there has been little research into managing bereavement following the sudden or unexpected death of a child, guidelines for care (Cook *et al.* 2002) recommend the following:

Key elements of a bereavement meeting

- Bereavement meetings should be delayed for 8–12 weeks following the death of a child.
- All new information should be discussed with the family, and an opportunity given to review any of their clinical questions/concerns.
- Issues related to childhood death, such as support for siblings or professional help needed by families, should be specifically discussed.
- Revisiting the ward/department where a child died can be of particular importance, especially if some family members were unable to visit during the child's illness.
- Staff undertaking bereavement meetings need to recognise signs of 'pathological' grief.

A useful list of resources and organisations available to families who have had a sudden bereavement is listed at the end of this chapter.

Conclusion

Outcome from cardiac arrest in children is poor. It is important that nurses recognise the different causes of cardiac arrest in children compared with those in adults. The child is more likely to have suffered a cardiac arrest as a consequence of respiratory failure than from circulatory failure in the main. There are important anatomical and physiological differences to be taken into account when resuscitating children. Intraosseous access is recommended in the collapsed child with no patent intravenous access in place. Post resuscitation management of the patient aims to achieve and maintain homeostasis in order to optimise the chances of recovery. Early recognition of the seriously ill child is the key to a successful outcome.

However, not all resuscitation interventions have a successful outcome which clearly raises the need for staff to support the family during this traumatic time. It is essential that resources are put in place to help and care for the family through their grieving process.

Appendix 1   Resources and organisations available to families who have had had a sudden bereavement (following the death of their child)

Box 9.3   UK sources of information and/or support

Babyloss
Website with pages that have been collated to provide information and support online for bereaved parents whose baby has died during pregnancy, at birth or shortly afterwards.

Bereavement
Factsheet from the Royal College of Psychiatrists.

Befriending Network
Established to help improve the quality of life for people living at home with a terminal or life-threatening illness. Trained volunteers offer emotional and practical support through their regular visits. The person who is being befriended decides with the volunteer how the relationship is to develop.

Child Bereavement Network
An excellent resource for information on young people's bereavement services.

Child Bereavement Trust
Aims to improve the care offered by professionals to grieving families in the immediate crisis and in the many months following the death of someone important in their lives.

Child Death Helpline
Freephone telephone for all those affected by the death of a child.

Compassionate Friends
TCF is an organisation of bereaved parents and their families offering understanding, support and encouragement to others after the death of a child or children. TCF also offers support, advice and information to other relatives, friends and professionals who are helping the family.

Cruse Bereavement Care
Cruse Bereavement Care is the largest bereavement charity in the UK, with 150 local branches. It offers help to people bereaved by death, in any way, whatever their age, nationality or belief.

Cardiac Risk in the Young (CRY)
A charity which offers help, support and counselling to families where there has been a sudden cardiac death of an apparently fit and healthy young person (sudden death syndrome). Has expert medical information about heart conditions provided by doctors.

Dignity
Offers a wealth of information to people experiencing bereavement, planning for their future, or people who would simply like to find out more about the bereavement process. Information covers topics such as funeral etiquette, cremation, what to do when someone dies, grief, and eight other titles. The site also has a Dignity Funeral Director finder and a range of information on arranging a funeral, funeral planning and memorials etc.

Epilepsy Bereaved
Help for people bereaved through epilepsy.

Families of Murdered Children
An organisation offering support, information, advice, and advocacy to those families who have lost a loved one as a result of murder.

Laura Centre
A Family Bereavement Counselling Centre offering support to: anyone affected by the death of a child at any age and from any cause; any school age child/young person affected by the death of a parent/carer, grandparent, sibling or other significant adult.

Learn and Live
Represents bereaved parents who have lost youngsters in road accidents. Lobbies for common-sense measures to make learning to drive a safer process and save other families from losing a beloved son or daughter.

London Association of Bereavement Services
Information about grief and bereavement, lists of services for bereaved people in London and the UK, links to Internet resources worldwide on the subject of bereavement and related issues plus special resources on the themes of race and culture and attachment.

Box 9.3 (Continued)

Nottinghamshire Bereavement Trust

Offers freephone helplines every evening of the year between 6 pm and 10 pm to give 'a sympathetic listening ear' to those suffering the pain of a bereavement.

Papyrus

A voluntary organisation committed to the prevention of young suicide and the promotion of mental health and well-being. Aims include: to promote public awareness of the risk of mental or emotional distress during adolescence and young adulthood, and to help to remove the stigma of such occurrences; to provide useful information for the parents of suicidal young people; and where a suicide has already occurred, to encourage the provision of appropriate support, either voluntary or professional, for those closely and traumatically affected.

Roadpeace

Provides practical and emotional help to those newly bereaved and injured as a result of a road crash.

Ruby Care Foundation

A registered charity dedicated to the care of the terminally ill, companionship of the dying, and support and counsel for the bereaved. They work towards the best possible mental, emotional and spiritual back-up and care for everyone involved when death and dying are near.

SADS – sudden arrhythmic death syndrome

Information for the family and relatives of a young person who has died of sudden arrhythmic death syndrome – SADS sometimes called sudden adult death syndrome.

SAMM – Support After Murder & Manslaughter

Understanding and support to families and friends, who have been bereaved as a result of murder and manslaughter. See also SAMM South East (The Gatwick Group).

Scottish Cot Death Trust

The Trust has three main aims: to raise funds for the research into the causes and, hopefully, the prevention of cot death; to improve and extend the support available to bereaved families; to educate the public and health care professionals about cot death.

Stillbirth and Neonatal Death Society

A national self-help organisation. It has a network of over 200 groups and contacts. All people involved in the network are volunteers and their purpose is to befriend and support bereaved parents and their families, who have suffered a stillbirth or neonatal death.

Sudden Death Support Association

An organisation to help relatives and close friends of people who die suddenly.

The Way Foundation

Provides a self-help social and support network for men and women widowed under the age of 50, and their children.

Winston's Wish

Helps bereaved children and young people rebuild their lives after a family death. Offers practical support and guidance to families, to professionals and to anyone concerned about a grieving child.

UK Funerals Online

Website to create awareness of funerals and how the industry works, general advice, help contacts, directory of funeral directors and monumental masons.

References

Advanced Paediatric Life Support Group (APLS) (2004) *Advanced Paediatric Life Support: The Practical Approach*, 4th edn. BMJ Publishing Group, London.

American Heart Association (2000) Pediatric Advanced Life Support. *Resuscitation*, **46**(1–3), 343–399.

Appleton, G.O., Cummins, R.O., Larson, M. & Graves, J.R. (1995) CPR and the single rescuer: at what age should you 'call first' rather than 'call fast?' *Annals of Emergency Medicine*, **25**, 492–94.

Bernard, S.A., Jones, B.M. & Horne, M.K. (1997) Clinical trial of induced hypothermia in comatose survivors of out of hospital cardiac arrest. *Annals of Emergency Medicine*, **30**, 146–153.

Bingham, R. (2001) Evidence Based Paediatric Resuscitation. *Paediatric Anaesthesia*, **11**(1), 1–2.

Byrne, E. & Phillips, B. (2003) The physiology behind resuscitation guidelines. *Current Paediatrics*, **13**(1), 1–5.

Castle, N. (2002) Paediatric resuscitation: advanced life support. *Nursing Standard*, **17**(11), 47–52.

Cook, P., White, D.K. & Ross-Russell, R.I. (2002) Bereavement support following sudden and unexpected death: guidelines for care. *Archives of Disease in Childhood*, **87**, 36–38.

European Resuscitation Council. European Resuscitation Council Guidelines for Resuscitation 2005. *Resuscitation*, **67**(Suppl. 1), S1–S190.

European Resuscitation Council and Resuscitation Council UK (2005) *European Life Support Course: Provider Manual for use in the UK*. Resuscitation Council (UK), London.

Evans, R.J., Jewkes, F., Owen, G., McCabe, M. & Palmer, D. (1995) Intraosseous infusion, a technique available for intravascular administration of drugs and fluids in the child with burns. *Burns*, **21**(7), 552–553.

Hampson-Evans, D.C. & Bingham, R. (1998) European Resuscitation Council Guidelines. *Care Of The Critically Ill*, **4**(6), 188–193.

Hazinski, M.F. (1992) *Manual of Pediatric Critical Care*. Mosby, New York.

Jesudian, M.C., Harrison, R.R., Keenan, R.L. & Maull, K.I. (1985) Bag-valve-mask ventilation: two rescuers are better than one. *Critical Care Medicine*, **13**, 122–123.

Jewkes, F. (1998) Paediatric advanced life support. *Prehospital Immediate Care*, **2**, 83–89.

Kern, K.B., Hilwig, R.W., Berg, R.A., Rhee, K.H., Sanders, A.B., Otto, C.W. & Ewy, G.A. (1997) Post-resuscitation left ventricular systolic and diastolic dysfunction: treatment with dobutamine. *Circulation*, **95**, 2610–2613.

Kinney, S.B. & Tibballs, J. (1999) An analysis of the efficacy of bag-valve-mask ventilation and chest compression. *Resuscitation*, **43**, 115–120.

Kuisma, M., Suominen, P. & Korpela, R. (1995) Paediatric out-of-hospital cardiac arrests – epidemiology and outcome. *Resuscitation*, **30**(2), 141–50.

Mackway-Jones, K., Molyneux, E., Phillips, B. & Wieteska, S. (1997) *Advanced Paediatric Life Support. The Practical Approach*, 2nd edn. BMJ Publishing Group, London.

Maybloom, B., Chapple, J. & Davidson, L.L. (2002) Admissions for critically ill children: where and why? *Intensive and Critical Care Nursing*, **18**, 151–161.

McCarthy, G. & Buss, P. (1998) The calcaneum as a site for IO infusion. *Journal of A&E Medicine*, **15**(6), 421–429.

McKissock, M.A. & McKissock, D.R. (1991) Bereavement: a 'natural disaster'. Responses and Adaptations. *Medical Journal of Australia*, **154**(10), 677–681.

Morton, R.J. & Phillips, B.M. (1992) *Accidents and Emergencies in Children*. Oxford University Press, Oxford.

Murphy, S.A., Johnson, L.C., Cain, K., Das Gupta, A., Dimond, M., Lohan, J. & Baugher, R. (1998) Broad-spectrum group treatment for parents bereaved by the violent deaths of their 12 to 28 year old children: A randomized controlled trial. *Death Studies*, **22**, 209–235.

NHS Executive (1997) *Paediatric Intensive Care: a framework for the future*. Report from the National Coordinating Group on PIC. NHS Executive, Leeds.

Orlowski, J.P., Porembka, D.T., Gallagher, J.M., Lockrem, J.D. & Van Lente, F. (1990) Comparison study of IO, central IV and peripheral IV infusions of emergency drugs. *American Journal of Disease in Childhood*, **144**, 112–117.

Phillips, B., Mackway-Jones, K. & Jewkes, F. (2000) The European Resuscitation Council's Paediatric Life Support Course 'Advanced Paediatric Life Support'. *Resuscitation*, **47**(3), 329–334.

Resuscitation Council UK (RC UK) (2005) *Resuscitation Guidelines 2005*. RC UK, London.

Richman, P.B. & Nashed, A.H. (1999) The aetiology of cardiac arrest in children and young adults: special considerations for ED management. *American Journal of Emergency Medicine*, **17**, 264–270.

Rubel, R. (2004) A Review of Death, Dying and Bereavement: Providing Compassion during a Time of Need. Western Schools, Brockton, MA.

Saunders, A.B., Ewy, G.A. & Taft, T.V. (1984) The prognostic and therapeutic importance of the aortic diastolic pressure in resuscitation from cardiac arrest. *Critical Care Medicine*, **12**, 871–873.

Seidal, H.M., Ball, J.W., Dains, J.E. & Benedict, G.W. (2003) *Mosby's Guide to Clinical Examination*. Mosby, New York.

Thompson, S.W. (1990) *Emergency Care of Children*. Jones & Bartlett, Boston.

Walsh, C.K. & Krongrad, E. (1983) Terminal cardiac electrical activity in pediatric patients. *American Journal of Cardiology*, **51**, 557–561.

World Health Organization (WHO) (2005) *The World Health Report 2005*. World Health Organization, Geneva.

Young, K.D. & Siedal, J.S. (1999) Pediatric cardiopulmonary resuscitation: a collective review. *Annals of Emergency Medicine*, **33**, 195–205.

Zaritsky, A., Nadkarni, V., Getson, P. & Kuehl, K. (1987) CPR in Children. *Annals of Emergency Medicine*, **16**, 1107–1111.

Chapter 10 **Emergency Care and Management of Children with Acute Respiratory Illness**

Janet Kelsey and Gill McEwing

Introduction

Respiratory disorders are the most common cause of illness in infants and children. They remain a significant cause of mortality in children under the age of 16, although mortality rates due to all respiratory illnesses have fallen over the past few decades, with pneumonia and cystic fibrosis accounting for the highest levels of mortality (Panickar *et al.* 2005). The principal cause of 'paediatric medical' attendances at emergency departments are associated with 'breathing difficulties' (Armon *et al.* 2001; Kibirige *et al.* 2003; Stewart *et al.* 1998). The Office for National Statistics (2004) has revealed that the prevalence of asthma has decreased; although a national study examining asthma trends in young people aged 12–14 found that self-reported symptoms were high in this age group, with evidence of substantial under-diagnosis and treatment (Kaur *et al.* 1998). Many children with asthma present to hospital accident and emergency departments, a high proportion of whom are subsequently admitted to hospital (Partridge *et al.* 1997).

Acute respiratory failure can result from any airway, pulmonary or neuromuscular disease that impairs oxygen exchange or elimination of carbon dioxide (Mackway-Jones *et al.* 1997), resulting in the need for emergency treatment. This chapter begins by considering the anatomical differences between children and adults, outlining their significance in the manifestation of respiratory illness. It then reviews commonly encountered respiratory illnesses and the principles of management within the paediatric accident and emergency setting. For a full account of the principles of assessment of respiratory distress and associated circulatory deterioration please refer to Chapter 8 (the critically ill child) and Chapter 9 (paediatric resuscitation) respectively. Rotta and Wiryawan (2003) also provide an authoritative summary of respiratory emergencies in children.

The anatomy and physiology of the respiratory tract in infants and children

The human body cannot function without a supply of oxygen; children due to their metabolic rate have an increased need for oxygen, which demands that their respiratory system is functioning effectively. The primary function of the respiratory system is the exchange of gases between the environmental air and the blood. The three steps in this process are:

- the movement of air in and out of the lungs
- the movement of gases between air spaces in the lungs and the blood
- the movement of blood from the capillaries surrounding the lungs to the body's organs and tissues.

The first two processes are the functions of the respiratory system, the third is performed by the cardiovascular system (McCance & Huether 2002). The anatomy and physiology of the respiratory and cardiovascular systems of young children differs from that of adults. This influences the emergency care given and must therefore be considered when assessing and managing children with respiratory problems. These differences and their significance have been summarised in the previous chapters, but are summarised again in Table 10.1.

Table 10.1 The differences in the anatomy and physiology of the respiratory and cardiovascular systems of children and their influence on emergency care (Cosby 1998 cited by Dolan & Holt 2000; Hazinski 1992; Mackway-Jones *et al.* 1997)

Factor	Nursing considerations
Airway	
Large head, short neck, inability to support head	Assistance required to maintain position of comfort
Large tongue	Airway is easily obstructed by tongue; proper positioning is often all that is necessary to open the airway
The floor of the mouth is easily compressible	Care is required when positioning of the fingers when holding the jaw
Infants less than 6 months old are obligate nose breathers	Obstruction of the nasal passages by mucus can compromise the infant's airway
Smaller diameter of all airways (in a 1-year-old child tracheal diameter is less than the child's little finger)	Small amounts of mucus or swelling easily obstruct the airways Child normally has increased airway resistance
The epiglottis is horseshoe-shaped and projects posteriorly at 45°	Tracheal intubation can be more difficult
The larynx is high and anterior	A straight blade laryngoscope is used, cricoid pressure may be necessary to facilitate intubation
The trachea is short and soft (the cricoid cartilage is the narrowest portion of neck)	Airway of infant can be compressed if neck is flexed or hyperextended Tube displacement is more likely Provides a natural seal for endotracheal tube
The cricoid ring is lined by pseudostratifed ciliated epithelium loosely bound to areolar tissue	Particularly susceptible to oedema Uncuffed tubes are preferred in pre-pubertal children
Breathing	
Infants rely mainly on diaphragmatic breathing. The ribs lie more horizontally in infants and contribute less to chest expansion Their muscles are more likely to fatigue compared with adults	Children are more prone to respiratory failure Anything that impedes diaphragm contraction or movement e.g. abdominal distension can contribute to the development of respiratory failure
Sternum and ribs are cartilaginous Chest wall is soft	Infant's chest wall may move inwards instead of outwards during inspiration (retractions) when lung compliance is decreased
Intercostal muscles are poorly developed	Greater intrathoracic pressure generated during inspiration The compliant chest wall may allow serious parenchymal injuries to occur without rib fracture
Increased metabolic rate (about twice that of an adult) Increased respiratory demand for oxygen consumption and carbon dioxide elimination	Respiratory distress increases oxygen demand, as does any condition that increases metabolic rate, e.g. fever
Lung compliance and high chest wall compliance in the neonate	Respiratory function inefficient during episodes of respiratory distress
Smaller amount of elastic and collagen tissue in the paediatric lung	May contribute to the increased incidence of pulmonary oedema, pneumomediastinum and pneumothorax in infants
Circulation	
Child's circulating blood volume is larger per unit of body weight (70–80 ml/kg) but absolute volume is relatively small	Blood loss considered minor in an adult may lead to shock in a child Decreased fluid intake or increased fluid loss quickly leads to dehydration

Table 10.1   (Continued)

Factor	Nursing considerations
70–80% of a newborn's body weight is water, compared with 50–60% of an adult's body weight; about half of this volume is extracellular	Acute blood loss produces symptoms when 20–25% of circulating volume has been lost Dehydration will compromise peripheral perfusion when 7–10% of the infant's or child's body weight and 5–7% of the adolescent's or adult's body weight is lost
Stroke volume is small and relatively fixed in infants Cardiac output is directly related to heart rate By the age of 2 years the myocardial function and response to fluid is similar to that of an adult	Stroke volume cannot increase to improve cardiac output; response to volume therapy is therefore blunted Tachycardia is the child's most efficient method of increasing cardiac output However ventricular rates >180–220 beats/min compromise diastolic filling time and coronary artery perfusion
Systemic vascular resistance rises after birth and continues to do so until adulthood	Children's normal values for blood pressure increase with age

Respiratory assessment and examination of the chest

Thomas (1996) states that there are three parts to a paediatric assessment:

- The across room assessment
- The physical assessment
- The patient's medical history.

The diagnosis of acute respiratory disease in childhood is largely a clinical one. It rests on history and examination with the aid of chest radiograph when necessary. The clinical signs of respiratory failure include those demonstrating evidence of a significant increase in the work of breathing and may manifest as:

- Severe retractions or grunting
- Inadequate ventilation rate
- Apnoea or gasping
- Reduced or absent inspiratory breath sounds
- Alterations in level of consciousness
- Evidence of compromise in systemic perfusion (e.g. significant tachycardia, bradycardia and extended capillary refill).

Alert: Central cyanosis is a late sign of severe hypoxia and requires urgent treatment (Hazinski 1992; Morton & Phillips 1992).

Respiratory problems that may be encountered in the accident and emergency department

Respiratory infections and asthma are major causes of morbidity in children and a common reason for admission to hospital (Meadow & Newell 2002). Respiratory tract infections in children are common but they are not usually serious. Frequent infections occur in children because the immune system has not been exposed to common pathogens and therefore infections tend to develop with each new exposure. Some respiratory problems are more common at certain ages. The same organism can cause different illnesses at different ages such as respiratory syncytial virus (RSV), which commonly causes bronchiolitis in infants but only a sore throat/cold in older children (Meadow & Newell 2002). Most of these infections do not cause a serious problem to the child; however children are particularly vulnerable to respiratory problems because of their relatively high oxygen requirements and the immaturity of their respiratory system (Neill & Knowles 2004). Respiratory disease in early childhood can interfere with the development of the lungs and cause permanent lung damage.

Upper respiratory tract problems

Apnoea

Apnoea is the temporary cessation of breathing, which can be the result of central respiratory depression or from mechanical obstruction. It can occur in the first two days of infections particularly RSV and pertussis (Meadow & Newell 2002). When apnoea is associated with cyanosis or unconsciousness then possible causes that need to be considered are seizures, congenital heart disease or airway obstruction.

Acute laryngotracheobronchitis (croup)

Croup is a common cause of upper airway obstruction in young children; it is usually mild but can (rarely) result in life threatening airway obstruction. It is acute inflammation of the upper and lower respiratory tract that occurs in children aged 6 months to 4 years usually occurring in the winter months. Table 10.2 lists the characteristics of croup.

Table 10.2   Characteristics of croup (Rudolf & Levene 1999)

- Usually preceded by an upper respiratory tract infection
- Rhinorrhoea
- Coryza
- Low grade fever
- Sudden onset – often at night

Presenting with
- Inspiratory stridor
- Barking cough
- Harsh cry, hoarseness

If obstruction is severe
- Tachypnoea
- Stridor
- Intercostal, supraclavicular, substernal and suprasternal inspiratory retractions

As condition worsens
- Cyanosis
- Increased respiratory effort
- Restlessness
- Reduced stridulous sound

These symptoms are a result of oedema of the larynx and trachea triggered by recent infection with the parainfluenza virus. The incidence of croup is 1.5–6% of children under 6 years, of which 1.5–31% may be admitted to hospital (Ausejo *et al.* 1999).

Treatment

The priority is to maintain a patent airway – less than 5% require intubation; when this is required it is usually due to gradual deterioration rather than acute obstruction. Nebulised and or oral glucocorticoids (Ausejo *et al.* 1999) usually nebulised budesonide and oral dexamethasone (Maill *et al.* 2003) are the most effective treatments, providing relief within 6 hours of treatment commencing, resulting in shorter hospital stays and fewer return visits and/or re-admissions (Russell *et al.* 2003). Inhaled steroids reduce upper airway oedema (Rudolf & Levene 1999) which has a rapid and sustained effect (D'Amore & Campbell-Hewson 2002). Cold humidified air (mist therapy) is *not* effective in improving clinical symptoms in children presenting to the emergency department with moderate croup (Neto *et al.* 2002). Oxygen therapy, ongoing assessment and monitoring throughout the child's stay in the emergency department are essential.

Epiglottitis

Epiglottitis is mainly seen in children aged 2–6 years. The infection is usually caused by *Haemophilus influenzae B* (HIB) and has therefore become increasingly rare following the introduction of the HIB immunisation of infants (Tanner *et al.* 2002). It is, though, a life threatening condition and there is concern that medical and nursing personnel may not recognise the onset of epiglottitis as they are increasingly less likely to have experienced cases in their career histories. The infection causes inflammatory oedema of the supraglottic area, which includes the epiglottis and the pharyngeal structures. Unlike children presenting with croup, those presenting with epiglottitis are likely to have had a sudden onset of illness, are systemically unwell, drool and extend their neck (Tanner *et al.* 2002). Table 10.3 provides an overview of the characteristics of epiglottitis.

Table 10.3   Characteristics of epiglottitis

- Short history
- Fever
- Stridor
- Dyspnoea
- Systemically unwell – pale, toxic, lethargic
- May drool and be unable to swallow but have minimal cough (Tanner *et al.* 2002)
- Child often adopts the characteristic posture of sitting upright, mouth open and chin thrust forward (Rudolf & Levene 1999)
- Extreme anxiety

If epiglottitis is suspected examination of the mouth is avoided as acute or total airway obstruction could result; examination should only be undertaken in the presence of an experienced anaesthetist in case intubation is required (Rudolf & Levene 1999).

Alert: Do not lie the child down because this forces the epiglottis to fall backwards leading to complete airway obstruction.

Radiography of the neck is only justified if diagnosis is in doubt and should only take place if the child is stable; radiography in lateral position may also precipitate respiratory arrest due to complete airway obstruction (Tanner *et al.* 2002). It is also not advisable to perform any procedure that may increase the child's anxiety as this could precipitate airway spasm and cause death, for example, taking a blood specimen (Porth 1994).

Treatment
Maintaining airway patency is the priority, through positioning, and if necessary emergency intubation should be performed to protect the airway. High flow (100%) oxygen should be administered, nebulised adrenaline 5 ml of 1:1000 can help with severe obstruction but will not treat the underlying cause (Tanner *et al.* 2002). Intravenous antibiotics are required immediately following intubation, usually chloramphenicol or ampicillin (Rotta & Wiryawan 2003; Rudolf & Levene 1999). Recovery is usually rapid once the airway is established and antibiotic therapy given.

Lower respiratory tract problems

Aspirated foreign body
Aspiration of foreign bodies usually occurs in toddlers who are (in line with expected stage of development) increasingly mobile and inquisitive; consequently they are more likely to put small objects in their mouths. Small beads, coins and foodstuffs (particularly dry foods such as nuts, crisps, biscuits and cereal) are the most common objects aspirated. Aspiration of peanuts poses particular problems, both due to the potential of nut allergy, and because peanut oil is an irritant to the respiratory mucus causing inflammation and oedema. They also swell in the airway becoming firmly embedded and difficult to remove because they fragment (Rudolf & Levene 1999). Initially the child may suffer from acute choking but the aspiration of a foreign body may not be recognised until the child subsequently presents, possibly with a history of recent onset of high fever and cough. The characteristics associated with the aspiration of foreign bodies are outlined in Table 10.4.

Rotta and Wiryawan (2003) note that a foreign body lodged in the extrathoracic airway typically causes inspiratory or biphasic stridor, an intrathoracic foreign body is associated with expiratory or biphasic wheezing.

Management
Bronchoscopy under general anaesthetic and removal of foreign body is likely to be required.

Table 10.4   Characteristics of aspirated foreign body (Rudolf & Levene 1999)

- Acute onset
- Respiratory distress
- Wheeze often unilateral
- Persistent cough
- Asymmetry of chest
- Mediastinal shift
- Dull percussion if collapse has occurred

It is important that this is performed as soon as possible to prevent coughing, which can lead to movement of the foreign body back up into the trachea which may lead to more severe obstruction of the airway (Mackway-Jones *et al.* 1997).

Bronchiolitis

Bronchiolitis is the commonest cause of severe respiratory infection in infancy, usually occurring as winter epidemics. It is a viral infection, 75% of cases are due to respiratory syncytial virus, but other viruses such as adenovirus, parainfluenza and rhinovirus have been found to be causative agents (Mackway-Jones *et al.* 1997). By the age of 2 years 90% of children are immune to respiratory syncytial virus (Meadow & Newell 2002).

In bronchiolitis the infection causes inflammatory obstruction of the small airways and necrosis of the cells lining the lower airways. The infant is often able to inhale but has difficulty exhaling; air becomes trapped below the obstruction and interferes with gaseous exchange. Hyperinflation of the lungs and collapse of alveoli can result. Hypoxia and, in severe cases, hypercapnia may occur (Porth 1994). Table 10.5 outlines the characteristics of bronchiolitis.

Table 10.5 Characteristics of bronchiolitis (Mackway-Jones *et al.* 1997; Meadow & Newell 2002)

- Initial coryza
- Fever
- Tachycardia
- Tachypnoea
- Irregular breathing, recurrent apnoea
- Cough
- Subcostal and intercostal recession
- Irritability
- Poor feeding
- Widespread wheeze and crepitations
- Hyperventilated chest
- Cyanosis/pallor

Alert: Cyanosis, pallor, listlessness and reduction or absence of breath sounds may precede respiratory failure (Porth 1994).

Management

As with other respiratory illnesses, airway patency and management of breathing are the priority. The most commonly used therapies used in a previously well infant or young child are supportive care, including administration of humidified oxygen, nasal suctioning and supplemental fluids (Patel *et al.* 2004). Bronchodilators such as beta$_2$ agonists and anticholinergic agents are often used to relieve symptoms although the evidence to support the use of anticholinergic drugs is not wholly convincing (Everard *et al.* 2002). Similarly the use of glucocorticoids, while routinely practised, does not appear to have a clinically significant effect on the outcome and course of acute viral bronchiolitis (Patel *et al.* 2004).

Asthma

Asthma is the commonest medical condition of childhood (Phelan 1994). It affects approximately 10% of children; changes in prevalence of asthma in children are difficult to determine owing to changes in diagnostic practice (Magnus & Jaakkola 1997). However, defined asthma and wheezing in children increased dramatically over the latter part of the 20th century (Kaur *et al.* 1998) with a recent decline noted (ONS 2004). The increase previously seen is thought to be due to environmental factors (Caldwell 1998), with evidence of under-diagnosis and treatment a further possible contributory factor (Kaur *et al.* 1998). There are approximately 2000 deaths (adults and children) each year in Britain; 80% of these are thought to be preventable.

The British Thoracic Society (2004) adopts the definition of asthma provided by the National Heart, Lung and Blood Institute (1992) which defines asthma as 'a chronic inflammatory disorder of the airways . . . in susceptible individuals. Inflammatory symptoms are usually associated with widespread but variable airflow obstruction and an increase in airway response to a variety of stimuli. Obstruction is often reversible either spontaneously or with treatment'. Asthma can be difficult to diagnose in young children, but should be suspected in any child with wheezing, ideally heard on auscultation, and distinguished from upper airway noises (British Thoracic Society 2004).

The British Thoracic Society (2004) guidelines provide guidance for the management of childhood asthma in the emergency department, based on the presenting symptoms, and assessment of asthma severity. These are accessible from the following website (annex 5) http://www.britthoracic.org.uk/iqs/sid.04977940755929847709666/Guidelinessince%201997_asthma_html.

Principles of asthma management

When a child attends the emergency department with asthma, airway patency is the first priority. Having established this, maximising the child's breathing and oxygenation is then the goal, with the British Thoracic Society (2004) guidelines for emergency care providing a good basis to work from. Over 90% of asthmatics take all the medications they require by inhalation. Asthma guidelines recommend that drug delivery to children should be through metered dose inhalers with spacers – across all age groups (British Thoracic Society 2004; NICE 2000, 2002). However, the guidelines also note that the method of delivery should be acceptable to the patients; for older children (aged 5 years or over), bulky spacers are not always practicable (or 'cool'), thus dry powdered inhalers may also be used for school aged children. It is of note, though, that research indicates that children do not always know how to use inhaler devices appropriately, for example Child *et al.* (2002) found that of 1444 children using asthma inhalers a large proportion were given inhalers they could not use.

Inhaled street drugs

Inhaled street drugs are abused pharmacological agents that are toxic to the respiratory system. These illegally obtained drugs are frequently combined with additional substances that promote airway injury because of their toxic nature (Cruz *et al.* 1998). Recognising the signs and symptoms of airway involvement from inhaled street drugs is difficult because the clinical presentation is similar to other acute respiratory disorders. They include wheezing, shortness of breath, chest pain and haemoptysis. The cause of the respiratory problem being linked to inhaled street drugs is usually made from the history taken from the patient or their friends (Cruz *et al.* 1998).

The management of the pulmonary complications related to inhaled street drugs is principally supportive. All patients should be carefully monitored and supplemental oxygen administered. Specific therapeutic measures are offered on an individual basis, such as ventilator support for respiratory failure and chest tube placement for clinically significant pneumothorax.

The two drugs that cause the most significant respiratory effects are crack cocaine and inhaled heroin.

Crack cocaine

The pulmonary complications from the use of crack cocaine occur in up to 25% of users and range from cough and shortness of breath to fatal pulmonary haemorrhage (Tashkin *et al.* 1996). The respiratory symptoms usually develop acutely within minutes or hours of use. The cough may be productive of characteristic black sputum accompanied by wheezing and dyspnoea. The black sputum is attributed to inhalation of the carbonaceous residue from butane- or alcohol-soaked cotton sponges used to ignite the cocaine (Klinger *et al.* 1992). Haemoptysis is reported to occur in up to 25% of crack users; overt alveolar haemorrhage is observed in 30% of users at autopsy in those experiencing sudden death from cocaine overdose.

Crack smoking has been known to cause acute exacerbations of pre-existing asthma and has been reported with near fatal and fatal acute bronchospasm in patients with a previous history of asthma (Cruz *et al.* 1998).

Management

Symptomatic relief of wheezing and dyspnoea should include oxygen therapy and, when appropriate, beta$_2$ agonists. Sputum should be obtained when available and examined for routine, community-acquired and opportunistic organisms, because many patients are, or have been, intravenous drug abusers, and crack smoking is considered a risk factor for acquired human immunodeficiency virus (Cruz *et al.* 1998).

Heroin

Inhaled heroin produces respiratory symptoms including shortness of breath, wheezing, and upper-airway obstruction from oedema; acute eosinophilic pneumonia has also been reported (Cruz *et al.* 1998).

The most serious pulmonary complication from inhaling heroin fumes is the provocation of severe and even fatal exacerbation of asthma. Opiates are powerful releasers of histamines, which can produce inflammation and oedema. This can be particularly problematic in asthmatics that are atopic. Another potential danger of heroin use in acute asthma is the central respiratory depression effect of opiates. This consequence of heroin may compromise the normal compensatory respiratory responses to an asthmatic attack.

Management

Management should include administering naloxone, an opiate antagonist, whenever the systemic manifestation of ventilatory depression from opioid use is suspected (Cruz *et al.* 1998).

Conclusion

This chapter has presented an overview of the most commonly presenting acute respiratory problems in children and young people. Many children do, though, also attend with non-specific viral upper respiratory tract infections and the more seriously ill infants and children may also present with pneumonia, which is commonly secondary to another underlying problem such as cystic fibrosis or AIDS. Whatever the underlying pathology the immediate assessment and management of these children follows the same principles, with the mnemonic ABCDE a useful reminder. These are fully outlined in the chapters on the critically ill child and paediatric resuscitation for further reference. Below are two scenarios which may be considered typical of a presentation to the emergency department; these can be used as a basis for testing your knowledge and response to the presentation of an acutely unwell child with respiratory distress, drawing on information from this and Chapters 8 and 9.

Scenario 1   Acute laryngotracheobronchitis (croup)

It is 6 a.m. and an 8-month-old baby boy weighing 8.2 kg is brought to the assessment unit by his parents following an emergency visit by his general practitioner.

The baby has a history of having had a runny nose for 2 days and being off his feeds for the last 24 hours. His parents report that he felt hot all day yesterday. Last night his cough got worse, he was making funny noises when he was breathing and didn't seem to be able to get his breath. Mum tried giving him some water to drink to calm him down but this seemed to make his breathing worse. For the last hour he has been a lot quieter but mum is worried because he doesn't seem right.

Consider the following:

1   How would you assess the current physiological status of this child?
2   What observations would you carry out?
3   What would you expect these observations to be and why?
4   From the given history which statements would you pick out as giving you concern?
5   What care would you initiate?

Scenario 2   Asthma

Mohammed is a 5-year-old asthmatic brought to the accident and emergency department by his mum after being unwell since he walked home from school earlier. Mohammed always likes to run ahead of mum with his friend and today it is particularly cold outside. Mum has already administered Mohammed's usual asthma medication but it is now 8 p.m. and mum is worried that he has not improved enough to go to bed.

1   What observations would you expect to carry out on Mohammed?
2   What are the normal ranges for these observations for Mohammed?
3   What medications would you expect mum to have administered?
4   What treatment would you initiate?

Scenario 2   (Continued)
5   What criteria would you use to decide if Mohammed requires admitting to the paediatric ward?
6   Before discharging from the department what would you consider important to discuss with mum and Mohammed?

References

Armon, K., Stephenson, T., Gabriel, V., MacFaul, R., Eccleston, P., Werneke, U. & Smith, S. (2001) Determining the common medical presenting problems to an accident and emergency department. *Archives of Disease in Childhood*, **84**, 390–392.

Ausejo, M., Saenz, A., Pham, B., Kellner, J., Moher, D. & Klassen, T. (1999) The effectiveness of glucocorticoids in treating croup: meta-analysis. *British Medical Journal*, **319**, 595–600.

British Thoracic Society (2004) *British Guidelines on the Management of Asthma: A National Clinical Guideline*. British Thoracic Society. Scottish Intercollegiate Guidelines Network, available at: http://www.britthoracic.org.uk/iqs/sid.0497794075592984770 9666/Guidelinessince%201997_asthma_html.

Caldwell, C. (1998) Management of acute asthma in children. *Nursing Standard*, **12**(29), 49–54.

Carter, B. (1995) Nursing support and care: meeting the needs of the child and family with altered respiratory function. In: *Child Health Care Nursing*. B. Carter & A.K. Dearman (eds). Blackwell, London. pp. 275–305.

Child, F., Davies, S., Clayton, S., Fryer, A.A. & Lenney, W. (2002) Inhaler devices for asthma: do we follow the guidelines? *Archives of Disease in Childhood*, **86**, 176–179.

Cruz, R., Davis, M., O'Neil, H., Tamarin, F., Brandstetter, R. & Karentzky, M. (1998) Pulmonary manifestations of inhaled street drugs, heart and lung. *Journal of Acute and Critical Care*, **27**(5), 297–307.

D'Amore, A. & Campbell-Hewson, G. (2002) The management of acute upper airway obstruction in children. *Current Paediatrics*, **12**, 17–21.

Everard, M.L., Bara, A., Kurian, M., Elliott, T.M. & Ducharme, F. (2002) Anticholinergic drugs for wheeze in children under the age of two years. *Cochrane Database of Systematic Reviews*. 2002 Issue 1. No.: CD001279.

Hazinski, M. (1992) *Nursing care of the critically ill child*, 4th edn. Mosby, St Louis.

Kaur, B., Anderson, H.R., Austin, J., Burr, M., Harkins, L., Strachan, D. & Warner, J.O. (1998) Prevalence of asthma symptoms, diagnosis, and treatment in 12–14 year old children across Great Britain (international study of asthma and allergies in childhood, ISAAC UK). *British Medical Journal*, **316**, 118–124.

Kibirige, M.S., Edmond, K., Kibirige, J.I. & Rahman, S. (2003) A seven year experience of medical emergencies in the assessment unit. *Archives of Disease in Childhood*, **88**, 125–129.

Klinger, J.R., Bensadoun, E. & Corrao, W.M. (1992) Pulmonary complications from alveolar accumulation of carbonaceous materials in cocaine smokers. *Chest*, **101**, 1171–1173.

Mackway-Jones, K., Molyneux, E., Phillips, B. & Wieteska, S. (1997) *Advanced paediatric life support. The practical approach*, 2nd edn. BMJ Publishing Group, London.

Magnus, P., & Jaakkola, J.J.K. (1997) Secular trend in the occurrence of asthma among children and young adults: critical appraisal of repeated cross sectional surveys. *British Medical Journal*, **314**, 1795–1803.

Maill, L., Rudolf, M., & Levene, M. (2003) *Paediatrics at a glance*. Blackwell Science, Oxford.

McCance, K. & Huether, S. (2002) *Pathophysiology – The biologic basis for disease in adults & children*. Mosby, London.

Meadow, R. & Newell, S. (2002) *Lecture notes in Paediatrics*, 7th edn. Blackwell Science, Oxford.

Morton, R.J. & Phillips, B.M. (1992) *Accidents and Emergencies in Children*. Oxford University Press, Oxford.

National Heart, Lung and Blood Institute (1992) National Institute of Health. Maryland 20892. International Consensus Report on the Diagnosis and Treatment of Asthma. Publication No: 29-3091. March 1992. *European Respiratory Journal*, **5**, 601–641.

National Institute for Clinical Effectiveness (2000) *Guidance on the use of inhalers for under 5's with asthma*. http://www.nice.org.uk/ (accessed).

National Institute for Clinical Effectiveness (2002) *Inhaler devices for routine and chronic asthma in children*. http://www.nice.org.uk/ (accessed 8 April 2005).

Neto, G.M., Kentab, O., Klassen, T.P. & Osmond, M.H. (2002) A randomized controlled trial of mist in the acute treatment of moderate croup. *Academic Emergency Medicine*, **9**, 873–9.

Office for National Statistics (2004) *The Health of Children and Young People*. ONS, London.

Panickar, J.R., Dodd, S.R., Smyth, R.L. & Couriel, J.M. (2005) Trends in deaths from respiratory illness in children in England and Wales from 1968 to 2000. *Thorax*, **60**, 1035–1038.

Partridge, M.R., Latouche, D., Trakao, E. & Thurston, J.G. (1997) A national census of those attending UK accident and emergency departments with asthma. The UK National Asthma Task Force. *Journal of Accident and Emergency Medicine*, **14**(1), 16–20.

Patel, H., Platt, R., Lozano, J.M. & Wang, E.E.L. (2004) Glucocorticoids for acute viral bronchiolitis in infants and young children. *The Cochrane Database of Systematic Reviews 2004*, Issue 3. Art. No.: CD004878. DOI.

Phelan, P.D. (1994) Asthma in children: Epidemiology. *British Medical Journal*, **308**, 1584–1585.

Porth, C.M. (1994) *Pathophysiology – Concepts of Altered Health States*, 4th edn. Lippincott Company, London.

Rotta, A.T. & Wiryawan, B. (2003) Respiratory emergencies in children. *Respiratory Care*, **48**(3), 248–258.

Rudolf, M. & Levene, M. (1999) *Paediatric and Child Health*. Blackwell Science, Oxford.

Russell, K., Wiebe, N., Saenz, A., Ausejo, M., Segura, M., Johnson, D., Hartling, L. & Klassen, T.P. (2003) Glucocorticoids for croup. *The Cochrane Database of Systematic Reviews*. 2003, Issue 4. Art. No.:CD001955. DOI:10.1002/14651858.CD001955.pub2.

Stewart, M., Werneke, U., MacFaul, R., Taylor-Meek, J., Smith, H.E. & Smith, I.J. (1998) Medical and social factors associated with the admission and discharge of acutely ill children. *Archives of Disease in Childhood*, **79**, 219–224.

Tanner, K., Fitzsimmons, G., Carrol, D., Flood, T. & Clark, J. (2002) Haemophilus influenzae type b epiglottitis as a cause of acute upper airways obstruction in children. *British Medical Journal*, **325**, 1099–1100.

Tashkin, D.P., Kleerup, E.C., Koyal, S.N., Margues, J.A. & Goldman, M.D. (1996) Acute effects of inhaled and iv cocaine on airway dynamics. *Chest*, **110**, 904–910.

Thomas, D.O. (1996) Assessing children – it's different. *RN*, **59**, 4.

Chapter 11 The Assessment and Management of Paediatric Fever in the Emergency Setting

Karen Cleaver

Introduction

Fever or elevated temperature is documented as a common experience of childhood and an area of concern for parents and health professionals (Armon *et al.* 2001; Kai 1996). There are a number of causes of fever, but most commonly its basis is infection. Similarly there are numerous infections that, partly due to their immaturity, children are susceptible to. However, as parental and health care professionals' anxieties around fever are largely concerned with the possibility of meningitis, this chapter will focus on the recognition and early management of meningitis. The recognition and management of all infections including urinary tract infections are beyond the scope of this chapter, but plenty of informative sources are available. The evidence base of fever management is also reviewed. The chapter concludes with a scenario that is used to summarise the key points of the chapter.

Fever phobia

It is not uncommon to find children attending an emergency department with fever, as it accounts for 20–30% of all acute episodes (Armon *et al.* 2001; Browne *et al.* 2001; Watts *et al.* 2003). This rate of attendance reflects the fact that parents themselves worry about fever, seeing it as a disease rather than a symptom (Crocetti *et al.* 2001). The anxiety that fever in children provokes has led to writers on the subject coining the term 'fever phobia' (Schmitt 1980), with evidence that this phenomenon still exists today (Crocetti *et al.* 2001; Karwowska *et al.* 2002). For example, Crocetti *et al.* (2001), in their study of 340 caregivers, found that 56% were worried about the potential harm of fever, with 44% considering a

temperature of 38.9°C to be a 'high' fever. Ninety-one per cent of caregivers believed that fever could have harmful effects, including brain damage (21%) and death (14%). Karwowska *et al.* (2002) found similar concerns among parents but also found that health care professionals shared these too. A study undertaken by Poirier *et al.* (2000) specifically looked at emergency nurses' perspectives on fever in children and found that 31% of respondents were unsure as to what would constitute a temperature that would be dangerous to a child. Fifty-seven per cent of these nurses also considered seizures to be the primary danger, with 29% stating that permanent brain injury or death could occur; the authors thus concluded that 'fever phobia' was inherent within the sample of nurses surveyed.

Studies have, though, found that parents will manage fever at home prior to seeking medical help. For example, Kallestrup and Bro (2003) in their study of 153 parents presenting to an out-of-hours GP clinic found that 52% of parents had sought advice from family, friends, day care staff and others before seeking medical help. Twenty-one per cent had tried over the counter remedies prior to the consultation. Having exhausted these avenues the parents then resorted to the out-of-hours clinic, in the expectation that their child would be physically examined. Contrary perhaps to our expectations, 71% of the parents did not expect a prescription for antibiotics. The worries the parents have centre on their concerns about failing to recognise a serious problem, notably meningitis (Kai 1996). As a (likely) consequence there is evidence that fever is treated aggressively at home by parents and caregivers (Crocetti *et al.* 2001; Kinmonth *et al.* 1992) with aggressive treatment also evident in the approach taken by health care providers (Karawowska *et al.* 2002; Poirier *et al.* 2000). This is despite the fact that there is little evidence that fever is dangerous, and paradoxically may have a beneficial effect (Kluger 1980, 1992).

Physiological aspects of fever

From a biomedical perspective it has been determined that fever most commonly results when the hypothalamic set point is raised due to the action of cytokines, released in response to the presence of viral or bacterial pathogens. Once reset the thermoregulatory centre maintains a high temperature through cutaneous vasoconstriction, heat conservation or shivering thermogenesis (Browne *et al.* 2001). Less commonly fever can also occur as a result of excessive heat production which exceeds heat loss that can occur due to excessive environmental temperature, but also hyperthyroidism, malignant hyperthermia and salicylate poisoning (Browne *et al.* 2001). Defective heat loss mechanisms, as manifested in ectodermal dysplasia, heat stroke and poisoning from anticholinergic drugs also result, less commonly, in fever (Browne *et al.* 2001).

Determining what constitutes fever is not consistent within the medical and nursing literature, and thus studies that consider aspects such as the interventions and the management of fever are difficult to systematically evaluate, as many take a different starting point in relation to what a fever is. As noted above both parents and health care providers lack consistency in what they deem to be a 'significant' temperature, which is further exemplified in other studies in this area. For example Edwards *et al.* (2001) identified that nurses have a 'temperature' at which they consider a child febrile which is between 37.2–39°C. Similar findings were reported in a study which surveyed emergency nurses. Thomas *et al.* (1994) found a wide variation in the range of what emergency nurses considered the norm – from 37.8 to 40.6°C, while Watts *et al.* (2003) concluded from a systematic review that, in respect of oral temperatures, fever onset was considered to have occurred with a temperature

of 37.6–37.8°C. It is generally agreed that an infant's normal temperature is likely to be higher than the older child's, and can as a norm be as high as 37.8°C. It is also agreed that a child with a temperature of >41°C is at a higher risk of serious illness.

Children presenting at the emergency department or clinic with a temperature do so with variable histories of fever. Studies which have investigated causes of fever have determined that approximately 80% of cases will have infection as a basis for fever, including fever of prolonged (>14 days) and unknown origin (Cogulu *et al.* 2003). The cause of fever is commonly viral, particularly over the winter months, when respiratory syncytial virus (RSV) is more prevalent. A number of clinical markers have been identified that have been validated and found to increase the accuracy with which acute/serious illness in children is diagnosed:

- Presence/level of drowsiness
- Decreased level of activity
- Alteration in respiratory pattern, including presence of respiratory grunt
- Colour/pallor
- Poor feeding
- Decreasing urinary output
- Presence of vomiting, including bile stained vomit
- Presence of a lump >2 cm and temperature (Hewson *et al.* 2000).

However, predicting which children presenting with fever may have a serious illness can be difficult (Finkelstein *et al.* 2000; Nademi *et al.* 2001), with the degree of temperature and white blood count (WBC) found to be poor predictors of serious disease. For example, Finkelstein *et al.* (2000) reviewed the cases of a random sample of 5000 children from a cohort of 20 585 children who presented with temperatures >38°C. They found that among 3819 initial visits of an illness episode, 41% of the children had no diagnosed bacterial or specific viral source, concluding that the majority of children in the study were diagnosed with a bacterial infection and treated with an antibiotic appropriately. However further laboratory testing was not warranted in order to screen for meningitis, as it was unlikely to affect the overall detection rate (Finkelstein *et al.* 2000).

In their study Hewson *et al.* (2000) found bronchiolitis to be the most commonly occurring diagnosis (n = 418), although only 13.2% were found to have a serious illness, whereas the numbers presenting with meningitis were comparatively low (n = 12) but all of these children were seriously ill. As noted above a key concern for parents whose children have a fever is the fact that they may miss a serious illness in their child, particularly meningitis, which is also of concern to health care professionals in the emergency department. Parents are likely to be aware of the significance of a non-blanching rash due to prominence given to parental advice on the 'glass test'. As a consequence a parent whose child has fever with a non-blanching rash is likely to seek medical advice promptly. However, as Wells *et al.* (2001) suggest from their research, the presence of a non-blanching rash in children, confined to the distribution of the superior vena cava is unlikely to be meningococcal infection. It is also of note that five of the children in their study who had a diagnosis of meningococcal disease presented with a temperature below 37.5°C. However, Pollard *et al.* (1999) report that meningococcal infection should be suspected in any child who presents with a non-blanching rash as 80% of bacteriologically proved cases would develop purpura or petechiae.

Bacterial meningitis

El-Bashir *et al.* (2003) report that bacterial meningitis can be difficult to diagnose, as the symptoms and signs are often non-specific, especially in young children. They report that symptoms of bacterial meningitis may include:

- High temperature
- Poor feeding
- Vomiting
- Lethargy and irritability.

Clinical signs may include:

- Bulging fontanelle
- Fever

- Drowsiness
- Apnoeas
- Convulsions
- Purpuric rash (although note above).

The specific signs associated with meningitis, Kernig and Brudzinski, are noted to be unreliable in children, a factor borne out in a study undertaken by Oostenbrink *et al.* (2001), who concluded that in infants bacterial meningitis is more likely to be associated with irritability and bulging fontanelle. El-Bashir *et al.* (2003) advise that analysis and culture of cerebrospinal fluid obtained through lumbar puncture remains the definitive method for diagnosis of meningitis, assuming that it is not contraindicated in the case concerned. However, Pollard *et al.* (1999) advise that in the presence of meningococcal disease and septicaemia, lumbar puncture is not recommended, and note that it adds little additional information to aid diagnosis.

Once a diagnosis of bacterial meningitis is made, it is imperative that parenteral treatment is commenced in the emergency department as this has been found to reduce mortality (Pollard *et al.* 1999), with retrieval to a specialist tertiary centre required if specialist services are not available locally. Protocols for the management of acute bacterial meningitis should have been developed; and the meningitis organisation (www. meningitis.org) have devised an algorithm for the early management of meningococcal disease in children, based on that presented in the original paper by Pollard *et al.* (1999). The algorithm can be accessed as a PDF file from the above site.

Temperature taking

A further area of debate is which method of temperature taking/thermometry leads to the most accurate measurement of fever, with variations in terms of tympanic thermometry versus digitally recorded axillary or rectal temperatures apparent in the literature. For example, while Jirapaet (2000) recommends that infrared tympanic thermometers should not be used as a substitute for rectal temperatures in healthy term and preterm neonates, Bailey and Rose (2001) conclude from their study that they are safe, accurate, easy to use, and comfortable for the healthy preterm neonate. Smith (1998) compared mercury, digital and IVAC tympanic thermometers and found significant differences in recording between the three devices. Duce (1996) found that electronic digital and disposable crystal thermometers are as accurate and consistent as glass mercury, while infrared tympanic thermometers with an 8 mm probe were found to be inaccurate, inconsistent and an insensitive method of measuring core temperature. The axillary site was found to be inaccurate and inconsistent in children over 1 month of age. Nevertheless this systematic review also identified that while neonates, infants and children did not exhibit any preferences, infrared tympanic thermometry was the most preferred type of thermometer for both staff and parents, due to its speed, hygiene and safety. He concludes that the optimal method of temperature measurement is disposable crystal, mercury glass and electronic digital at the rectal site until the child is old enough to cooperate with oral temperature measurement. However, this route of temperature measurement is both increasingly culturally unacceptable and also, within an emergency department, impractical. Arguably child and parental choice should be the key factor but as the axillary site is inaccurate, infrared tympanic thermometry (with a 4 mm probe if available) is probably the most appropriate for the emergency care setting.

Fever management

Having determined the presence of fever, and ruled out any serious underlying pathology or sepsis, the most acceptable methods of fever management need to be determined and agreed with the child and their parents/carers. As noted above, from a biomedical perspective fever can be viewed by physicians as an important marker of the body's normal physiological response. There is some debate within the literature as to whether the treatment of low grade fever (<38.5°C) is warranted or desirable, as fever provides an environment which facilitates destruction of invading micro-organisms. However, as noted above, most parents will have already implemented fever reducing methods, and are

likely to wish to continue to do so, partly based on concerns about the potential damage of high fever, and because of the associated concerns that fever may lead to convulsions. With regard to the latter, the evidence for the use of pharmacological agents such as paracetamol as a means of preventing convulsions is not convincing (Purssell 2000; Watts et al. 2003).

Concerns have been raised about the use of paracetamol, with some cases of hepatotoxicity reported, although Kramer et al. (1991) found that the clinically relevant hazards and benefits of paracetamol antipyresis have been exaggerated. In the UK it remains the favoured pharmacological treatment, and is routinely prescribed with ibuprofen (alternating two-hourly) when temperature is elevated. A systematic review has revealed that while there is little evidence at present to support the use of paracetamol, its continued use should be recommended until further studies can confirm its therapeutic effect (Meremikwu & Oyo-Ita 2002). Moreover, even where paracetamol or ibuprofen may not be indicated due to the core temperature not being significantly elevated, its value in rendering additional comfort to a child is recognised and particularly appreciated by concerned parents, with the longer action of ibuprofen making it preferable in some circumstances (Purssell 2004).

Conclusion

The following scenario illustrates the concerns of many parents whose child has a fever. It is typical of many cases that parents or carers initially attempt to manage their child's fever at home, through both pharmacological and non-pharmacological cooling methods. However, anxiety that a fever may be indicative of an underlying serious condition which could result in brain injury or death (largely due to concerns about the presence of meningitis) are common. This results in parents seeking medical help and the aggressive treatment of fever by both parents/caregivers and health care professionals. Parents and caregivers will have selected their own chosen methods of temperature measurement and management, which while not necessarily the most effective (temperature measurement), is seen by them as

Scenario

Molly, aged 4 years, attends the emergency clinic, accompanied by her mother who is particularly anxious as Molly is irritable, is complaining of a severe frontal headache and has a fever, which is causing her to be delirious, and preventing her from sleeping. Molly's mother has been managing the fever at home for two days; she has been measuring the temperature using a tympanic thermometer and managing the temperature using paracetamol (Calpol) and tepid sponging; she is concerned though about the quantity of Calpol Molly is having and following the advice on the bottle is now seeking medical advice. She is also concerned that because the fever is not resolving this may result in a convulsion, or that Molly has meningitis.

On examination Molly is very pale and tired looking. There is no evidence of rash, there is no history of vomiting or diarrhoea and she has no respiratory symptoms. Molly is able to tuck her chin on her chest and is not light sensitive. Following a full examination the doctor reassures the mother that she probably has a viral infection, and that the reason for her headache is dehydration due to increased insensible loss. Molly's core temperature is 38.8°C. The doctor notes that Molly is indoors wearing a fleece, and only removed her outdoor coat for the examination. The doctor advises the mother that she should ensure that Molly drinks plenty of fluids, can safely continue with Calpol alternating this with ibuprofen, and that she should be cooled, by removing excess clothing.

Initial assessment of Molly to include:

Information to obtain during initial assessment	Rationale
Temperature on arrival	Provide a base-line Determine significance of the temperature; 38.8 is raised but not on its own a marker of serious illness (Nademi *et al.* 2001)
Day of onset	Even fever of prolonged duration is likely to be caused by infection (Cogulu *et al.* 2003) but other causes if prolonged need to be excluded (Browne *et al.* 2001) Indication of extent to which carers have been managing fever themselves (Kallestrup & Bro 2003) Prolonged fever, with evidence of bacteraemia may need parenteral treatment
Trends (i.e. time of day when temperature is raised)	May be clinically significant in determining type of infection/causative agent
Fever management methods employed by carers	Fever management by carers may have been aggressive due to 'fever phobia' (Crocetti *et al.* 2001; Kinmonth *et al.* 1992) Provides opportunity for educative strategies in the appropriate management of fever – in this case regarding clothing and fluids, as well as medication management Method of temperature measurement employed and accuracy of (Smith 1998), acceptability of fever measurement device by parents should influence choice in department – in this case tympanic thermometry
History of febrile convulsions	Relatively common with a recurrence rate of 30% (Hopkins 1991) Evidence for the use of antipyretics for preventing febrile convulsions has been found to be unconvincing (Purssell 2000; Watts *et al.* 2003)

Scenario (Continued)	
Colour/pallor	Marker of serious illness when associated with fever and the presence of other markers (Hewson *et al.* 2000)
Fluids in over 24 hours versus fluids out	Decreased oral intake and urinary output markers of serious illness (Hewson *et al.* 2000) Insensible loss will increase in presence of fever, leading to early signs of dehydration, including headache, as is the case in this scenario Parents/carers can then be reassured as to the possible cause of headache and irritability
Presence of rash	Depending on type of rash can indicate specific viral illness/infection such as measles Purpura and petechial rash likely to occur in 80% of cases of meningococcal disease and septicaemia (Pollard *et al.* 1999)
Perfusion	Check capillary refill. Septic shock is an early indicator of meningococcal disease arising from loss of circulating plasma due to increased vascular permeability, maldistribution of intravascular volume, and impaired myocardial function (Pollard *et al.* 1999)
Health of close family and family contacts (i.e. school and nursery)	Presence of infection in other close family members or friends is indicative of infectious illness. Many viruses notably RSV occur during winter epidemics
History of recent travel	A history of recent travel could suggest infectious illness, and if relevant, malaria and other tropical diseases not commonly seen would need to be considered

the most acceptable. The phenomenon of 'fever phobia', it is argued, can be reduced through education of parents (Crocetti *et al.* 2001), and also, judging by the literature, of health care professionals too. Nurses and doctors working in the accident and emergency setting are well placed to inform and advise parents about what constitutes a high temperature, the importance of fluids, and the use of cooling methods; these can all be addressed with parents whose children, while not seriously ill, have presented with fever.

References

Armon, K., Stephenson, T., Gabriel, V., MacFaul, R., Eccleston, P., Werneke, U. & Smith, P. (2001) Determining the common medical presenting problems to an accident and emergency department. *Archives of Disease in Childhood*, **84**, 390–392.

Bailey, J. & Rose, P. (2001) Axillary and tympanic membrane temperature recording in the preterm neonate: a comparative study. *Journal of Advanced Nursing*, **34**(40), 465–474.

Browne, G.J., Currow, K. & Rainbow, J. (2001) Practical approach to the febrile child in the emergency department. *Emergency Medicine*, **13**(4), 426.

Cogulu, O., Koturoglu, K., Kurugol, Z., Ozkinay, F., Vardar, F. & Ozkinay, C. (2003) Evaluation of 80 children with prolonged fever. *Pediatrics International*, **45**, 564–569.

Crocetti, M., Moghbeli, N. & Serwint, J. (2001) Fever phobia revisited: Have parental misconceptions about fever changed in 20 years? *Pediatrics*, **107**(6), 1241–1246.

Duce, S.J. (1996) A systematic review of the literature to determine optimal methods of temperature measurement in neonates, infants and children. *Database of Abstracts and Reviews of Effects 2004 Issue 4*. University of York, York.

Edwards, H.E., Courtney, M.D., Wilson, J.E., Monaghan, S.J. & Walsh, A.M. (2001) Fever management practices: What paediatric nurses say. *Nursing and Health Sciences*, **3**(3), 119–130.

El-Bashir, H., Laundy, M. & Booy, R. (2003) Diagnosis and treatment of bacterial meningitis. *Archives of Disease in Childhood*, **88**, 615–620.

Finkelstein, J.A., Christiansen, C.L. & Platt, R. (2000) Fever in pediatric primary care: occurrence, management and outcomes. *Pediatrics*, **105**(1pt 3), 260–266.

Hewson, P.H., Poulakis, Z., Jarman, F., Kerr, D., McMaster, D., Goodge, J. & Silk, G. (2000) Clinical markers of serious illness in young infants: A multicentre follow-up study. *Journal of Paediatrics and Child Health*, **36**, 221–225.

Hopkins, A. (1991) Guidelines for management of convulsions with fever. *British Medical Journal*, **303**, 634–636.

Jirapaet, V. (2000) Comparisons of tympanic membrane, abdominal skin, axillary, and rectal temperature measurements in term and preterm neonates. *Nursing and Health Sciences*, **2**, 1–8.

Kai, J. (1996) What worries parents when their preschool children are acutely ill, and why; a qualitative study. *British Medical Journal*, **313**, 983–986.

Kallestrup, P. & Bro, F. (2003) Parents' beliefs and expectations when presenting with a febrile child at an out-of-hours general practice clinic. *British Journal of General Practice*, **53**, 43–44.

Karawowska, A., Nijssen-Jordan, C., Johnson, D. & Davies, D. (2002) Parental and health care provider understanding of childhood fever: a Canadian perspective. *Canadian Journal of Emergency Medicine*, **4**(6), online.

Kinmonth, A.L., Fulton, Y. & Campbell, M.J. (1992) Management of feverish children at home. *British Medical Journal*, **305**, 1134–1136.

Kluger, M.J. (1980) Fever. *Pediatrics*, **66**, 720–724.

Kluger, M.J. (1992) Fever revisited. *Pediatrics*, **90**, 846–850.

Kramer, M.S., Naimark, L.E., Roberts-Brauer, R., McDougall, A. & Leduc, D.G. (1991) Risks and benefits of paracetamol antipyresis in young children with fever of presumed viral origin. *Lancet*, **337**(8741), 591–594.

Meremikwu, M. & Oyo-Ita, A. (2002) Paracetamol for treating fever in children. *The Cochrane Database of Systematic Reviews 2002*. Issue 2. Art No. CD003676.DOI:10.1002/14651858.CD003676.

Nademi, Z., Clark, J., Richards, C.G., Walshaw, D. & Cant, A.J. (2001) The causes of fever in children attending hospital in the North of England. *Journal of Infection*, **43**(4), 221–225.

Oostenbrink, R., Moons, K.C.W., Theunissen, C.C.W., Derksen-Lubsen, G., Grobbee, D.E. & Moll, H.A. (2001) Signs of meningeal irritation at the emergency department: How often bacterial meningitis? *Pediatric Emergency Care*, **17**(3), 161–164.

Pollard, A.J., Britto, J., Nadel, S., DeMunter, C., Habibi, P. & Levin, M. (1999) Emergency management of meningococcal disease. *Archives of Disease in Childhood*, **80**, 290–296.

Poirier, M.P., Davis, P.H., Gonzalez-del Rey, J.A. & Monroe, K.W. (2000) Pediatric emergency department nurses' perspectives on fever in children. *Pediatric Emergency Care*, **16**, 9–12.

Purssell, E. (2000) The use of antipyretic medications in the prevention of febrile convulsions in children. *Journal of Clinical Nursing*, **9**, 473–480.

Purssell, E. (2004) Treating fever in children: paracetamol or ibuprofen? *British Journal of Community Nursing*, **7**(6), 316–320.

Schmitt, B.D. (1980) Fever phobia; misconceptions of parents about fevers. *American Journal of Disease in Childhood*, **134**, 176–181.

Smith, J. (1998) Are electronic thermometry techniques suitable alternatives to traditional mercury in glass thermometry techniques in the paediatric setting? *Journal of Advanced Nursing*, **28**(5), 1030–1039.

Thomas, V., Riegel, B., Andrea, J., Murrray, P., Gerhart, A. & Gocka, I. (1994) National survey of pediatric fever management practices among emergency department nurses. *Journal of Emergency Nursing*, **20**(6), 505–510.

Watts, R., Robertson, J. & Thomas, G. (2003) Nursing management of fever in children: a systematic review. *International Journal of Nursing Practice*, **9**(1), S1–S8.

Wells, L.C., Smith, J.C., Weston, V.C., Collier, J. & Rutter, N. (2001) The child with non-blanching rash; how likely is meningococcal disease? *Archives of Disease in Childhood*, **85**, 218–222.

Chapter 12 Emergency Care of Children with Sickle Cell Disease: One Family's Experience

Priscilla Dike

Introduction

Specialised and comprehensive medical care decreases morbidity and mortality associated with most illnesses, but especially for sickle cell disease (SCD), a group of complex chronic blood disorders characterised by haemolysis, unpredictable acute complications that rapidly become life threatening. Timely and appropriate treatment of acute illness in children with SCD is critical so as to prevent deterioration, the development of chronic organ damage and other related morbidity, and ultimately possible mortality associated with this debilitating condition. It is therefore imperative that every child with sickle cell disease has 24-hour access to appropriately resourced emergency and acute in-patient paediatric care, in order that rapid assessment and treatment can be initiated.

This chapter aims to provide the reader with some insight into the experiences of one family whose youngest child has SCD. During his early childhood our son's illness rendered him seriously ill, culminating in a bone marrow transplant. Throughout this period he required rapid access to emergency care and paediatric services. These were provided by skilled and knowledgeable staff that were able to provide us with the information and support we needed to enable us to cope with, and manage, our son's illness. On this basis this chapter provides an overview of what I, as his mother, and my family members, have come to know and understand about SCD, as this has ultimately helped us make sense of our son's illness.

We have discovered that there are as many definitions and terms for SCD as there are authors on the subject. The term sickle cell anaemia is restrictive and has a tendency to portray the pathology of the condition while sickle cell disease tends to denote illness and infectivity. Even terms such as sickle cell disorder are a misrepresentation of the condition as an abnormality or minor ailment, and hence do not make explicit the variable nature of this condition. At times, the nature of the condition is confused in the sophistication of the terms of definition. Thus I present a broad definition that encapsulates the vital realms of this condition, based on broad reading and my personal experience:

'Sickle cell condition is a family of genetically inherited recessive haemoglobin disorders in which the beta-globin (β-globin) (a protein that aids oxygen transportation in the blood) make abnormal versions of haemoglobin: the chains of β-globin develop sticky patches, stretching the red blood cell into a characteristic sickle shape, which get stuck in blood vessels and obstruct blood flow, thereby causing painful crises, anaemia, tissue/organ damage and stroke.'

In terms of a blanket description of haemoglobinopathy conditions, Adams (1996) offers a broad definition as follows:

A term used to describe any one of a group of hereditary disorders where there is abnormality of haemoglobin, which during oxygenation of the red blood cells, creates shape distortion, thus blocking the microcirculation and causing severe pain and infarction to surrounding tissues.

Various types and descriptions of the condition abound; some of these are presented in Table 12.1.

Table 12.1 Classification and description of haemoglobinopathies

Types of sickle cell disease	Descriptions
HbSS: Sickle cell disease/condition	The inheritance of HbS from both parents
HbSC disease	The inheritance of HbS and HbC from either parent, known as SC disease/condition
HbCC	The inheritance of HbC from both parents. This is a relatively benign (milder form) of the condition, producing a mild haemolytic anaemia and splenomegaly (spleen enlargement)
HbSβ thalassaemia	Sickle beta thalassaemia. The inheritance of HbS and beta-thal from one parent and beta-thal from the other parent
HbSD Punjab disease	Haemoglobin SD Punjab disease. A variant of sickle cell disease found mainly in Punjabi communities
HbSO Arab disease	Haemoglobin SO Arab disease. A variant of sickle cell disease found mainly in Arab communities
HbSE disease	Haemoglobin SE disease is extremely common in South East Asia. In some areas, it is as common as HbA (normal haemoglobin). Conversely, it is a relatively benign (milder form) of the condition, producing a mild haemolytic anaemia and splenomegaly (spleen enlargement)
HbS Lepore Boston	Haemoglobin S Lepore Disease. A variant of sickle cell disease found mainly in Lepore Boston

Homozygous SCD (HbSS) is said to be the most common type of sickle cell disease (Davies & Oni 1997). There are estimated to be between 6000 and 10 000 people with SCD and around 600 with thalassaemia in the UK (Atkin *et al.* 1998; Laird *et al.* 1996). These figures suggest that about 6% of the UK population and 10% of all births are in 'at risk' groups for haemoglobinopathy disorder (DoH 1993).

Sickle cell conditions mainly affect people who are descended from families where one or more members originate from parts of the world where falciparum malaria was, or still is, endemic (Anionwu & Atkin 2001). Hence, it is often controversially portrayed as a 'black disease' in an attempt to categorise the population groups affected (Dyson 1999; Tapper 1999). In fact, the sickle gene is spread widely throughout Africa, the Caribbean, the Middle East and Southeast Asia, as well as Mediterranean countries including southern Italy, northern Greece and southern Turkey (Atkins & Anionwu 2001; Davies & Oni 1997; Serjeant 1997). Migration of at-risk populations to different parts of the world has caused

an unintended redistribution of the condition to western countries including northern Europe and America. Racial intermixing through marriages and reproductive relationships invariably increases the prevalence rates among Caucasians. For example, US national screening programmes have noted mean prevalence rate of 242–258:100 000 for sickle cell trait in whites and 1–72:100 000 for sickle cell disease (Sickle Cell Disease Guideline Panel 1993). It is estimated that at least 5% of the world's population are carriers for one or other of the most serious types of sickle cell (Anionwu & Atkin 2001) and that over 300 000 infants are born each year with the major sickle cell and thalassaemia syndromes. It is of note, though, that a majority die undiagnosed, untreated or undertreated (Angastiniotis & Modell 1998). It is estimated that 3000 babies are born annually in England with sickle cell trait and about 2800 carry thalassaemia trait (Hickman *et al.* 1999).

The onset, frequency and severity of complications associated with SCD are varied and unpredictable. Vaso-occlusion and tissue ischaemia can result in acute and chronic injury to any organ of the body in varying degrees, and are attributable in children to factors such as acidosis, exhaustion, infection, stress, sudden changes and extremes of temperature, weather conditions, reduced amount of oxygen (for instance in high altitudes), poor ventilation and poor living conditions, and dehydration (Newland & Evans 1997). In the older child factors such as smoking and other associated lifestyle choices such as alcohol also cause complications. These complications manifest in different ways and are often the provoking factor(s) which results in a family attending for emergency care; they are therefore key stressors in the lives of parents and children with SCD and are discussed briefly below.

Pain

Painful crisis is the most common manifestation of sickle cell conditions and often the reason for seeking emergency medical assistance. Pain resulting from blockage of blood vessels can range from mild to, at times, excruciating. Many uncomplicated episodes of pain can be successfully managed at home with oral fluids, mild to moderate analgesia or by comfort measures such as massage and heated pads. Dick (2004) recommends paracetamol (12 mg/kg/4-hourly) and ibuprofen (10 mg/kg 8-hourly) for mild to moderate pain; codeine phosphate (0.5–1 mg/kg/dose) is recommended in severe pain.

Where these measures fail to alleviate pain, it is essential that the patient receives rapid triage in an emergency department and is assessed by a paediatric haematologist for appropriate monitored morphine-based analgesia. At times hospitalisation is necessary to enhance regular review and the prevention/early detection and management of life threatening complications. Pain has been reported to occur on up to 30% of days per year (Shapiro *et al.* 1995) with a loss of 10% of school days over one year (Fuggle *et al.* 1996). Yet pain management remains the most controversial and problematic aspect of sickle cell conditions care (Elander *et al.* 2004) partly due to poor pain assessment and management in children generally, but also due in part to social stereotypes and prejudices associated particularly with young black males. Adolescent males

with sickle cell condition face a turbulent transition to adulthood in terms of tackling the common uncertainties of puberty and combating health care professionals' disablist marginalisation and racism (Atkin & Ahmad 2001). In this regard, it has been acknowledged that services for young people with sickle cell disease have major shortcomings and often do not reflect the specific health and other needs of young children and families (Royal College of Paediatrics and Child Health 2003).

Fever

Fever is often associated with infection such as septicaemia, pneumococcal meningitis and osteomyelitis (Dick 2004; Sickle Cell Society 1981). In the presence of spleen dysfunction, SCD patients are at risk of septicaemia and meningitis with pneumococci and other encapsulated bacteria (Zarkowsky *et al.* 1986). As a result, urgent triage and physical assessment and prompt administration of broad spectrum parenteral antibiotics are recommended (Davies 1997; Lane *et al.* 2000; Serjeant 1997; Sickle Cell Disease Guideline Panel 1993). Other acute complications such as acute chest syndrome, splenic sequestration and aplastic crisis need to be excluded during febrile illness (American Academy of Paediatrics 2002).

Anaemia

This is a significant feature of SCD due to rapid haemolysis, defective erythropoiesis and recurrent infections (Anionwu & Atkin 2001). Death of the nipple-shaped protuberance of the kidney (renal papillary necrosis) may cause a drop in haemoglobin and therefore may exacerbate anaemia. To enhance haemodynamics, healthy nutrition, prevention and prompt management of infections, and antibiotic therapy and blood transfusion (as necessary) are vital measures. Iron deficiency is a feature of SCD but iron therapy is inappropriate unless iron deficiency is proven. Blood transfusions are administered to support erythropoiesis and provide normal red cells to maintain the percentage of the patient's cells at less than 30% (National Heart, Lung, and Blood Institution 2002).

'Sickling'

This is where 'clogging' of the deformed red cells in the blood capillaries results in the formation of knots of red cells that block blood flow and cause tissue infarction (Anionwu & Atkin 2001; Serjeant 1997). Lack of oxygen to the surrounding tissues causes pain and organ damage, and as the brain in children is particularly vulnerable to hypoxia, tissues infarct can ensue, causing stroke in early childhood. **Hence any neurological symptom other than a mild headache requires urgent medical evaluation.** In the eyes, itchiness, swelling and visual impairment is not uncommon during sickling crisis. Acute chest syndrome (sickling in the lungs) caused by viral and bacterial infections including mycoplasma, pulmonary infarction and pulmonary fat embolism represent severe sickling crisis (Vichinsky *et al.* 2000). Therefore, early recognition and aggressive treatment with oxygen, analgesia, antibiotics and exchange transfusion are essential, and may be life-saving (National Heart, Lung, and Blood Institute 2002; Quinn & Buchanan 1999; Vichinsky *et al.* 2001) as deterioration is often rapid with progression to pulmonary failure and death (American Academy of Paediatrics 2002).

Splenic sequestration

This is an acute sickling crisis and is characterised by spleen enlargement and a drop in haemoglobin (less than 2 g/dl of patient's baseline) and varying degrees of thrombocytopenia (low platelets), which causes large quantities of sickled erythrocytes to pool in the splenic pulp. The manifestations are left upper quadrant pain, exacerbated anaemia and, often, hypotension. In children, a large fraction of the circulating blood volume is frequently sequestered. Splenic sequestration crisis is a medical emergency that demands prompt and appropriate treatment. Parents should be familiar with the signs and symptoms of splenic sequestration crisis. Children should be seen as speedily as possible in the emergency room. Prompt recognition and treatment with red blood cell transfusions may be life-saving (Vichinsky 2001) as severe cases progress rapidly to hypovolaemic shock and death (American

Academy of Paediatrics 2002). Sequestration in the liver causes liver dysfunction.

Aplastic crisis

This is a potentially deadly complication of sickle cell disease that develops when erythrocyte production temporarily drops. Infection with parvovirus B19 is frequently the cause of aplastic crises, is characterised by anaemia associated with decreased reticulocyte count (American Academy of Paediatrics 2002) and makes the bone marrow unable to produce red blood corpuscles. Red blood cell transfusions are often needed to prevent heart failure (Vichinsky 2001).

Priapism

This is a prolonged painful erection of the penis common in children and adolescents with SCD, affecting about 40% of post-pubertal males (Serjeant 2001). The affliction often occurs in association with spontaneous nocturnal erections. Episodes of priapism can last from several hours to several days. One group of investigators reported a 90% actuarial probability of at least one episode of priapism by age 21 years (Mantadakis *et al.* 1999). Severe episodes require urgent medical evaluation and treatment that may include hydration, analgesia, aspiration, irrigation by an urologist and sometimes blood transfusion (Mantadakis *et al.* 2000).

Dactylitis

Dactylitis is a swelling of fingers, hands and feet in children due to sickling of blood capillaries in the peripheries of the limbs. This results from necrosis of metabolically active bone marrow, causing pain and swelling of the small bones in the hands and feet of children under 5 years (Serjeant 2001). Similar pathology affecting the joints, particularly ankle, hips and shoulders, as well as the bones of the spine, ribs and sternum in older children and young adults causes painful crises (Anionwu & Atkin 2001).

Osteomyelitis

Osteomyelitis is infection of the bone, usually by pus-forming bacteria. All bacterial osteomyelitis starts as acute infection. If untreated or unsuccessfully treated after 6 weeks, by definition, it becomes chronic osteomyelitis. In sickle cell disease, it is a result of recurrent bone crisis.

Enuresis

Nocturnal enuresis is common among boys with sickle cell anaemia.

This has been linked to insufficient oxygen in the blood (hypoxaemia) (Brooks & Topol 2003), and can cause physical and psychological problems especially when mismanaged. Sensitive care is demanded of staff and carers in this aspect.

Ulcers

Ulcers occur mainly on the hands and feet due to stasis of blood flow to the skin. The ulcerations often have no clear-cut antecedent trauma and progress over a period of weeks to the point that the lesions extend into the dermis, and often into the underlying subcutaneous tissue. With the breakdown in the protection provided by the integument, patients are susceptible to infections and other complications. Treatment of ankle ulcers should be conservative. Rest, elevation and dry dressings with antimicrobial ointments are the best approaches to this problem. Attempts at skin grafting are frequently thwarted by the poor blood flow to the affected region. Healing usually takes weeks to months. The area should be protected against trauma when the patient is up and about (Wethers *et al.* 1994). Anecdotal reports exist of enhanced healing of ulcers in patients placed on chronic transfusion therapy. The evidence that zinc supplementation aids the healing of ankle ulcers is controversial. However, the benign nature of zinc supplementation makes it a reasonable option in patients with this terribly debilitating and often unmanageable condition.

The parental perspective

From a parental perspective, SCD can be seen as a chronic illness with disabling consequences, as it is characterised by a steady state of well-being with erratic periods of severe ill health. Unpredictable episodes of severe pain on affected parts of the body are characteristic of SCD. In our situation many episodes of mild to moderate pain

were managed at home with analgesia such as paracetamol, distalgesic, codeine and diclofenac sodium (Voltarol). Oral fluids and comfort measures such as a soothing bath, heated pads or tepid sponging (during pyrexia) also proved invaluable.

When home management measures failed to resolve our son's pain or crises, admission into hospital via the emergency department was an open option. This was vital to us as a family, as our son's condition was classified as being severe. We also frequently found that GP care was not an option in our situation, as when immediate care was required, the appointment system often meant being unable to access a GP when we needed a doctor most. This in effect added to the stresses of coping with a chronic condition, as well as undermining our family's own coping strategies. Reliance on the emergency department gave us direct access to paediatric haematologists, specialist nurses, anaesthetists and other health care professionals, who we felt knew more and were better equipped to manage our son's crises. Doctors and nurses working in the GP surgery acknowledged that they were unable to provide for these urgent needs of our son, as they would usually refer him straight to an emergency department, thereby reinforcing our views. However, the GP's role in prescribing regular medications and repeat prescriptions was invaluable in maintaining our son's health and well-being.

Our son, like most infants with SCD, was born healthy and was taken home from hospital on the second day following diagnosis. We had been advised that he was not expected to be symptomatic of the condition until later in infancy or childhood, after his fetal haemoglobin (HbF) levels decreased. However, at exactly 7 days old, the community midwife expressed concerns over his distended abdomen and referred us to a local children's hospital where he was diagnosed with 'dilated intestines'. No apparent cause for this was evident as he was totally breastfed at this point, and had been well. No treatment was given but medical review in 3 days was recommended. Although high levels of fetal haemoglobin hindered confirmation of his sickle status at this point, he suffered recurrent bouts of abdominal distension, which heralded the commencement of oral penicillin prophylaxis and folic acid at 1 month old.

Our son was 6 months old when we had our first official visit to an emergency department, as he had become irritable, had a temperature, was lethargic, not feeding, and was generally pale and quiet. We were triaged as requiring urgent medical attention and were seen within minutes by a paediatrician, who subsequently admitted our son to a neonatal ward where he spent almost a month and his first Christmas. His condition deteriorated so rapidly that, by evening of the admission date, he was peripherally shutdown as a result of severe anaemia, with haemoglobin of only 4.1 g/dl and oxygen saturation of 93% for most of the period. He was transfused 160 ml of packed red cells, which brought his haemoglobin level to 7.4 g/dl.

This admission was to form the pattern of our lives and experiences with emergency departments for many years. By our son's first birthday, we had made numerous visits to various emergency departments with various recurrent symptoms including unexplained constipation leading to rectal biopsy, upper respiratory tract infections, fever, jaundice, croup, pneumonia and lung/splenic sequestrations, leading to various exchange and full blood transfusions, and cardiac failure, for which we spent a few days in high dependency unit/intensive care unit. By his third birthday our son had been seen by almost every medical officer in the local emergency department, and the medical opinions varied as often as the conditions and symptoms. There were numerous episodes of microplasma bacterial infection with debilitating chest infections, and the resultant shortness of breath. Splenomegaly and hepatomegaly became common features of his SCD complications. These were further complicated by adenoiditis and tonsillitis, as well as some unavoidable accidental injuries resulting in surgery. Each operation demanded full blood transfusion, or a partial exchange transfusion; the potential complications associated with all anaesthesia is greater for children with SCD in terms of the interaction of anaesthetic drugs and hypoxia associated with anaesthesia.

The optimism and faith of the entire family was tried and tested, especially on the occasion when he suffered laryngeal spasm during intubation prior to surgery, and on another occasion when septicaemia almost claimed his life. Our family remained on tenterhooks each time any of his symptoms manifested, and felt every bit of the agony of the numerous intravenous cannulation attempts. At times, more than ten attempts were made by various personnel within the department, before finally calling on the skills of the anaesthetist. What do you tell a 3-year-old who looks you in the eye with the most expressive sorrow in his own eyes begging, 'Mommy don't let the doctors hurt me any more, and they've hurt me enough'. Anguish and terror over our son's life remained a constant feature in our daily lives until the age of 5 when bone marrow transplant was indicated to cure his condition. Similarly, the anguish of families like ours nurturing a child through this condition is inexpressible and unspeakable.

Living with SCD has similarities with living with other forms of disability and chronic conditions (Thomas 1994). The long-standing nature of the condition and its features and clinical complications impact on daily living, social relationships and self-identity. Consequently, it is not possible to focus solely on the needs of the child in isolation from the family. The great majority of families living with a child who has SCD experience the same emotions, bonds, joys and pleasures of family life, as well as the pains, conflicts and disappointments. They also have and share the same aspirations and worries as the 'general population' and should be supported in every way possible to achieve a balance in all aspects of life and to come to terms emotionally with the condition and any limitations it imposes. Equally, care providers should help the family cope with feelings of isolation, dependence, fear of death/illness, and disruption/withdrawal from normal relationships with peers, as well as poor self-image and depression.

Of course disparity exists in the care individuals with this condition receive, with negative experiences documented (Anionwu & Atkin 2001; Atkin et al. 1998). These authors have found that not only were some parents perceived by some staff as 'interfering' and 'demanding', but they were at times undermined by prejudiced attitudes and unreasonable restrictions imposed on them by staff. My family and I know only too well the consequences of these negative attitudes and behaviours on the part of staff, and therefore did our utmost to abide by every rule and restriction. Our caution did not however deter the negative and irrational/insensitive approaches of some ignorant staff. Health care staff should appreciate the important role parents play in the life of a child with SCD. Caring may involve less physical tending but there are still the emotional and psychological consequences for parents and siblings. It is demanding dealing with the child's frustrations and helping him/her to cope with the condition; having then to cope with staff stress and frustrations can prove overwhelming to the family.

Poor quality service provision can and does impede parents' coping and worsen the stress of caring. It is burdensome to feel that one has to fight constantly in order to obtain appropriate care for a sick child, or to be confronted by staff insensitivity or prejudice at the height of anxiety. At times parents are labelled difficult or hysterical when advocating the (sometimes neglected) needs of their child. Negative and unsympathetic responses from professionals can also be anxiety provoking and exacerbate feelings of isolation, inadequacy and helplessness among parents (Anionwu 1993).

Our family did not feel that we were victims at the mercy of the condition and the care system. Rather, we were active agents struggling against difficulties imposed by the condition as well as balancing other competing social roles and confronting the battles of daily life. Thankfully, there were a number of health care personnel whose care and support (beyond the call of duty) helped boost our coping mechanisms and enabled us to survive the worst episodes of the illness and the process of bone marrow transplantation. My family remain indebted to them and the medical profession as a whole. We are ever willing to share our experiences of this condition with any interested party in a totally unbiased manner. The education we received about preventative care,

temperature monitoring, spleen/liver palpation, and ways of recognising other manifestations of the condition/symptoms of life threatening complications helped us immensely, and served to avert disaster by informing us as to when to seek medical attention appropriately and promptly.

For families affected by SCD, a service that can respond to the needs of the most marginalised section of society and is better able to cater for all its users is best. One cannot over-emphasise the importance of this in aiding the coping abilities of families affected by SCD. However, SCD care provision is caught up in the general struggle for more equitable provision faced by minority ethnic groups.

> 'SCD as a "black condition" is not accorded the same priority as other genetic illnesses such as cystic fibrosis or haemophilia; specific shortfalls include inadequate information, unsupportive, unsympathetic and poorly informed service providers and teachers, inappropriate treatment, racist assumptions informing attitudes of some staff, insensitivity to the individuals' and families' worries, and failure to meet their needs. These problems occur across health and social care agencies in the UK' (Anionwu & Atkin 2001, p. 110).

In conclusion therefore, policy and practice needs to ensure that the difficulties faced by families with children with SCD are addressed adequately. These measures may include improved training of frontline practitioners and better provision of information to enhance parents' role as prime carers, as well as the incorporation of empathy and respect to parents' concerns, and acknowledging them as expert on their child's condition. I am hopeful that the information contained in this chapter, and the account of my own family's experiences, will enhance your understanding of the needs of children and families coping with sickle cell disease and will enable staff to provide adequate and effective care for them, within an accident and emergency setting.

Acknowledgement

My sincere gratitude to David Dike for the consent to narrate his experience of this condition through this medium, and for all we've learned together as a family about this condition. Your love of life and your determination to be well is astounding and commendable. As a family, we are indebted to your sister Darlene who wished to do so much to change your predicament with this condition and inadvertently became your bone marrow donor. Many thanks to Professor Irene Roberts and her team at Hammersmith Hospital for their professionalism beyond the call of duty. David is now free of sickle cell disease after his successful bone marrow transplant.

References

Adams, S. (1996) Sickle cell disease in pregnancy: caring for the pregnant woman with sickle cell crisis. *Professional Care of Mother and Child*, **6**(2), 34–36.

American Academy of Paediatrics (2002) Health supervision for children with sickle cell disease. *Paediatrics*, **109**(3), 526–535.

Angastiniotis, M.A. & Modell, B. (1998) Global epidemiology of haemoglobin disorders. *Annals of the New York Academy of Sciences*, **850**, 250–269.

Anionwu, E.N. (1993) Sickle Cell and Thalassaemia: Community Experiences and Official Response. In: *'Race' and Health in Contemporary Britain*, W.I.U. Ahmad (ed). Open University Press, Buckingham.

Anionwu, E.N. & Atkin, K. (2001) *The Politics of Sickle Cell and Thalassaemia*. Open University Press, Buckingham.

Atkin, K. & Ahmad, W.I.U. (2001) Living a 'normal' life: young people coping with thalassaemia major or sickle cell disorder. *Social Science Medicine*, **53**, 615–626.

Atkin, K., Ahmad, W.I.U. & Anionwu, E.N. (1998) Screening and counselling for sickle cell disorders and thalassaemia: the experience of parents and health professionals. *Social Science Medicine*, **47**(11), 1639–1651.

Brooks, L.J. & Topol, H.I. (2003) Enuresis in children with sleeping apnoea. *Journal of Paediatrics*, **142**, 515–518.

Davies, S.C. & Oni, L. (1997) Fortnightly review: management of patients with sickle cell disease. *British Medical Journal*, **315**, 656–660.

Department of Health (1993) *Report of Working Party of the Standing Medical Advisory Committee on Sickle Cell, Thalassaemia and other Haemoglobinopathies*. DoH, London.

Dick, M. (2004) Management of Sickle Cell Disease in Childhood. In: *Practical Management of Haemoglobinopathies*, I. Okpala (ed). Blackwell Publishing, London.

Dyson, S. (1999) Genetic screening and ethnic minorities. *Critical Social Policy*, **19**(2), 195–215.

Elander, J., Lusher, J., Bevan, D. *et al.* (2004) Understanding the Causes of Problematic Pain Management in Sickle Cell Disease: Evidence That Pseudoaddiction Plays a More Important Role Than Genuine Analgesic Dependence. *Journal of Pain Management*, **27**(2), 156–169.

Fuggle, P., Shand, P.A.X., Gill, L.J. & Davies, S.C. (1996) Pain, Quality of Life and Coping in Sickle Cell Disease. *Archives of Disease in Childhood*, **75**, 199–203.

Hickman, M., Modell, B., Greengross, C. *et al.* (1999) Mapping the Prevalence of Sickle Cell and Thalassaemia in England: Estimating and Validating Ethnic-specific rates. *British Journal of Haematology*, **104**, 860–867.

Laird, L., Dezateux, C. & Anionwu, E.N. (1996) Fortnightly Review: Neonatal Screening for Sickle Cell Disorders: What about the Carrier Infant? *British Medical Journal*, **313**, 407–411.

Lane, P.A., Buchanan, G.R., Hutter, J.J. *et al.* (2000) *Sickle Cell Disease in Children and Adolescents: Diagnosis, Guidelines for Comprehensive Care, and Protocols for Management of Acute and Chronic Complications*. Mountain States Genetics Network and Texas Genetics Network, Denver, CO.

Mantadakis, E., Ewalt, D.H., Cavender, J.D., Rogers, Z.R. & Buchanan, G.R. (1999) Outpatient Penile Aspiration and Epinephrine Irrigation for Young Patients with Sickle Cell Anaemia and Prolonged Priapism. *Blood*, **95**, 78–82.

National Heart, Lung, and Blood Institute (2002) *Management and Therapy of Sickle Cell Disease*, 4th edn. National Institute of Health, Bethesda, MD.

Newland, A.C. & Evans, T.G.J.R. (1997) ABC of Clinical Haematology: Haematological Disorders at the Extremes of Life. *British Medical Journal*, **314**, 1262.

Quinn, C.T. & Buchanan, G.R. (1999) The Acute Chest Syndrome of Sickle Cell Disease. *Journal of Paediatrics*, **135**, 416–422.

Royal College of Paediatrics and Child Health (2003) *Bridging the Gaps: Health Care for Adolescents*. Royal College of Paediatrics and Child Health, London.

Serjeant, G.R. (1997) *Sickle Cell Disease*, 2nd edn. Oxford University Press, Oxford.

Serjeant, G.R. (2001) Historical review: The emerging understanding of sickle cell disease. *British Journal of Haematology*, **112**, 3–18.

Shapiro, B.S., Dinges, D.F., Orne, E.C. *et al.* (1995) Home Management of Sickle Cell-related Pain in Children and Adolescents: Natural History and Impact on School Attendance. *Pain*, **61**, 139–144.

Sickle Cell Disease Guideline Panel (1993) *Sickle Cell Disease: Screening, Diagnosis, Management, and Counselling in Newborns and Infants: Clinical Practice Guideline* (Number 6). US Department of Health and Human Services, Rockville, MD.

Sickle Cell Society (1981) *Sickle Cell Disease: The Need for Improved Services.* Sickle Cell Society, London.

Tapper, M. (1999) *In the Blood: Sickle Cell Anaemia and the Politics of Race.* University of Pennsylvania Press, Philadelphia, PA.

Thomas, R.J. (1994) Stability and Change in Psychological Adjustment of Mothers of Children and Adolescents with Cystic Fibrosis and SCD. *Journal of Paediatric Psychology,* **19**(2), 171–188.

Vichinsky, E.P. (2001) Transfusion-related Iron Overload in Sickle Cell Anaemia. *Seminar Haematology,* **38**(Suppl. 1), 1–84.

Vichinsky, E.P., Haberkern, C.M., Nuemayr, L. *et al.* (2000) Causes and Outcomes of Acute Chest Syndrome with Sickle Cell Disease. *New England Journal of Medicine,* **342**, 1855–1865.

Wethers, D.L., Ramirez, G.M., Koshy, M., Steinberg, M.H., Phillips, G. Jr, Siegel, R.S., Eckman, J.R. & Prchal, J.T. (1994) Accelerated Healing of Chronic Sickle-Cell Leg Ulcers treated with RGD Peptide Matrix. RGD Study Group. *Blood,* **84**(6), 1775–1779.

Zarkowsky, H.S., Gallagher, D., Gill, F.M. *et al.* (1986) Bacteraemia in Sickle Cell Haemoglobinopathies. *Journal of Paediatrics,* **109**, 579–585.

Further reading

Ahmad, W.I.U. & Atkin, K. (2000) Primary Care and Haemoglobin Disorders: A Study of Families and Professionals. *Critical Public Health,* **10**(1): 41–53.

Department of Paediatrics (2003) *Paediatric Emergency Manual: Sickle Cell Anaemia.* http://www.vnh.org/paediatrics emergencymanual/sicklecell.html.

Hall, F.J. (2002) Screening for Sickle Cell Disorders: Part 1. *British Journal of Midwifery,* **10**(4), 232–237.

Mandell, E. (2000) Care Coordination for Patients with Sickle Cell Disease. http://sickle.bwh.harvard.edu/coordination.html.

Steinberg, M.H. (1999) Management of sickle cell disease. *New England Journal of Medicine,* **340**(13), 1021–1030.

Streetly, A. (2000) A National Screening Policy for Sickle Cell Disease and Thalassaemia Major for the United Kingdom. *British Medical Journal,* **320**, 1353–1354.

Thomas, V.N., Wilson-Barnett, J. & Goodhart, F. (1998) The role of cognitive-behavioural therapy in the management of pain in patients with sickle cell disease. *Journal of Advanced Nursing,* **27**, 1002–1009.

Weatherall, D.J. (1997) Fortnightly Review: The Thalassaemias. *British Medical Journal,* **314**, 1675–1682.

Chapter 13 Emergency Care of Children and Young People with Diabetic Ketoacidosis

Camille Roddam

Pathophysiology of Type 1 diabetes

The term 'diabetes mellitus' is an ancient word describing the flowing over of sweet urine; there are many other terms used to describe the disease such as juvenile diabetes or insulin-dependent diabetes mellitus. However, in 1998 the World Health Organization (WHO) agreed the international term 'Type 1 diabetes', and is the term that is adopted in this chapter.

Type 1 diabetes is one of the most frequently seen chronic diseases in children and young adults affecting 1.8 million worldwide (WHO 1999). Moreover it would seem that in many parts of the world the incidence has increased by 3.5% per annum (ISPAD 2000). A recent survey suggested that 16 000 children and young adults are attending diabetic paediatric clinics in England, of which 95% have Type 1 diabetes (National Collaborating Centre for Women and Children's Health 2004).

There has been, over the years, an investment into research to determine possible causes of Type 1 diabetes. It has been linked to a genetically determined predisposition that leads to an auto-immune response by the body. However, we know that not all children with this genetic predisposition go on to develop the disease. An example of this is found in identical twins where there is less than a 35% chance of both twins developing the disease (Atkinson & Maclaren 1994), thereby indicating that an environmental trigger factor is involved. However, researchers have yet to identify exactly what this is, although there has been some indication towards viruses such as mumps, coxsackie B virus and intrauterine rubella (Williams & Pickup 2004). Certain food components have also been associated, an example

is cow's milk but researchers have not as yet been able to provide enough established evidence to support these theories (www.diabetes.org.uk 2000).

Once the disease process commences, auto-antibodies named GAD and islet cells are produced that target the beta cells of the islets of Langerhans in the pancreas, destroying them all over a period of time (Hanas 1998). The beta cells produce a hormone called insulin that is responsible for the metabolic utilisation of glucose to be used for immediate energy or to be stored in the liver as glycogen and as fat. The stored glucose is required when the body is subjected to stress or illness (Williams & Pickup 2004). Without the presence of insulin the body feels that it has been starved and resorts to using other methods to provide it with the energy it requires; this process will be discussed in more detail in this chapter.

The early symptoms of diabetes develop due to the excessive glucose in the blood known as hyperglycaemia; there is insufficient plasma insulin to activate the insulin receptors that are found in tissue cells so glucose is unable to diffuse across the cell wall. Hyperglycaemia leads to an increase in osmotic diuresis; glucose is excreted in the urine along with excess fluid, known as polyuria, leading to mild dehydration. To help replace fluid the child or young adult will become thirsty and want to drink excessively, this is known as polydipsia. Both polyuria and polydipsia are the early presenting symptoms of Type 1 diabetes; if a child or adolescent presents with these early symptoms the urine should be tested for glucose and ketones followed by a 'finger prick' glucose test. A random blood glucose of a level of 11.1

mmol or more or a fasting glucose of 7 mmol or more is diagnostic of diabetes (WHO 1999).

If the early symptoms of Type 1 diabetes are not recognised the disease process continues and the symptoms of ketoacidosis manifest. Low insulin levels and excessive amounts of counter-regulatory hormones stimulate hepatic conversion of amino acids into glucose (glucose neogenesis), and fatty acids into ketone bodies (ketogenesis). The symptoms cause the child to feel lethargic, and a dramatic weight loss may be observed (Hanas 1998; Williams & Pickup 2004). Ketone bodies are water-soluble and cross over the cell wall providing the brain and other major organs with an alternative source of energy. However, hydrogen ions are a by-product of ketogenesis and it is these ions that cause acidosis (pH < 7.3 mmol). In normal pathophysiology, insulin levels would increase to switch off ketogenesis, but in Type 1 diabetes there is an insufficient level of plasma insulin so the production of ketones continues. The build-up of ketones causes abdominal pain and induces central vomiting making it more difficult for the body to replace any fluid loss caused by increased diuresis. Blood glucose continues to rise increasing the osmotic diuresis and resulting in intravascular and intracellular dehydration that causes a reduction in tissue perfusion and an electrolyte imbalance. A child presenting under these circumstances will now be experiencing severe symptoms of diabetic ketoacidosis (DKA). Kussmaul respiration may be observed (deep rapid breathing) along with hypovolaemic and cardiogenic shock. Neurological changes may be noted due to central nervous system depression; this can lead to coma and death if left untreated (ISPAD 2000).

Causes of diabetic ketoacidosis

Diabetic ketoacidosis (DKA) in diabetic patients under the age of 20 is still the most common cause of death (Inward & Chambers 2002; Williams & Pickup 2004). This medical emergency is caused by the absence of insulin, and is more frequently seen in children and young adults who are presenting with undiagnosed Type 1 diabetes (Harrop *et al.* 1999). It can though also be present in children and young adults with established disease when they are unwell. This is because during an episode of acute illness the body demands more energy; hormones such as adrenaline, noradrenaline and glucagon stimulate the conversion of glycogen into glucose (gluconeogenesis). In normal circumstances insulin levels would increase to facilitate extra glucose entering the cells to provide more energy to help cope with the increased metabolic demand that occurs during illness. However, due to the altered physiology associated with Type 1 diabetes, the beta cell cannot respond to the body's demands for more insulin and the subcutaneous insulin is not sufficient to cope with the onset of illness; the body therefore resorts to the production of ketones to provide energy (Williams & Pickup 2004).

DKA may also occur when insufficient exogenous insulin has been given via subcutaneous injection, this can be as a result of a mistake or due to non-adherence to treatment. Adolescents may have personal conflict with regard to dealing with their diabetes (Eiser 1993); they may feel different from their peers, often denying the existence of the disease (Williams & Pickup 2004). Missing injections and inducing weight loss has an appealing effect for some young adults, who fail to realise that the acute side-effects can be life threatening (National Collaborating Centre for Women and Children's Health 2004).

Junior doctors and nurses working in acute paediatric settings such as emergency care will come across children and young adults with DKA especially as the incidence of Type 1 diabetes is increasing (ISPAD 2000). Clinical presentation may not always be clear and can be misleading. The level of management will also differ from one patient to another and health care professionals will require an efficient and versatile approach to decision making to ensure the specific needs of the child and family are met. Diabetes care for children and young adults within the primary care setting has had its challenges, with reports of professionals misdiagnosing the early symptoms of diabetes (polyuria and polydipsia) as urinary tract infection

(UTI) or psychogenic drinking (ISPAD 2000). This therefore has implications for emergency care staff, who may then receive a child whose disease has progressed as outlined below, or is referred by the GP with suspected UTI. It is imperative therefore that guidelines for diabetic management in paediatrics should be available to all emergency care staff either in the format of protocols or integrated care pathways.

In order to illustrate the variations that emergency care staff may encounter, two case studies from the author's experiences are presented. The first involves a 9-year-old girl who was initially diagnosed by her GP, and who was then referred for urgent assessment and treatment. The second involves a Somalian boy, whose presentation was atypical. Both children have been given fictitious names to assure confidentiality.

Case study 1

Samantha presented with a 3-week history of polyuria and polydipsia; she had also felt tired and had been finding it difficult to take part in her PE lesson at school; her teacher had also commented that her levels of concentration had deteriorated in class. A relative had recently visited the family home and remarked on how much weight Samantha had lost and suggested that her mother took her to the GP. The family attended the GP the following day, where a full examination was undertaken and history obtained. Urinalysis revealed the presence of (8%) glucose and a moderate amount of ketones. This then prompted the GP to carry out a finger-prick blood glucose test that measured 22 mmol. Both tests are inexpensive and fairly non-invasive and the GP was able to give a provisional diagnosis of Type 1 diabetes. The GP contacted the on-call paediatric registrar and arrangements were made for the family to come to the hospital.

In line with good practice guidelines Samantha was triaged as an urgent case. Wherever possible it is recommended that children should be transferred to a paediatric assessment unit or directly to the ward to enable the early intervention and initiation of the treatment regime (DoH 2003). On arrival Samantha was initially clinically well;

she had no underlying illness. She was examined and bloods were taken for full blood count, urea and electrolytes, blood gases, plasma glucose, bicarbonate, GAD and islet cell antibodies, and antibodies for coeliac and thyroid disease (ISPAD 2000; National Collaborating Centre for Women and Children's Health 2004). The results of the blood test were within normal parameters apart from an elevated glucose thus confirming the diagnosis of Type 1 diabetes. It was agreed that Samantha would be transferred to the paediatric ward and given a subcutaneous insulin injection 30 minutes before her evening meal. She was commenced on a mixed insulin regime at a starting dose of 0.5 units/kg in 24 hours with two-thirds of the dose to be given a.m. and one-third p.m.

The next day the paediatric diabetes nurse visited the family and the education programme commenced; diabetes provides individuals with a lifelong learning curve. However, it is essential that initial skills of injection technique, blood glucose monitoring and recognition and management of hyper- and hypoglycaemia are developed in order to ensure and maintain the safety of the child. Samantha and her family learnt quickly and were able to go home within 24 hours. Twenty-four hour telephone support was available from the diabetes team; a home and school visit followed enabling Samantha to resume her normal routine as soon as possible.

Our local community is culturally and ethnically diverse, thus as health care professionals we need to be responsive and alert to the varying needs this diversity brings. In some cases English may not be a family's first language and therefore communication may not be wholly effective. Without the help of an interpreting service it may be difficult to obtain a full clinical history resulting in misdiagnosis (Flores *et al.* 2003). The National Service Framework (DoH 2003) and NICE guidelines (National Collaborating Centre for Women and Children's Health 2004) emphasise the importance of having access to interpreting services to help facilitate communication. The following case history illustrates some of the challenges posed under such circumstances.

Case study 2

Abdul, whose family recently arrived from Somalia, is $2^1/_2$ years old. He presented at accident and emergency with a vague history of being unwell for a week with flu-like symptoms; he had more recently seemingly deteriorated having also developed 'breathing difficulties', hence the mother's decision to come to the hospital. He was triaged by the nurse who felt that Abdul required an assessment by the paediatric team. On examination by the senior house officer, Abdul had a low grade fever, was restless and his respirations were elevated. However, the doctor found it difficult to obtain an accurate clinical history, as the mother had limited spoken English, and there was no interpreter available that spoke Somalian. On the basis of the presenting picture, a provisional diagnosis of a chest infection was made. Abdul was referred to the paediatric registrar, but meanwhile Abdul's breathing continued to deteriorate; the mother was obviously distressed but could not verbally communicate her concerns about her son. Abdul had now vomited, and was increasingly lethargic, with his respiratory rate further elevated. At this point the nurse performed a finger-prick blood glucose test which revealed a glucose level of 24 mmol, well over the diagnostic guidelines of diabetes (WHO 1999). Abdul was immediately taken to a high dependency bay within the resuscitation area where he received one to one nursing. His neurological status was assessed each hour using the modified Glasgow Coma scale. These observations were carried out with the aim of detecting any early signs of neurological deterioration due to acidosis, or raised intracranial pressure indicating the early presentation of cerebral oedema.

Cerebral oedema is a rare condition (occurring in 1% of DKA cases) but is seen in young, and more frequently, in newly diagnosed diabetic children, and accounts for between 57–87% of all DKA deaths (Dunger *et al.* 2004). Cerebral oedema can be present on admission (Durr *et al.* 1992) but typically occurs 4–12 hours after treatment is initiated (Dunger *et al.* 2004). It has been suggested that the child's condition initially improves but can then suddenly deteriorate quickly (Brown 2004). The pathophysiology and aetiology is still unclear. Some researchers would argue that it is associated with rapid rehydration and/or overzealous use of insulin, causing an imbalance in the osmolar gradient between the serum and that of the brain leading to swelling of the brain cells and resulting in herniation if not diagnosed and treated effectively. However there are other theories and Brown (2004) presents a good review of the literature. Although the cause of cerebral oedema is still debatable many consultants rehydrate the child in DKA more slowly to avoid this life threatening condition (ISPAD 2000) than the European guidelines for paediatric advanced life support suggest (Felner & White 2001). The treatment for cerebral oedema is outlined in the BSPAD algorithm and is available at: http://www.bsped.org.uk/professional/guidelines/index.htm.

Abdul's oxygen saturation was 92% so oxygen was administered via a facemask to improve tissue oxygenation and to help reverse lactic acidosis. He had dry mucous membranes and was peripherally cold; it was estimated that he was more than 5% dehydrated. Bloods were taken but, as advocated, the doctors did not wait for the results before proceeding with treatment. Two intravenous cannulae were inserted, one to take regular bloods and the other to administer intravenous fluids and insulin. Fluid replacement and insulin regime were established using the Diabetes UK (2003) guidelines to ensure that best practice was adhered to. Once Abdul's immediate safety was assured he was transferred to a high dependency area on the ward where he received one to one nursing. Regular bloods were taken for blood glucose, urea and electrolytes and blood gases 2–4-hourly and peripheral blood glucose was obtained hourly. His fluids and insulin regime were adjusted accordingly, following clear guidelines. If Abdul's condition had deteriorated further or he had developed signs of cerebral oedema, emergency treatment would have been required and he would have been retrieved to a hospital with a paediatric intensive care unit (BSPED 2004). As soon as it was physically possible a Somalian speaking interpreter was requested and the diabetic specialist nurse was able to explain the diagnosis and what future treatment would be required. Abdul made a full recovery and is doing well at home with his parents managing his care, support being provided by the diabetes team and the interpreting service.

If an interpreter had been immediately available, communication could have been facilitated

Case study 2 (Continued)

more effectively and the doctor would have been able to obtain a more detailed clinical history from the family and might have made the diagnosis sooner. As Abdul waited in the department his condition was deteriorating, as his buffer systems (serum bicarbonate) would have been trying to correct the acidosis. He would not have been able to maintain this for long as the acidosis would have become overwhelming, leading to eventual collapse, thus illustrating why a swift diagnosis and efficient management is required for these children.

However, there are lessons to be learnt from this episode of care. A more efficient procedure to enable access to interpreters would have provided the doctors with a clearer history. However, resources and finance have implications on the accessibility to 24-hour interpreting services and this does not facilitate the ability to be culturally aware and sensitive to others' needs if we cannot communicate with them. A steering group is now in place within the hospital; part of its remit is to develop an integrated care pathway. Blood glucose has been included as part of the triage assessment of children who present to the emergency department with abdominal pain, breathing difficulties, respiratory distress and who are critically ill. The objective of this is to detect DKA as soon as possible even if the clinical signs and the history may be misleading. This then endeavours to reduce the clinical risk for the child and provides a better outcome.

Conclusion

In summary, therefore, when triaging and assessing a child who has presented with symptoms suggestive of Type 1 diabetes with associated DKA the following is recommended:

- Confirm characteristic history – polyuria and polydipsia, weight loss, fatigue, abdominal pain, vomiting, Kussmaul respiration.
- Biochemical confirmation of suspected glycosuria, ketonuria.
- Serum/plasma potassium as hypokalaemia is commonly seen in DKA. In severe cases DKA ECG monitoring may be warranted to

assess T waves for evidence of hyper- or hypokalaemia (Dunger *et al.* 2004).
- Height and weight if the child's condition allows.
- Calculate severity of dehydration. Assess capillary refill time.
- Determine whether there is evidence of severe acidosis – hyperventilation, SaO_2, blood gases, serum bicarbonate.
- On-going monitoring should include the following when DKA has been diagnosed:
  — hourly heart rate, respiratory rate and blood pressure
  — frequent accurate recording of fluid intake and output
  — capillary blood glucose monitored hourly (cross-checked against laboratory venous blood glucose)
  — hourly or more frequent observation of neurological status to detect warning signs of cerebral oedema which may include the following:
    — headache
    — inappropriate slowing of heart rate
    — recurrence of vomiting
    — change in neurological status (i.e. restlessness, drowsiness, irritability, incontinence)
    — rising blood pressure
    — decreased oxygen saturation (Dunger *et al.* 2004).
- Careful and slow rehydration following national and international guidelines.
- Commencement of insulin regime.

References

Atkinson, M.A. & Maclaren, N.K. (1994) The pathogenesis of insulin dependent diabetes. *The New England Journal of Medicine*, **331**, 1428–1436.

Brown, T.B. (2004) Cerebral oedema in childhood diabetic ketoacidosis: is treatment a factor? *Emergency Medical Journal*, **21**, 141–144.

BSPED (2004) *Recommended DKA Guidelines*. Available at: http://www.bsped.org.uk/professional/guidelines/index.htm.

Department of Health (2003) *National Service Framework for Diabetes Delivery*. HMSO, London. Available at: http://www.doh.gov/planning2004-2006/index.htm.

Diabetes, U.K. (2003) Guidelines for the management of diabetic keto-acidosis in children and adolescents. *Diabetic Medicine*, **20**, 786–807. Available at: http://www.diabetes.org.uk.

Dunger, D.B., Sperling, M.A., Acerini, C.L., Bohn, D.J., Daneman, D., Danne, T.P.A., Glaser, N.S., Hanas, R., Hintz, R.L., Levitsky, L.L., Savage, M.O., Tasker, R.C. & Wolfsdorf, J.I. (2004) ESPE/LWPES consensus statement on diabetic ketoacidosis in children and adolescents. *Archives of Disease in Childhood*, **89**, 188–194.

Durr, J.A., Hoffman, W.H., Sklar, A.H., el Gammal, T. & Steinhart, C.M. (1992) Correlates of brain edema in uncontrolled insulin dependent diabetes mellitus. *Diabetes*, **41**(5), 627–632.

Eiser, C. (1993) *Growing up with a chronic disease: The impact on children and their families.* Jessica Kingsley, London.

Felner, E.I. & White, P.C. (2001) Improving management of diabetic ketoacidosis in children. *Pediatrics*, **108**(3), 735–740.

Flores, G., Laws, M.B., Mayuo, S.J., Zuckerman, B., Abreu, M., Medina, L. & Hardt, E.J. (2003) Errors in medical intervention and their potential clinical consequences in pediatric encounters. *Pediatrics*, **111**(6 part 1), 1495–1497.

Hanas, R. (1998) *Insulin dependent diabetes in children, adolescents and adults.* Class Publishing, London.

Harrop, M., Thornton, H. & Woodhall, C. (1999) Improving paediatric diabetes care. *Nursing Standard*, **13**(51), 38–43.

Inward, C.D. & Chambers, T.L. (2002) Fluid management in diabetic keto-acidosis. *Archives of Disease in Childhood*, **86**, 443–444.

ISPAD (2000) *Consensus Guidelines.* Available at: www.ispad.org.

National Collaborating Centre for Women's and Children's Health (2004) *Type 1 Diabetes: Diagnosis and management of type 1 diabetes in children and young people.* RCOG Press, London.

Williams, G. & Pickup, J.C. (2004) Epidemiology and aetiology of Type 2 diabetes. In: *Handbook of Diabetes*, 3rd edn. Blackwell Publishing, Oxford.

World Health Organization, Department of Non-communicable Diseases (1999) *Definition, diagnosis and classification of diabetes mellitus and its complications. Report on a WHO consultation Part 1: Diagnosis and classification of diabetes mellitus.* World Health Organization, Geneva.

Index

Note: page numbers in *italics* refer to figures, those in **bold** refer to tables.